ETHICS
of Health Care

Benedict M. Ashley, OP
Kevin D. O'Rourke, OP

The Catholic Health Association OF THE UNITED STATES **CHA**

Nihil Obstat:
        Dennis R. Zusy, OP

Imprimatur:
        +Edward J. O'Donnell, DD
        Auxiliary Bishop of St. Louis
        April 29, 1986

Library of Congress Cataloging-in-Publication Data

Ashley, Benedict M.
  The ethics of health care.

  Rev. ed. of: Health care ethics / Benedict M. Ashley. 2nd ed. ©1982.
  Bibliography: p.
  Includes index.
  1. Medical ethics. 2. Medicine and Christianity. 3. Christian ethics—Catholic authors. 4. Pastoral medicine—Catholic Church. I. O'Rourke, Kevin D. II. Ashley, Benedict M. Health care ethics. III. Title. [DNLM: 1. Ethics, Medical. 2. Pastoral Care. 3. Religion and Medicine. W 50 A817h]
  R724.A738   1986   241'.642   85-29133

ISBN 0-87125-111-6

CONTENTS

Introduction

Our book, *Health Care Ethics: A Theological Analysis* (1978; revised edition 1982), was an effort at a comprehensive treatment of the subject and has been widely used both as a general treatise and as a textbook. Written primarily for health care professionals, its length and detailed documentation made it less suitable for teaching purposes. We have had many requests to produce a version designed especially for courses in medical ethics or for the general reader who desires an introduction to the subject. The present work is aimed at meeting this need.

With the help of Robert Barry, OP, and other college teachers who have made use of our original volume in their ethics courses, we have revised the original, stressing the essentials that apply to the ethics of health care. Hence, instead of the detailed documentation of the original version, a current bibliography of works easily accessible to students has been added, as have cases and questions for study and discussion. In an effort to simplify the text, we have included only a minimum of footnotes, realizing that readers can refer to our more detailed work if they seek additional information. We have retained the social perspective of health care because it is essential for ethical study. Ethics cannot be discussed thoroughly without a knowledge of health care and responsibility. However, the treatment of ethical principles and of concrete ethical problems that are matters of controversy today have been retained in full.

We have entitled this work *Ethics of Health Care* rather than "Medical Ethics" or "Bioethics" because the former is too narrow to cover all the topics that concern health care today and the latter too broad. Those concerned with helping people care for their health must think about social issues that exceed the limits of professional competence of physicians and nurses, but they need not deal with all the bioethical questions involved, for example, the industrial uses of genetic engineering or the humane treatment of animals. We have omitted the subtitle of the original version, "A Theological Analysis," nevertheless, we have retained its Christian and Catholic orientation because we believe that the Christian tradition has something unique to contribute to current ethical discussion and that Catholics have a responsibility to witness human dignity in the profession of health care. At the same time we have tried to show that a Christian approach to health care issues need not be exclusive of other traditions, including that of nontheistic humanism, but can play an inclusive and reconciling role. In an effort to be ecumenical in our thinking, while not mitigating Catholic teaching, we seek to follow the inspiration of the Second Vatican Council, which encouraged Catholics to take an active role in offering solutions to the ethical issues raised by science and technology.

As we seek to explain the *Ethics of Health Care*, some fundamental questions concern us: (1) What is health and who is responsible for it? (2) What are the ethical principles of health care? and (3) How should these principles be applied to ethical issues? Hence the plan of the book is as follows:

1. Since adequate health and health care require the cooperation of many people, we must ask: What are the different roles and ethical responsibilities of the health care team? (Chapter 1 and Chapter 12). Chapter 1 considers the

fundamental question: Who and what is the human *person* whose health is to be cared for? Chapter 2 asks: What is human *health*? Chapter 3 considers the personal responsibility of health care professionals. In Chapter 5 we ask the question: What are the responsibilities of society for the health care of its citizens? Finally, in the concluding Chapter 12 the question is asked: What are the pastoral, religious responsibilities in the healing process?

2. Since every ethical decision ought to be based on *good reasons* that are not merely subjective and arbitrary but that can be rationally defended, Chapter 6 (which is the heart of this book) deals with the question: What are the ethical principles on which health care decisions should be based? In this chapter the ethical principles of the Christian, Catholic tradition are compared with other points of view that enter into current controversies about ethical dilemmas.

3. After considering the responsible persons involved in health care decisions and the principles on which they make these decisions, it is necessary to ask how these principles should be effectively applied to the chief controversial issues of today. Hence in Chapter 7, issues on human experimentation in research and the fair use of limited resources are treated because these are general problems in health care. In Chapter 8, problems of reproduction and, in Chapter 9, problems of the surgical and genetic reconstruction of the human body are dealt with, since in these matters modern medicine has achieved remarkable new powers, the proper use of which is highly controversial. Since the psychological aspect of health is often the source of ethical problems, in Chapter 10 issues of psychotherapy are treated; in Chapter 11 the care of the suffering and dying person whose needs are often more psychological than medical is discussed.

The cases and study questions at the end of each chapter are intended to illustrate the problems raised in the chapter and to stimulate the internalization of ideas presented in the text. The text includes a basic bibliography which will enable the reader to pursue any of these topics in greater breadth and detail.

We wish to thank the many colleagues at Aquinas Institute of Theology and St. Louis University Medical Center who encouraged us as we prepared this book for publication.

Chapter 1
The Person and Health Care

1.1 The Notion of Person

Health care professionals have the knowledge and skill to make technical decisions, but every health care decision involves human needs and human values and therefore is also an *ethical* decision. Ethics concerns the needs and values of human persons in all matters of human concern, including that very common concern we call "health." Nothing is more human, more personal, than health. Concern about health goes far beyond physical well-being. The World Health Organization has declared: "Health is a state of complete physical, mental, and social well-being and not merely the absence of disease or infirmity."

To understand human health and to make ethical decisions about how to care for human health in a way that protects human values, we must be aware of the true worth and dignity of human persons. But today there is much confusion about what it means to be a person. We live in a technological age in an artificial environment, and we view the world through scientific eyes. Scientific training equips us to deal well with facts, but it does little to clarify the meaning of values. Yet in ethical decisions the issues have to do with values.

Perhaps the best way to find a working definition of person in the ethical context of this book and in a way that will go beyond questions of fact to questions of value is to begin with the notion of human *need*. The human being is not definable merely as a static entity, but rather as a dynamic system of needs. Although humans have many of the same needs as plants and animals, they also have distinctively human needs, some of which are acquired through nurture and culture, but others which are genetically innate. Anything that fulfills a human need, whether that need is innate or created by us, is called a value. A disvalue is anything that makes it impossible to fulfill a human need. For example, nutritious food is a value because it meets a basic human need; but so is a symphony concert for one who has learned to enjoy classical music. Junk food and music out of time and tune to sensitive ears are disvalues. Faithful friendship is a value; teachery is a disvalue.

Determining which human needs and capacities are genetically determined and common to the whole human species and which have been created by human culture is not easy. But it is obvious that human beings stand out among all animals in their capacity and need to use symbols, to invent tools, to communicate by speech with a variety of invented languages, to create and modify social and political systems, and to understand and control the world through science and technology. We human beings actually create some of our own values as we create needs, yet we do so because creativity, by which needs are created, is a value we did *not* create for ourselves. Creativity is a value *innate* to human persons. We are creative animals and so, unlike any other animals, we have developed culture.

Satisfying Needs

We are indeed bodily, biological, animal beings with inherent needs for food, shelter, and reproduction; but our intelligence makes it possible and even necessary for us to choose from a vast range of ways to satisfy these needs. Culture is only the expression of our nature, which is to be intelligently free from fixed patterns of behavior, free to create our own lives of intelligent choices among many options. This *embodied intelligent freedom*, by which we create some needs and choose the ways to satisfy needs, defines us as human and gives unity and continuity to the human family across time and space. When we discuss needs and values in relation to other members of the human family, we speak about *rights*. By insisting upon a recognition of rights, we make it possible to pursue our own needs and values as well.

Because we are beings who make intelligent and free choices about the methods of fulfilling human needs, and because we live with other human beings, we are ethical beings. Ethics is the discipline that helps human beings and human communities to choose among values and so fulfill innate or created needs wisely. Thus ethics determines which values are truly human, that is, which actions or things help us fulfill truly human needs whether innate or created, and helps us decide what to do when values seem to be in conflict. When we move into consideration of how to protect our ability to pursue needs and how to respect the ability of others to do the same, we move into the field of rights and law. Law then is based upon ethics, not vice versa, because rights are based upon legitimate human needs.

When we talk of human needs and human rights we have to ask: Who is a member of the human family? When considering who the human family comprises, some philosophers today raise the question: Is every human being a human person? Or, is every member of the human species, as science defines that species factually, necessarily a human *person*? Some prefer to define a person as a moral agent, a human being mature enough to make free moral decisions. Others want to add qualifications such as "conscious," "able to form interpersonal relations," "having feelings." Therefore they conclude that an infant is only *potentially* a person, and a severely defective infant who will never be a moral agent, or a senile or irreversibly comatose adult who will never recover the ability to be a moral agent is a human being but not a person. Since *rights* belong to persons, it follows that according to this view such immature, defective, or senile humans have no inalienable rights. Paradoxically, some of these same thinkers claim that animals have the same kind of rights as humans! Thus they end up defending the rights of animals, while denying rights to the unborn and old people. Unquestionably animals should not be abused, but abuse of children and aged adults is surely something far more serious.

This effort to deny that all human beings are also persons rests on confusing two sets of terms. First, some people fail to distinguish between the terms *person* and *personality*. Personality in current usage refers to those traits, genetic or learned, which persons develop as they mature and which express their uniqueness as persons. An infant is too immature to have much personality, and seriously mentally defective or senile persons are too handicapped to express personality. Nevertheless, we would never develop a personality unless we were first of all persons, that is, members of the human species, who differ from other animals by the innate capacity to mature into intelligent and free personalities. That the seriously defective child will never actually be able to develop in this way does not mean it lacks the innate capacity to do so if medical science ever finds a way to release this capacity. One only has to think of the famous case of Helen Keller, who seemed like a little animal until her skillful and patient teacher found a way to release her hidden potentialities so that she could become the marvelous "personality" we all admire. As for senile persons, their intelligence and freedom have been clouded over by the depredations of age, but until death they still retain a personal identity.

The second confusion consists in saying that a child is only *potentially* a person, when what is really meant is that he or she is *actually* a person, but a person whose full *potentialities* have not yet matured. Of course none of us have yet realized our full potentialities for growth and learning, but this does not mean that we are only potentially persons. Only a very static conception of personhood overlooks the fact that to be a person is to be always in the process of growth unless that growth is pathologically hindered. We ought to maintain, therefore, that every human being is a person at every stage of maturation or dying.

Christian View of Person

The Christian view of the worth of the human person is based on the Biblical teaching that each human being is created by God in his own image and likeness, differing from the animals in the possession of a spiritual intelligence and free will (Gn 1:26-31). Although God produces the human body through the cooperation of human parents, the creation of the human soul is a direct act of God (Gn 2:7; 2 M 7:22-23) which calls each person into existence in relation to God himself (Ps 22:10-11). Each person is unique and irreplaceable (Mt 10:29-31), and all are called not only to maturity but to eternal life (1 Tm 2:4). The differences of sex, race, or individual talents in no way detract from this basic equality of all human beings (Rm 2:11; Ga 4:38; Ep 6:9).

God does not give his gifts equally to all, since each person is unique and the good of the community in which all share is enhanced by the complementarity of different gifts (1 Co 12). The extreme inequality between persons we see in our world today, however, is not the work of God, but of human sin through which the stronger and less moral oppress the weak and more innocent (Rm 3:9-18). The defects of health that contribute to this inequality are due in part to chance and natural causes, but they are also due to unjust social conditions and the pollution of the environment resulting from human ambition, greed, and neglect. God wills only good for us, including good health (Ws 1:12-15), but he gives us as stewards of his creation the responsibility of using natural resources intelligently (Gn 2:15) so as to overcome disease and preserve health.

The worth of human persons was confirmed when God sent his Divine Son to take on human nature and to share our life with us, including the miseries wrought by human sin (Heb 4:14-16). In recalling us to our dignity and restoring to us the hope of perfect happiness, which God intended when he created us, Jesus Christ worked miracles of healing (Mk 1:32-39) to encourage us to use

God's gifts for the health care even of the most neglected and powerless members of society (Mt 26:31-46).

Our first conclusion, therefore, is that[*a human person is a being with a radical capacity for embodied intelligent freedom, whether that capacity is still undeveloped or has been frustrated by accident, disease, or neglect, and thus has inalienable rights that should be ethically respected, including those rights which relate to health care.*]

1.2 The Person in the Community

Every ethical problem about health care ultimately is reduced to our conception of what it is to be human and to actualize personhood. This must not, however, lead to either the error of collectivism or individualism. Aristotle, who first formulated the definition of a human being as "a rational animal" (that is, having embodied intelligent freedom) also insisted that "a human being is a political animal," that is, a being who needs the company of other people. No person can exist long apart from the human community. Each of us has parents and no one can develop either physically or psychologically without constant human relationships. The human brain cannot develop fully without language; and language is a cultural, social creation.

This correlation of person and community is not merely superficial. People need a community not just because it supplies them with certain instrumental needs (food, housing, clothing, defense), but also because their personalities can be fulfilled only in the act of communication and sharing. If personhood is embodied intelligent freedom, it can be fulfilled only in the free acts of knowing and loving. This means that a health care professional cannot understand a patient or diagnose his or her ailment as if the patient were a thing, because the patient is a person whose whole mode of health or sickness is relational.

In our twentieth century world two extreme views about the relation of person to community are in constant competition. One is *collectivism*, which prevails in the communist world, but which also was fostered by the Fascists and Nazis. Generally, collectivism favors a socialist economic system in which the state closely regulates the production and distribution of wealth. Collectivism teaches that the welfare of individual persons must be strictly subordinated to the welfare of the total community, so that the rights of persons can be sacrificed to the interests of the nation. Thus the Khmer Rouge in Cambodia, under the leadership of Pol Pot, declared a "Year Zero" in which a new social order would be instituted for the young, and the old who could not adjust to this fine new system would simply be wiped out.

The other extreme, *individualism*, is a system to whose evils we in the United States are more likely to be blind than to the more glaring evils of collectivism. We often hear individualism called "the democratic way of life." To many it is identified with the free enterprise system—capitalism—in which the economic system is regulated by the free market, which in practice often means competition between a few private corporations. Many argue that the goal of government is to protect the maximum of individual freedom in the face of the growing influence of the collectivism of the communist states, so that any restrictions on this freedom, including any regulation of the economy, is believed to be an attack on the survival of the nation.

The meaning of this radical individualism is summed up in the principle, "I have a right to live my own life as I please as long as I don't hurt anybody else." Here *hurt* means direct harm by bodily injury or damage or theft of private property. According to this ethic, society exists only as a means to protect one individual from another, so as to leave each to pursue his or her private purposes. Ethical behavior becomes the consistent pursuit of self-interest with a minimal code of law and contract enforcement. Proponents of this ethic often argue that (1) in fact, people really act this way and therefore other ethics are hypocritical, and (2) this system of laissez faire actually produces more economic prosperity and human progress than do collectivist ethics.

Oddly, in the United States our familiar political polarization between conservatives and liberals only conceals the fact that although conservatives often call liberals "socialists" (that is, collectivists) and liberals often call conservatives "fascists" (that is, collectivists), both are actually radical individualists. Conservatives oppose government intervention in the business affairs of individuals (for example, they advocate deregulation and no income tax) except to maintain the conditions of competition. Liberals oppose government intervention in the private lives of individuals (for example, they advocate free choice in abortion) except to further certain social programs they favor.

Christian Perspective

The Christian point of view, which also has support in many other religions and philosophies of life, rejects both collectivism and individualism (whether that individualism be conservative or liberal). Christianity rejects collectivism because the community exists to serve persons and not persons to serve the community as if it were a superperson. On the other hand, it rejects individualism because Christianity teaches that the highest and most important goods of the person are not private property but are spiritual goods, which can be achieved and fully enjoyed only by sharing with others. Because modern states, both collectivistic and individualistic, are oriented to maximizing material goods and military power, rather than maximizing spiritual goods, the struggle between person and community has become chronic.

The Christian point of view is neither idealistic nor altruistic. The words of Jesus were, "Treat others the way you would have them treat you; this sums up the law and the prophets" (Mt 7:12); and "You shall love your neighbor as your self" (Mt 22:39). According to this teaching we are not asked to love our neighbor and *not* love ourself, but to love our neighbor as our self. In other words, if we really love ourselves, not selfishly, but intelligently, we will realize that we cannot be happy in isolation, because we were created as *social* beings. We can be truly happy only by sharing in a community of happy people, and that means that we each must not only respect the rights of others in a negative sense, but must be actively concerned to promote each other's welfare. Therefore both collectivism and individualism are self-defeating. We can see that in the communist countries the ruthless subordination of persons to the collectivity in the name of equality has made the citizens equally slaves. In the so-called democratic countries individualism in the name of freedom has left many people poor and unemployed. Both types of nations have seen an increase in crime and the disintegration of the family.

The social teaching of the Catholic Church, derived from the teaching of Jesus, insists therefore that the human community, including its government, be actively concerned in promoting the health and welfare of every one of its members so that each member can contribute to the common good of all.[1] This concern cannot be a matter of a mere trickle-down by which the weak live on the leavings of the powerful, but must be aimed directly at enabling the weak to share in the goods of life. The Christian remembers that God has called us all to share in his own life, the community of Father, Son, and Holy Spirit, in which there is nothing that is not common to all (1 Jn 1:3).

Thus our second conclusion is that *the human community and its government exist to promote the welfare, including the health, of all. Moreover, each member of the community, according to abilities and resources, must contribute generously to this common welfare.*

1.3 Developing Common Values

Human community is difficult when there is no agreement on common values. At least there must be the possibility of dialogue toward common values. The Second Vatican Council insisted that the spirit of dialogue must extend beyond the Christian family to other religions.[2] Do we have values in common with non-Christians? Judaism and Islam believe in the same personal God as do Christians and also have the same fundamental convictions about the dignity of the human person in relation to God.

The religions of India and China are becoming more popular in American life. At first sight their outlook might appear incompatible with the Christian emphasis on the dignity of the human person in relation to a personal God, since they teach that the individual, after a series of reincarnations, is absorbed into the unity of the Absolute. Closer study, however, reveals that this Absolute is not subpersonal or impersonal, but superpersonal. Thus it becomes possible for monotheists to join with believers in these Eastern religions in a common search for authentic spiritual selfhood. Americans are beginning to appreciate how much these religions, with their meditative disciplines, can contribute to personal integration and total health. Thus Christians can learn a great deal from other world religions about ethical dialogue and the pursuit of true health.

Catholics should realize as well that they have something in common with humanists. According to the well-known *Humanist Manifesto* (1935), signed by a group of distinguished American thinkers under the leadership of a famous American philosopher, John Dewey:

> Religion consists of those actions, purposes and experiences which are humanly significant. Nothing human is alien to religion. It includes labor, art, science, philosophy, love, friendship, recreation—all that is in its degree expressive of intelligently satisfying human living....Religious humanism considers the complete realization of human personality to be the end of man's life and seeks its fulfillment and development in the here and now. This is the explanation of the humanist's social passion.

Thus humanism rejects the notion of an afterlife for man and his dependence on a God or an Absolute, but it does so precisely in the interest of human dignity, believing that the older religions tend to excuse man from full responsibility to create a good society here and now. In 1980 some humanists renewed their creed in *A Secular Humanist Declaration.* Most Christians would ascribe to 8 of its 10 principles, but the new document continues to belittle religion and divine guidance. In the opinion of many observers, humanism today is rapidly replacing Protestant Christianity as the predominant religion in American culture. While realizing the prevalence of the secular humanistic value system, Christians must respect the good will of humanists and seek common values that will enable all to build a peaceful, even though pluralistic, society.

Where humanism is not dominant, Marxism has become the contemporary equivalent of a religious system of values. Although Marxism shares many values with humanism, it has an even more materialistic conception of humanity according to which human beings emerge from nature by a struggle to control and refashion it (even their own nature) to suit their purposes.

Catholic Teaching

Many Catholics are under the impression that the Catholic Church, because it opposes communism, favors capitalism. They are unacquainted with the fully developed social teaching of recent popes, which must be considered in any Catholic approach to today's ethical problems, including those in the medical field. Thus Catholic teaching attempts to transcend the capitalist-communist impasse based in both camps on a materialistic conception of society. The popes urge us to work for a world community based on spiritual goods or values and economic cooperation. They link human health and world poverty as the most fundamental ethical problems of our time, problems which in the United States are often ignored by ethicists and health care professionals alike while attention is devoted to secondary problems such as eugenics and heart transplants.

Thus the kingdom of God begins here on earth with social justice, as Pope John Paul II has constantly preached, and no one will gain heaven who has neglected to work for social justice on earth. Jesus said, "I was hungry and you never gave me food...insofar as you neglected to do this to one of the least of these, you neglected to do it to me" (Mt 25:31-46). In the parable of Lazarus and the rich man (Lk 16:19-31) he taught the same lesson. Consequently a genuine Christian ethic cannot be written from the viewpoint of the status quo which in a sinful world tends to reflect the materialistic spirit of domination and possessiveness. It must also view the world from the side of the oppressed, whose needs have been ignored and neglected. Thus Jesus pointed to his preaching of the Gospel to the poor as the best sign of the authenticity of his own mission (Mt 11:5). Therefore a Christian politics of health care must be based on an option for the poor.

Christians, therefore, must join in common effort with all those who are sincerely concerned about human rights, including the right to health. This ecumenical search for ethical consensus in regard to human needs has its solid legal and political foundations in the United Nations' *Universal Declaration of Human Rights* (1948), signed by most of the countries of the world and supported by all the major religions as well as by humanists and Marxists (see Appendix). Catholics have been urged by all the recent popes to support this declaration as a sound basis for social justice. Thus in the twentieth century there are grounds for a basic consensus on the fundamental ethical values on which world peace and community must be based and on which health for all human beings must be sought. The aim of this book is to take that consensus very seriously without, however, glossing over the profound differences that continue to divide the Christian and secular communities and that challenge us to further research and dialogue.

Thus the third conclusion of this chapter is that *if human rights, including the right to health, are to be well served, we must strive through research and dialogue to broaden the consensus on ethical principles which respect the dignity of the human person.*

1.4 Priorities in Needs and Values

That the nations of the world at least nominally agree on a list of human rights or values is an important step toward increasing ethical consensus, but it is only a first step. Human beings must not only list agreed-upon rights or values, they must also deal with the question of priorities. What is the hierarchy of values? Which values are most important? These are key ethical questions. Some will reply that this question of emphasis and priorities is a wholly subjective matter about which rational discussion is impossible. Whether this is the case can be decided only if the concept of need-value and its relation to objective facts is examined more closely.

Above we defined ethics as a study of the satisfaction of the needs, whether innate or created, of persons in their lives as intelligent and free social beings. Anything that satisfies a need is a value. Thus a given value is always correlative to a human need, that is, it is a desire to satisfy the need. On the other hand, a negative value, or disvalue, is inimical to human need, and a neutral value neither satisfies nor obstructs a need. A value, therefore, can be something so trivial as a cup of coffee to satisfy thirst or so sublime as the philosophical truth needed to satisfy our thirst for meaning in the cosmos. The basic or the more important human values correspond to the basic human needs. In accord with ancient and modern philosophers and the psychologist Abraham Maslow, we can enumerate the following basic human needs.[3]

1. *Biological needs* (Maslow's physiological needs). Human beings share with all living organisms the need to maintain themselves homeostatically in a dynamic relation with their environment, to grow and mature to full biological development as individuals, and to continue the species through reproduction. This is the level of need dealt with by physicians.

2. *Psychological needs* (Maslow's safety needs and also his belongingness and love needs in their more emotional aspects). Human beings are psychic organisms who sense, imagine, and feel. This is the level of need generally dealt with by experimental psychologists and psychotherapists.

3. *Social needs* (Maslow's esteem needs, as well as the belongingness and love needs in their more developed aspects). This is the level of human free choice

within the limits of an existing culture. It comprises the need of the individual both for self-control and for social relationship beyond those determined by the family. This is the level dealt with by lawyers, political leaders, and clergy acting as moral counselors.

4. *Spiritual and creative needs* (Maslow's need for self-actualization, including needs to know and understand, to contemplate, and to create). Though many refer to this level as spiritual, we add the word *creative* because too many people confine the meaning of the word *spiritual* to our friendship with God. Actually this is the level of function where we also relate to other human beings and think, love, reflect on the past, and plan for the future. This is the level of commitment, creativity, and transcendence at which persons not only live within a culture, but also criticize it, transcend it, and contribute to it. It includes all activity with a creative element—in art or science or political innovation—and furthermore religious activity as it extends to ultimate, cosmic meaning. This is the level dealt with by the inspiring teacher and spiritual guide.

Each of these levels contains a complex of natural and cultural needs—the cultured needs being rooted in the natural needs but greatly expanding them. It cannot be emphasized too strongly that these four levels of needs are not stories in a building but *dimensions* of the human person which can no more be separated from one another than can the length, breadth, and height of a cube. Every human act or event has *all* four dimensions. A human spiritual activity, whether it be a creative, scientific, or artistic activity or the graced acts of faith, hope, or love is at the same time a biological, a psychological, and an ethical event.

Moreover, the reciprocity between these levels of the organization and function of the human personality are hierarchically ordered so that spiritual activities are the deepest, most central and the most integrating, biological activities are the least unified and the most peripheral, and the psychological and social activities have intermediate positions. At the same time the higher activities in this hierarchy are rooted in and depend on the lower in a network of interrelations. Nevertheless, each level has a certain genuine autonomy and differentiation in its structure and modes of functioning so that it is necessary that each be served respectively by the different professions of medicine, psychotherapy, ethical counseling, and spiritual direction using different healing and helping techniques.

St. Thomas Aquinas gave a somewhat different and simpler classification of basic needs as follows:[4]

1. The need to preserve life
2. The need to procreate
3. The need to know the truth
4. The need to live in society

Thus the ethical problems persons face are to plan their lives and to make decisions in such a way that *all* these basic needs are to a degree satisfied in an integrated and consistent manner. This obviously requires the adjustment of priorities in regard to both aims and objectives and of the practical steps to be taken. Moreover, it demands the subordination, and even sacrifice, of less important needs to greater ones. The exact mix or proportion will depend on both the culture and the individual.

1.5 Summary

Humanity differentiates human health from mere animal or vegetative health and from the functioning of a well-oiled machine. Our discussion on health and what it means to be a human person can be summed up in four statements:

1. Health care must serve persons. Human health is the physical, psychological, social, and spiritual well-being of a living organism of the human species, distinguished from other animals by its personhood, that is, by its capacity for intelligent freedom or ethical judgment, which can be actualized only in a truly human community.

2. A truly human community must be based primarily on the sharing of human values—the communication of truth and love—and only instrumentally on material values. The physical and mental health of persons, however, is a necessary basis not only for the acquiring and sharing of material, but also for the acquiring and sharing of spiritual values. The human community exists to enable its members to achieve all these values, and each member of the community is ethically obliged to share what he or she achieves with others.

3. To develop a truly human community, the community must not be restricted on the basis of nationality or race, but must extend to the whole human family resting on a consensus about basic human values. The existing basis of such a consensus is the United Nations' *Universal Declaration of Human Rights*, founded on the principle of human dignity. This consensus must be broadened and rendered practical by continuing patient research and dialogue.

4. All ethical decisions, including those in health care, should satisfy both the innate and cultural needs (biological, psychological, ethical, and spiritual) of every human person in each of the world's political communities.

Footnotes

1. United States Catholic Conference, "Catholic Social Teaching and U.S. Economy," *Origins* 14 (22/23), Nov. 15, 1984.

2. A. Flannery, editor, "Church in the Modern World," *Documents of the Second Vatican Council* (Collegeville, MN: Liturgical Press, 1975), p. 903ff.

3. Abraham M. Maslow, *Religion, Values, and Peak Experiences.* (Columbus, OH: Ohio State University Press 1964).

4. St. Thomas Aquinas, *Summa Theologica*, I-II, q. 94, a.2.

Study Questions

1. Explain each of the three terms in the definition of the human person: *embodied, intelligent, freedom.* How do the differences between the anatomy of a human being and a chimpanzee show evolutionary adaptation to the free, intelligent mode of human behavior? If we can approximate the capabilities of a human being by a computerized humanoid robot, what differences will remain?

2. Does human society exist to serve its members, or do the members exist to serve the society? Debate both sides of the question and then try to resolve the question.

3. Describe the value systems that might be typical of the following communities: (a) Evangelical Christians; (b) Orthodox Jews; (c) Muslims; (d) Buddhists; (e) Mexican-American Catholics; (f) Irish-American Catholics; (g) TV sit-com or soap opera writers; (h) the American Medical Association.

4. Debate the issue of whether the community confers personhood. How would you resolve this issue?

5. It is often said that "law should not impose morality" and that "religious groups should not impose their morality on others by lobbying for legislation." In what sense are such statements valid? Invalid?

Cases

1. St. Roch's Childrens Hospital is engaged in research in chemotherapy for leukemia in children. Experimental drugs are tested first on monkeys to determine possible side-effects and then, if they prove relatively safe, on human subjects with leukemia. A laboratory assistant notices that the monkeys are made very ill by some of these drugs, suffer a good deal, and finally die. In other cases they are permanently crippled. He wonders why it is ethically justifiable to cause this suffering to animals in order to help children who do not seem to suffer any more than the animals. Don't animals have rights too? What answer would you give him?

2. Jim Brown, a 10-year-old hemophiliac, has been diagnosed as a victim of AIDS incurred from the blood transfusions necessary for the proper management of his condition. Since it is still not certain whether AIDS can be transmitted in other ways than by transfusion, contaminated hypodermic injections, or homosexual intercourse, the parents of children attending Jefferson Public School demand that Jim be forbidden to attend it. Jim's parents hope that a cure may be found soon so that he may achieve adulthood and they do not want him to miss several years of school. If you were a member of the school board how would you formulate the principles that govern the rights of the *individual* vs. the rights of the *community* as these apply to this case?

3. Dr. Meyer attempts to persuade the Clarks to give permission for a blood transfusion for their child who is to undergo dangerous surgery. The Clarks are Jehovah Witnesses whose religious views forbid blood injections as a form of "eating blood" denounced in the Old Testament. The Clarks point out to Dr. Meyer, who is Jewish, that he has had his two sons circumcised although recent studies have shown that this ritual practice involves some medical risk. Dr. O'Brien enters the argument by saying that the risk of circumcision is not very great, while the need for a transfusion can be very great. The Clarks reply by asking Dr. O'Brien, a Catholic, whether he would perform an abortion on a woman with a heart condition for whom pregnancy is a serious risk. If you were involved in this discussion, how would you deal with these conflicts of value systems and the relation between medical and ethical values?

4. Samuel is a concert pianist who has suffered a serious accident to his left hand. He has consulted two physicians who differ in their opinions. Dr. A recommends immediate amputation not only because he predicts that the hand will be useless but also because it may develop life-threatening necrosis, symptoms of which seem already to be present. Dr. B agrees that the situation is very grave but would like to try a new and experimental therapy which has some promise of saving the hand and giving an opportunity for successful rehabilitation. Samuel says, "I would rather be dead than to give up my career. It is my whole life!" How would you help him make a decision?

Chapter 2
Defining Human Health

2.1 Concepts of Health and Disease

Many health care professionals know a great deal about disease, but often they are not able to define health. Unless one knows the meaning of "health" or of "illness" which indicates an absence of health, one will be unable to discuss the human values involved in health care and thus will not be able to make clear and accurate ethical decisions. The word *health* is related etymologically to the Anglo-Saxon word from which are derived not only *healing* but also *holiness* and *wholeness*. The root of that word denotes completeness. Such a whole can be considered statically as a structure with all its parts, each properly proportioned and all parts in their places. Thus a crippled child lacks wholeness or perfect health because some part of its anatomy is missing or deformed. But health can also be considered dynamically as a *functional* whole, in which all necessary functions are present and acting cooperatively and harmoniously. Thus some sicknesses do not involve any lack of an organic part or its deformity, but rather a dysfunction; that is, some needed function is suppressed or there is a lack of harmonious balance between functions, for example, if a person has diabetes or hyperthyroidism.

Briefly, "health is the state of being in which an individual does the best with the capacities he has, and acts in ways that maximize his capacities."[1] In the practice of medicine today health is most commonly defined in terms of standard physiological parameters—the vital signs, the presence of various chemicals in the blood, electroneurological readings, and so forth—as well as by gross anatomy and histology. Health, therefore, is often defined by a model of what is physiologically usual or average.

Such a physiological model, however, raises some problems. First of all, it is obvious that an exact, universal definition of human health in these terms is impossible and that only a range of usual values can be achieved. In the case of some values (temperature, for example) the range from one individual to another is small; in others (weight, for example) it is large; but in all cases what is identifiably healthy for one individual does not necessarily indicate a state of health for another person. How can the model of normality be determined? *Normal* is not identical with *average*, since it is quite conceivable that the majority of people today are not very healthy. The normal therefore is an ideal. How can such an ideal be determined in a way that is not arbitrary, but which has a sound empirical basis?

Health is better defined as optimal functioning. This implies that each organ and organ system are functioning well and together to form a single life process; the diverse functions are harmoniously interrelated yet differentiated phases. This concept of health is a consequence of considering a human being as an organism (etymologically a complex of instruments or organs), that is, a living whole composed of functionally differentiated parts. A human being is thus a dynamic or open system. A system is a complex of interacting elements. A living system is dynamic or open, that is, capable of maintaining homeostasis (dynamic stability) in relation to its environment by regulating the input and output of matter and energy.

Obviously, a definition of health in terms of optimal functioning of an open system must include the input-output of that system. A living thing cannot maintain itself in static existence; it must interact with the environment so as to modify it in its own interests. Thus animals build shelters and nests, fertilize plants on which they feed, and rid their environment of enemies. In fact, the present earth environment is largely the product of living things themselves, that have modified both the soil and the atmosphere in ways favorable to life.

Because humans are cultural as well as natural beings, their interaction with the environment is highly creative. They modify the environment with conscious purpose, so that civilization is the production of a city, that is, an increasingly synthetic environment. Today people are beginning to think about almost entirely artificial environments, for example, on the moon or even on constructed satellites where nothing will be natural except the basic raw materials from which the total environment will be constructed.

Even more significant is that human creativity is not limited to interaction with an external environment. Humans create not only external things, but also mental and emotional symbols to fulfill needs that cannot be fulfilled in ways that are merely objective, that is, outside conscience. Ultimately, human beings need to assimilate the whole order of the external environment. Thus scientists are constantly striving to re-create, as it were, the entire external cosmos in the form of symbols. The great importance of this human life process, from a personal point of view, is that such symbols provide communication between persons in the form of language. Human society ultimately uses this communication to get along within the same symbol universe.

In view of this concept of human functioning, we can see that human health means not only the capacity of the organism to maintain itself in its environment but also to create function within itself. This involves an ever-expanding culture, which is why the World Health Organization insists, "Health is a state of complete physical, mental, and social well-being and not merely the absence of disease or infirmity." Health in the broad sense of the World Health Organization definition is thus optimal functioning of the human organism to meet biological, psychological, social, and spiritual needs. However, the health care professions are concerned with health in the narrower sense as the optimal functioning at the biological and psychological levels, yet in the context of the integration of all four levels of need (see Chapter 1). Even though physicians specialize in biological or psychological functions, they must never neglect or ignore the ethical and spiritual needs of their patients if they wish to be truly concerned about human health.

Disease and Illness

Given the concept of health as structural and functional wholeness of the human organism in relation to itself and to its environment—a wholeness that extends even to the ethical and spiritual—the notion of disease can be more precisely defined. The World Health Organization definition maintains that disease and infirmity are not the exact contrary of health. Health, as we have defined it, is optimal functioning. For an organism to fall short of optimal functioning without actually being diseased or infirm is possible, because an organism can be healthy in a narrow sense without actually being used to its full capacity. However, less than optimal functioning soon leads to dysfunction. A man can be healthy in this narrow sense and yet be lazy, half-alive through lack of the full use of his capacity for living; but he will not stay healthy even in this minimal way for long because his faculties will atrophy.

The terms *disease, illness, sickness, malady, ailment, disorder, complaint* and many more synonyms have different connotations. Some seem to be more subjective, that is, they designate the feelings of the victim (illness, sickness, complaint); others are more objective (disease, malady, ailment, disorder). We, however, will use the term *disease* broadly to denote the opposite of health defined as optimal functioning.

Two Concepts of Disease

In the history of medicine the pendulum has constantly swung between two concepts of disease: the ontological and the physiological. The ontological concept regards diseases as separate entities (devils, contagions, morbid matters, bacteria, genetic defects, neuroses, psychoses) that can be classified and named like plants and animals. It supports the theory that the organism constantly fights to throw off such diseases as alien invaders which disturb its homeostasis. Those who think in these terms tend to diagnose disease as clearly classified and labeled entities and to treat them by seeking specific remedies (such as drugs or surgical procedures).

The opposite of the ontological concept, the physiological concept, views disease as a breakdown of the internal harmony of the organic system due to hyperfunctioning or hypofunctioning of an organ. Thus dysfunction opens the organism to attack by external agents such as bacteria, but the bacteria are not the primary cause of the disease. If the organism were functioning properly, it would resist such bacteria. Hence classifying or labeling diseases is dangerous because disease is essentially the condition of an *individual* who is internally maladjusted. The advocates of this position therefore tend to emphasize regimen or life style and to use drugs and surgery secondarily to assist in the adjustment of the individual organism.

The central tradition of medicine (usually identified with that of the Greek physician, Hippocrates) has always tried to reconcile the ontological and physiological concepts of disease. The physiologists are correct in thinking of health as an internal homeostasis or harmony within the organism and disease as an imbalance. The organism as a system is constantly adjusting to changes in the environment by means of feedback. These minor fluctuations are not diseases; rather they are health itself.

If the system fluctuates beyond a certain range, however, it cannot recover homeostasis without a major readjustment. This may be possible through the internal vital powers, but only at the cost of a period of sickness in which many normal functions must be minimized while the organism uses all of its energies to readjust. Such a disease is acute illness. Or the organism may readjust but at the cost of permanent diminishing of function or suppression of some functions. Then the disease becomes chronic, or permanent crippling or a handcap results. Finally, the adjustment may be greater than the organism can achieve, and death results.

From the physiological point of view, death is always the result of disease. Therefore death cannot be said to be natural if *natural* means, in the Greek's sense, the optimal functioning or health of the organism. Physiologically speaking, the organism seems to be made to live forever, always recovering from any malfunction. Hence death is due to injuries done to the organism from the environment, not from any intrinsic tendency.

But the ontological theory of disease sees death somewhat differently. A homeostatic system, by definition, is one that maintains itself perpetually when not disturbed. The human organism is an open system in constant interaction with the environment. The organism is homeostatic, but there are limits to its power of self-maintenance. Consequently, when the environment is altered beyond a certain normal range, the organism is unable to survive. Thus when the oxygen content of the air, the temperature, or the number of bacteria in the environment changes markedly, the human organism undergoes stress, then disorganization, and finally death.

Disease can be classified according to various external agents that tax the capacity of the organism to maintain itself in the environment. Diseases can be viewed as entities such as plague or pollution or radiation sickness that affect all the individual organisms in a given area. From the ontological point of view, disease and death are natural in the sense that the changing terrestrial environment is a part of the evolutionary process from which no individual, but only the species, is protected. The species itself ultimately yields to the rise of new species. Without disease and death, natural evolution cannot continue.

The organismic theory of health and disease has been central to Western medicine, but it has had strong competition from the mechanistic theory, which goes back to the Greek Democritus. Even today the thinking of many biologists and medical educators is influenced by the mechanistic theory. For a mechanist, the parts seem to be more significant and more practically controllable than the whole. Mechanists are more comfortable with anatomy or structure than with function or process. They tend to reduce process to quantitative measurements of results. Their diagnoses tend toward ontological views in which disease is the result of alien bacteria, of organic lesions, and so forth.

Maintaining an organismic view of disease in no way denies the mechanistic view, but includes it. The notion of the person as a dynamic system necessarily includes a detailed analysis of the parts, the interacting elements. To posit vitalistic or holistic forces apart from the interaction of the parts is unscientific. But an organismic view insists that the relationships among the parts are just as real, just as scientifically observable and intelligible, as the parts which are interrelated. Moreover, the parts themselves cannot be observed or understood in isolation, but only in the context of the system in which they exist. The eye or the kidney, the cell, and even the macromolecular gene cannot be understood except in the context of the whole organism of which they are parts. Medical specialization, therefore, can never be separated from a medical understanding of the whole person, nor can health or disease be defined except in terms of the whole and its parts.

Having defined human health as optimal functioning and having understood this as the satisfaction of innate and cultural needs, or the realization of potentialities, we have defined a norm by which the means to health can be discriminated from whatever tends toward disease and death, that is, the suppressing or disuse of functions. Now let us consider the various dimensions of human health.

2.2 Biological Health

This book cannot present even a sketch of the specifics of the biological level of human functioning. Biological and medical science are constantly making new discoveries about the tissues, organs, and secretions that constitute the human body, their chemical composition, structure, functional interrelations, and the control of their differentiation, development, and modification by environment and through individual biography. We, however, are concerned with discussing general biological function insofar as it contributes to integrated human behavior.

The important question for health care ethics is how the biological level of functioning can be considered truly human and personal, that is, as having ethical and spiritual significance. Dualistic theories of the human being have been present in all cultures throughout human history. According to these theories body and soul are in essential conflict with each other (that is, the biological and psychological levels of human functioning versus the ethical and spiritual levels). Generally the body is regarded as the negative factor and the soul as the positive factor.

Underestimating the plausibility of this dualistic anthropology is a mistake. The body is frequently experienced as a burden, as something negative, for two reasons. First, people cannot voluntarily control much of what goes on inside them physiologically. Biological life, often uncontrollable, becomes deranged and fails human purposes. People find themselves weary and exhausted, unable to do what they would like to do. Suffering from pain and disease, people are painfully conscious that eventually the body becomes subject to age and ultimate failure in death. Thus the body appears as a burden, a liability.

Second, the basic biological drives are urgent, constant, and inescapable—the need for sleep, the fear of insecurity, the demands of hunger and thirst, and the tension of sexual desire. They are so insistent that people feel them as compulsions, limiting their freedom and sometimes overwhelming them against their will.

Since the dignity of human personhood consists essentially in self-knowledge and freedom, we find it profoundly humiliating to be the helpless victims of our own bodies, with their limited energies, liability to pain, and their urgent and deterministic demands that arise from unconscious depths and disorganize our self-possession and freedom of action. Sexual drives have especially seemed demonic.

Thus it is understandable that dualism is so widespread. It is essential to certain religious systems (Buddhism, Gnosticism, Manichaeism) and has affected all of them (the Neo-Platonic influences in Jewish, Christian, and

Muslim theologies). It might seem though that such dualistic views are no longer common, since modern society emphasizes the value of sensual pleasure, the dependence of psychic functions on the body, and the equality of male and female. But some ethicists maintain that human biological structure and function, such as the body-soul unity, have no moral significance. Rather, these objective biological facts receive their moral meaning only from culture, that is, from subjective human choice.

Body-Soul Unity

Certainly it is fallacious to argue that the moral character of human behavior can be settled simply by asking biologists what is natural or unnatural to animals or even to human beings. The morality of any act must be considered in the context of the activity of the person as a whole, since the biological level of function is only one level of the total system. Conversely, however, this consideration means that the spiritual or ethical meaning of a human act cannot be indifferent or neutral to its biological character. Every human act is an act of the whole person, involving spiritual, social, psychological, and biological dimensions. Every human biological function has human (and therefore spiritual and social) significance; and, conversely, even the most spiritual activities involve the body and must respect the structure and functioning of the body.

Theologians of all the great monotheistic religions (Judaism, Christianity, Islam) have insisted that body-soul unity is a necessary implication of the doctrine of the creation of the human person by God and of the resurrection of the body. These theologians also have rejected the notion of reincarnation found in polytheistic religions because it seems to imply that the human person is a purely spiritual being and the body only its prison or a garment to be changed. Christianity goes even further by insisting on the Incarnation (through which God becomes truly a human being in bodily existence) and on the indwelling of the Holy Spirit in the human body as its temple, through which believers become members of the Body of Christ. This same principle leads to the sacramental concept of the human body by which the basic biological functions become signs of spiritual events; birth is reenacted in baptism, eating and drinking in the Eucharist, and sexual union in the sacrament of matrimony.

Catholic theology, however, recognizes a certain measure of truth in body-soul dualism that can be reconciled with the fundamental unity of the human person. The human person is a complex unity in which conflicts can arise, so the integration and self-individuation of any man or woman can be achieved only by discipline and a sane asceticism. Such asceticism, however, does not imply that the human body in its biological functions is evil or of little value, but rather that it shares in the spiritual dignity of the total person and therefore needs to be integrated with the other dimensions of human personality. Hence the body cannot be suppressed or ruthlessly sacrificed to higher values or even trivialized as of no moral significance. Instead Catholic theology has always been concerned to find a middle way between the dualistic extremes of asceticism and antinomianism (permissiveness) and to respect the intrinsic teleology of bodily structures and basic biological functions.

2.3 Higher Levels of Health

The development of modern psychotherapy and of psychosomatic medicine leaves no doubt that mental health, although it is intimately connected with physical health, is not identical with physical health. Mental disease is not describable in terms of physiological malfunction but only in terms of impairment of the characteristic human ability to deal with the environment by *symbolic* activity and communication. Human beings far surpass animals in the capacity to use symbols (images, feelings, words) which stand for realities but which can be combined and ordered in many ways different from the relatively fixed order of real things. The images and concepts by which people represent their world do so only imperfectly, but they can be verified and refined by using them as tools to change the world. Physical disease, especially dysfunctions of the central nervous system, can impair this symbolic activity; but the activity also can be disturbed by social and educational factors within the symbolic realm itself. For example, a physiologically healthy child can acquire prejudiced ways of perceiving reality and neurotic ways of reacting to it because of its social environment.

At this level of symbolic or psychic activity, however, are differentiated levels of health and disease that are too often lumped together. To reduce human psychic health to emotional adjustment and maturity is a common fallacy today, which we call *psychologism*. Psychologism assumes that a physically healthy person, who also is free from mental illnesses that are considered within the purview of psychotherapy, is entirely healthy. To avoid psychologism, one must realize that psychotherapy has the modest goal of helping patients acquire that degree of self-understanding and emotional integration which will free them from unconscious psychological determinisms that interfere with practical daily life. Psychologically healthy persons are "in touch with their feelings." They perceive the world of ordinary activity as most people do—without manifestly absurd illusions or projections. They are free to choose between practical alternatives, do not have unrealistic expectations, and are willing to assume responsibility for the consequences of their actions.

At this point of freedom from psychological determinisms a whole new level of human activity opens up: the level of free, responsible moral activity. Psychotics are incapable of moral action (at least within the area of the psychosis), and neurotics are severely limited in their freedom and responsibility. Only the free man or woman is a person fully capable of either moral good or evil.

It is also possible to fall into still another fallacy, however—that of *moralism*. This error reduces human failure to questions of right and wrong, attributes either mental or physical disease to the victims' sins, and attempts to heal them by moral exhortations. A more subtle form of this same fallacy is the assumption that the highest wholeness in the human personality is achieved at the level of practical ethical life. Some people identify the good person with the responsible, prudent, decent man or woman.

This fallacy ignores the deepest and most central fact of the human personality, namely, that which is spiritual, intuitive, and creative. Some psychotherapists of the Jungian and existentialist schools do concern themselves with this level, but only to free such activity from neurotic and psychotic impediments. To deal with this spiritual level of human existence in its own terms is the task of neither the psychologist nor the moralist, but of the philosopher, theologian, and spiritual guide. Spiritual health and disease, therefore, cannot be reduced simply to moral or psychological terms.

Even at this spiritual level it is possible to fall into the fallacy of what the philosopher Jacques Maritain called "angelism"—treating human persons as bodiless angels, or pure souls, as Plato and Descartes considered the true human self. Human problems cannot be treated in purely spiritual terms, in which the lower levels of human functioning—physiology, symbolic activity, and practical responsibility—are ignored. It would seem that this fallacy has influenced those mystical and religious enthusiasts who attempt to heal all bodily, psychological, and moral ills by purely spiritual means.

Thus trying to understand the fullness of human health requires being on guard against those reductionist fallacies which ignore the many dimensions of human health. For example, to determine whether alcoholism is a sickness without reductionist or arbitrary social construction, we must first define alcoholism in behavioral terms, and then four questions must be asked. First, is it a biological disease in terms of biological criteria, for example, a change in physiology that puts a strain on biological homeostasis? Second, is it a psychological disease in terms of psychological criteria, for example, a persistent emotional conflict that restricts the victim's capacity for intelligent free choice? Third, is it a moral disease in terms of social criteria, for example, free choice of behavior that is contradictory to the full actualization of the person in community? Fourth, is it a spiritual disease by spiritual criteria, for example, closure to intuition, creativity, commitment? Moreover, how are these different levels of functioning interrelated? The terms *disease* and *health* are used at each of these levels in very different but analogous ways.

2.4 Integrating Human Function

Human nature is an open system in which several hierarchical orders of functioning are integrated in the healthy person. The term *integrity* indicates that in a perfect whole each part must be fully differentiated and developed. Furthermore, each part must be fitted into the whole and harmonized with it by correct interrelations and interactions with the other parts of the whole. Integrity is lacking when a part is suppressed or unduly inhibited in function or when, on the other hand, one part is hypertrophied because of the injury of others.

In a hierarchical order some parts are said to be higher because they are necessary to the unification and integration of the whole in the performance of its most complex and specific functions (for example, the central nervous system). Other parts are said to be lower because their functions are more integrated than integrating. Yet the lower parts may be essential for the higher parts to function at all (such as, the liver and the kidneys). This concept is expressed in the saying, "He lives to eat, but should eat to live," which means that engaging in higher activities (living) requires eating. Consequently, eating is integral to human life. But eating is a lower activity, a means and not an end. When eating becomes an end, an absolute not measured by something higher, it destroys the integrity of human functioning.

It would be a mistake, however, to think that only the higher values in this hierarchy are human personal values. People share biological and psychological needs with other animals, but they share social and spiritual needs only with other persons. Nevertheless, all these needs and their correlative values, whether generically animal or specifically human, are equally needs and values of the human person, none of which can be destroyed without destroying personhood. People are human not only because they need love, but also because they need food.

This hierarchical yet interdependent ordering of the four levels of human functioning is true for any subsystem within each level. At the biological level the human body is divided into organ systems and then into organs, each having specific functions. The organ systems are commonly enumerated as follows: (1) nervous, (2) endocrine, (3) skeletal and muscular, (4) integumentary (skin), (5) alimentary, (6) respiratory, (7) circulatory, (8) excretory, and (9) reproductive. These systems are interrelated in very complex ways and not in any simple, linear hierarchy. Yet the nervous system (with the intimately related endocrine system) obviously coordinates the others and is the most directly involved in the psychological and higher functions. Also, the reproductive system has a special importance (1) because it is directly involved in the evolutionary process by which the human species came to be and is continued and (2) because it is the source of the family and hence of the communal character of the human person.

Greater unification of function occurs at the psychic level of personality. Yet psychic life is also composite. The external senses are differentiated by their organs; psychological functions, such as feelings and emotions, have some kind of localization in various parts of the brain, although they also involve other centers and the endocrine system as well.

At the rational and ethical levels still greater integration and unification of functions into the self-aware, conscious, free, self-controlling subject or person take place. Even at this level, what have been traditionally called the reason and the will are differentiated as distinct but ultimately correlative functions. Only at the spiritual level do the intellect and will come together in the top of the mind or "heart" (in the biblical, metaphorical sense) of the human person, in which peak experiences and basic decisions, commitments, and fundamental options take place to complete the total integration of the person.

2.5 Summary

Health is an analogous concept and applies to things and persons in different ways. But human health has a definite meaning: it is optimal functioning of the human organism to meet and integrate biological, psychological, social, and spiritual needs. Hence human health involves much more than biological functioning. How one assumes responsibility for health and enlists the help of others in this endeavor is the topic of the next three chapters.

Footnote

1. Henrik Blum, *Planning for Health Development and Application of Social Change* (New York: Behavioral Publishers, 1974), p. 93.

Study Questions

1. How do the *ontological* vs. the *physiological* concepts of disease apply to the common cold? To lung cancer? To cardiovascular disease in the U.S.?

2. If you were asked to select five men and five women from a specific population, who were the most healthy physically and mentally, what criteria would you use? If you were asked to select from this same population those who "ought to see their physician," what criteria would you use? How would you decide when someone who has been ill is now "well" and therefore no longer in need of medical care?

3. If you were interviewing a person "with a problem," what questions might you ask to determine whether the person should be referred to a physician, a psychologist, a lawyer, an ethicist, or a clergyman?

4. What are some examples of *psychosomatic* illnesses? Within the psychic realm give some examples of how spiritual, ethical, and psychological factors can affect health and are affected by it.

5. Many medical ethical controversies today make use of the concept of "quality of life." How would you evaluate the quality of life of an adult, a child, a very old person? What criteria would you use?

Cases

1. In the United States the average person is heavier for his or her height and body build than the average person in Japan where fewer people suffer from cardiovascular disease. How would you define *normal* weight? *Normal* caloric intake? *Normal* types of diet? *Normal* exercise?

2. A study of 47 prominent contemporary British artists by Kay Jamison, MD, a professor of psychiatry at the University of California at Los Angeles showed that more than half were manic-depressive compared to 6 percent of the general population. A study of writers by Professor Nancy Andreasan of the University of Iowa showed that 67 percent suffered from an emotional disorder, compared to 13 percent of a control group. If manic-depressive psychosis is a mental disease (probably with a physiological basis), why should it be associated with extraordinary creative abilities?

3. St. Augustine of Hippo, whose health was often poor, is considered one of the great saints and doctors of the Church. He is famous for his creative work as a theologian, and for his remarkable dedication, courage, self-sacrifice, and compassion for suffering. He also had extraordinary mystical experiences. Psychoanalytical studies based on his intimate *Confessions* have explained his career in terms of his Oedipus conflict, his love-hate attachment for his mother, Monica.

   Distinguish the spiritual, ethical, psychological, and biological dimensions of St. Augustine's life. Can the spiritual, ethical, and biological be explained by the psychological? Can the spiritual, ethical, and psychological be explained by the biological? Can the ethical, psychological, and biological be explained by the spiritual? What is the relation of Augustine's morality (as a young man he lived with a concubine, later lived as a celibate) to the other dimensions of his life?

4. After he nearly killed a pedestrian, John was arrested for the fifth time in three years for driving while intoxicated. As part of his treatment he was referred to a physician, a pastor, a lawyer, a psychiatrist, and a social worker. How might each of these professionals deal with his case? What proposals could they make for his rehabilitation and care? What is John's responsibility, presuming that alcoholism is in some sense a disease?

5. Oscar Wilde, a brilliantly witty writer, believed that beauty is the highest value and that an artist should sacrifice everything to achieve it. Consequently he felt that a bohemian life style, including homosexual affairs, was justified because it contributed to a range of experiences that would be useful to him as a writer. This eventually led to his imprisonment and social ruin. Some have praised him for his courage in sacrificing his life for his art. Others have suspected that he was driven by unconscious suicidal motives. On his death-bed he became a Catholic, an idea he had toyed with all his life.

   Was Wilde a kind of martyr? Was his case any different than that of Madame Curie who destroyed her own health in her successful efforts to discover radium? Is there a hierarchy of values in human life? How are the higher values dependent on the lower?

Chapter 3
Personal Responsibility for Health

3.1 Commitment to Life

The primary responsibility for a person's health rests on that individual, not on the community. This principle is clear because we maintain the intensely personal character of health in all its dimensions. Thus, the main ethical principle for health care ethics is that one must seek to preserve and maintain one's own health insofar as is possible. Biological health concerns that which is most individual and private to me, namely, my own body. My body, by its very materiality, its space-time limitations, is mine and mine alone. It identifies me as *not* anybody else. Someone can share a room with me, a table, a bed, even my clothes; but he cannot occupy my body. Ultimately, it is by reason of my body that I am alone in myself; yet it is also by reason of my body that I am in the world of things and persons.

My body is profoundly subjective not only because I possess it as my own and know it as myself, but because it is incommunicable. Much of what goes on in my body is hidden even from me; and even what I know of it I know for the most part in a thoroughly subjective way that I cannot express. When I consult a physician I experience the difficulty of relating how I feel. Bodily feelings are vivid, yet vague and hard to put into words. I am the final judge of whether I really feel well. When no medical test reveals anything wrong with me, but I do not feel well, then I am not well.

Even if my sickness is imaginary, it is real at the psychological level and therefore is a psychological illness. At the higher ethical and spiritual levels, health also depends on an individual's own conscience, or spiritual discernment. Thus no one but the person ultimately can judge his or her own well-being.

Furthermore, this subjectivity is true not only of diagnosis, but also of treatment. The psychotherapist constantly has to remind the client: "No one, ultimately, can help you if you refuse to help yourself." Even the spiritual counselor must say, "God will help you by his grace, but you must let yourself be opened to that grace."

Healing is a living process that must occur within the organism. It is true that near the end of life patients may be unconscious and completely passive about the surgery, medication, and injections thrust upon them, but these treatments seldom result in healing. Convalescence is an active process on the part of patients, and staying well is clearly something that they alone must do. No physician or nurse can make patients take pills, stick to a diet, or take necessary rest and exercise.

In a profound way the will to life and health is the fundamental element in all healing, and this will to life must be intelligent, that is, a realistic search for the means to health. Most physicians and nurses seem to believe that the patient's fighting spirit is a critical factor in recovering health.

Therefore, whether in working to prevent sickness, to maintain optimal health, to assist recovery from disease, or to rehabilitate oneself after a crippling trauma, a person must make a commitment to life and health. It might seem that no special commitment needs to be made, since everyone has an instinct to live. No doubt the need to live, to grow, and to function well is innate; it is within the very design of any organism. But in humankind, who at their innermost depths are not instinctive but free, this commitment is not a given; rather, it must be freely made.

The commitment to life, which overcomes commitments to death, such as violence, pollution of the environment, drug and alcohol addiction, treachery in human relations, is an affirmation of the value not only of pleasure, but also of freedom, intelligence, creativity, and love. As God says through Moses:

> I call heaven and earth today to witness against you. I have set before you life and death, the blessing and the curse. Choose life, then, that you and your descendants may live, by loving the Lord, your God, heeding his voice, and holding fast to him. For that will mean life for you, a long life for you to live on the land which the Lord swore he would give to your fathers Abraham, Isaac and Jacob (Dt 30:19-20).

Such a commitment to life has to proceed from the spiritual level, although it is ordinarily manifested at lower levels as well. This deep commitment can be so blocked that persons profoundly dedicated to life in their spiritual center can yet suffer from an unconscious will to die at the psychological level.

Judeo-Christian Teaching

The Old Testament presents the Jewish view as profoundly life affirming. It constantly emphasizes the idea that God gives his friends health, security, children, and long life and that God has created men and women for life and wishes to prolong it for them. In consideration of the fact that the just often suffer persecution and martyrdom, the last books of the Old Testament affirm that God will raise his friends from the dead to everlasting life (cf. 2 M 7:22-23). Jesus approved by saying, "God is God of the living, not of the dead" (Mk 12:27). St. Paul also teaches (Rm 5:12 ff.) that death (and by implication disease and aging) is somehow a consequence of sin (cf. Ws 1:13-15; see also Chapter 11, p. 193). Thus disease, aging, and death are not willed by God, but only permitted by him as a punishment (the inevitable consequence of the sin of the human race, which has committed itself to death rather than to life). St. Paul joyfully affirms that in Christ all may be born again to everlasting life.

When Jesus prayed in the garden, "O Father, you have the power to do all things. Take this cup away from me. But let it be as you would have it, not as I" (Mk 14:36), he was affirming his own commitment to life, but expressing his willingness to endure death if the Father in his transcendent wisdom knew that only through death could doubting men and women be convinced that God and his Son truly love them for their own sake and not for the sake of honor or power.

Thus a sound theology teaches that the Father and Christ desire only life, a desire which is fulfilled in the Resurrection. Following Jesus, who as St. Paul says was "never anything but 'Yes'" (2 Co 1:20), Christians must always affirm life while being willing to endure the evil of death (1) as witnesses to others that faith, hope, and love cannot be overcome by the fear and despair of death and (2) as sharers in Jesus' experience of death, by which we learn to be as unselfish, trustful, and hopeful as he was. The Christian, however, endures death serenely not because death is good, but because resurrection and eternal life are good and destroy death forever.

Thus it is essential to realize that Christian health care should never be directed to the passive acceptance of disease or death, as if they in themselves were somehow spiritual goods. In authentic Christian belief every individual has a responsibility to choose life and to fight for it. Christians must fight for a full and abundant life and must accept disease and death only as inevitable incidents in the battle, but not as its final outcome. Christian acceptance or resignation is not acquiescence, but rather a strategy by which good can be brought out of evil. Sometimes the enemy can be defeated only by patience, turning these evils into opportunities for growth and learning; but sickness and death should always be perceived as enemies. Christians should stand with St. Paul in condemning death as the ultimate evil ("and the last enemy to be destroyed is death" [Co 15:26]), especially if death is understood as the destruction of the human whole, that is, physical, psychological, moral, and above all spiritual death.

Spiritual death is nothing more than the commitment to personal death. Deliberately turning from the love of God and neighbor toward a false self-sufficiency is spiritual suicide. The self-sufficiency is so contradictory to the very nature of all persons and to their expansion into community, that this refusal to ask for any help can end only in prideful despair. Probably physical suicide seldom has this character of total death, since usually it seems to be an attempt to escape to some better life or at least to peace and sleep. But spiritual suicide is possible if a person shuts off all others and considers himself entirely self-sufficient.

The person who has made a spiritual commitment to life will strive to achieve wholeness in every dimension of personality. Some, of course, are so deceived by dualism that they do not realize that spiritual wholeness requires the integration of lower human functions. Thus some pseudo-mystics have neglected ethical development, moral people have neglected psychological and physical health, and people concerned about psychological health have not always perceived its intimate connection with both ethical and biological health. But a true understanding of the commitment to life leads to a balanced concern for the whole personality.

3.2 Preventive Medicine and Life Style

Personal responsibility for health is often thought of as just going to a physician, but this is only a part of it. The famous dictum attributed to Hippocrates was that the physician should prescribe "regimen, medicine, and surgery" in that order, meaning by *regimen* the person's life style of diet, rest, and exercise. Today medical technology emphasizes the curative aspect of medicine more than the preventive aspect. In the future perhaps the center of medical ethics will shift from the hospital (curative) to a center for teaching people how to improve their life styles and maintain health.

Current life styles, in terms of physiological and psychological norms, seem to foster extremely unhealthy people. First of all, modern life often leaves insufficient time for rest, not merely in the sense of lack of sleep, but also in the sense of too much stress. It might seem that people have more leisure because machines have relieved them of much hard, servile labor. But this relief is more than offset by the routine of urban life that forces us, for example, to spend hours a day driving to and from work in the hazards of traffic. Clearly, as individuals, people are powerless to escape this system, but within it they do have some freedom to make choices that will gradually give their lives greater simplicity and a more natural rhythm, free from excessive competition and the drive for success.

Reduced stress also contributes to moral and spiritual health by making room for a contemplative atmosphere, for service rather than for ambition for power, for solitude and silence, as well as for more time to give to persons and less to things. In the past, men and women suffered from the burden of manual work, from fear of enemies, from disease and hunger. Yet there was a natural rhythm of effort and of rest. Today these natural rhythms are often broken up by artificial pressures and hectic overstimulation.

A stressful life can lead to addiction, the enslavement of human beings to the pursuit of intense pleasure or anesthesia as an escape from the pain of life. This addiction can be to hard drugs, smoking, alcohol, and tranquilizers; in a milder form to the common addiction to overeating; and in a particularly corrosive way to the anxious twentieth century pursuit of sexual pleasure. In moderation, none of these things is unhealthy, but in addictive form they become obsessive and destructive to health.

Finally, modern people lack proper physical exercise. Although sports are highly cultivated, they are more watched than played by the average man and woman. The average person does little manual work and seldom walks or dances.

Assuming personal responsibility for health therefore requires a scientifically based knowledge of hygiene, good diet, rest, exercise, and moderation. These cannot be imposed from without. People need to design their lives to meet personal requirements, which differ greatly. To be healthy, people must express their personality in their life style—not a false one or a resignation to being half alive.

The problems of mental health are similar. People are overstimulated by sensation and passive imagination, but impoverished in active imagination, reflection, and meditation. They receive much input and information, but often little integration of symbols and feelings. They live at the top of their heads, out of touch with their feelings.

Concerning spiritual life, many persons live without clear commitments or goals and suffer from the emptiness, meaninglessness and absurdity of life, and loneliness, never seeking deep communication with others. Health therefore requires the courage to criticize the accepted norms of modern life and face the ethical dilemmas produced by modern technology. Perhaps it is futile to talk about a natural way of life, as counterculturists do. Has that point in human history arrived when nature must be replaced with a fabricated world, even with human beings who have fabricated themselves?

3.3 Stewardship

"The Lord God took the man and settled him into the Garden of Eden to cultivate and care for it" (Gn 2:15). Although humans are "masters" over lesser creatures, dominion over them and over themselves is only a stewardship for which human beings remain responsible to the one Lord.

Classical theology based Christian ethics on the conviction that God endowed all human beings with one common nature, which remains essentially the same throughout all history from Adam and Eve to the Last Judgment. Human beings are stewards of this nature as of the world in which God has placed them. By studying the God-given structure and dynamics of this nature, it is possible, so theologians in the past thought, to formulate unchanging moral norms that are binding for every time and culture. Stewardship demanded that human beings abide by these norms lest they destroy the garden of the world and the temple of their own bodies, which were given them to cultivate and care for.

Classical theology, in its account of human dominion, was too greatly influenced by the Old Testament image of the monarch God jealous of his supreme dignity and power. In New Testament perspective God is best revealed in Christ, who "though he was in the form of God, did not deem equality with God something to be grasped at, but rather he emptied himself and took the form of a servant (Ph 2:6-7). Thus God is not jealous of his power but calls men and women to share in his work of making all things new (Rv 21:51). Such cooperation is not merely filling in details in a finished "plan of God." Rather he has called human beings to use their own initiative and originality in completing his work.

In creative activity, however, people have to respect their own limits and the limits of the materials with which they must work. These limits are not set by God out of any concern for his own authority. God himself is "limited" only by his own wisdom and love, which forbid him to do what is contradictory to his own nature. Human beings are far more limited by the fact that their share in God's knowledge and love is finite. No matter how they may progress in science, freedom, and power, they dare not contradict their own human nature without destroying themselves.

At any given moment in history, people's limits are set by their knowledge. Once they understand some aspect of nature well, they can freely choose to improve nature and surpass it. But when they lack that understanding, their efforts to improve on nature may prove disastrous. The evils of modern technology are not the result of creative use of knowledge, but of rash exploitation of a nature little understood. Above all, people have failed to understand themselves, their authentic needs, and their potentialities. Research and experimentation, with all the risks involved, are necessary, but we must proceed with reverence for the persons and the environment at risk.

3.4 Making Responsible Decisions of Conscience

Given the limits just mentioned, the practice of modern medicine constantly involves both technological and ethical judgments. Practitioners must ask not only "Can it be done?" but also "Ought we do what can be done?" The claim of health care professionals that they can make autonomous decisions about medical therapy is invalid. That professional knowledge makes health care professional experts in the techniques of medicine does not imply that they are experts in the *use* of these techniques, since use involves social, political, and moral values for which the patient retains decision-making responsibility.

Thus individuals who seek the services of a medical professional cannot simply delegate to that professional all decisions about their health on the grounds that the doctor knows best. On the other hand, rarely is the individual competent to decide questions of medical therapy unless given adequate information about the medical aspects of the decision. So there is a dilemma in medical decisions: Who has the knowledge both of the ethical norms and of the medical facts to make a responsible decision? And how are these norms and facts to be related to each other? This dilemma requires a discussion of the problem of developing a well-formed conscience.

Christian theology has always insisted that when it comes to concrete ethical decisions each normal individual has the capacity and the responsibility to judge and to act on his or her own judgment. This responsibility cannot be delegated to anyone else or to any institution—not to custom, to the law, or to advisers and not even to civil or religious leaders. This is true in medical issues as well. The capacity to make practical judgment in matters involving ethical issues is called *conscience*. The Second Vatican Council (1965c) said of it:

> For the human being has in his or her heart a law inscribed by God. A person's dignity lies in observing this law, and by it he or she will be judged. Conscience is the person's most secret core and sanctuary. There the person is alone with God whose voice echoes in the person's depths. By conscience, in a wonderful way, that law is made known which is fulfilled in the love of God and one's neighbor. Through loyalty to conscience, Christians are joined to others in the search for truth and for the right solution to so many moral problems which arise both in the life of individuals and from social relationships. Hence, the more a correct conscience prevails, the more do persons and groups turn aside from blind choice and try to be guided by the objective standards of moral conduct.[1]

Thus, when making personal decisions "guided by the objective standards of moral conduct" about health care, people have the responsibility to follow *informed* conscience; that is, (1) obtain as much relevant information as possible about a situation, both the facts and the objective moral standards (principles) that apply to the situations, and (2) make and carry out a decision in accordance with this information. Sin is the failure either to inform the conscience or to follow the conscience after informing it.

In any question of health care people have the responsibility (1) to learn the facts about the medical condition, (2) to determine in accord with an objective value system the needs and rights of the people involved, and (3) to come to a concrete, personal decision in spite of disagreement or pressures from others.

Does having all the information before making a decision definitely determine what the decision is to be? If it did, then there would be no such thing as freedom. Human beings are free not simply because they are relieved from any external forces coercing their decisions, but for two other reasons. First, usually there are many alternative means to a goal, some of which are clearly inappropriate, but often many are appropriate, each with its advantages and disadvantages. Hence some value choices will be between two or more good actions. Second, it is possible for people to reconsider their goals and to redefine or even alter them in view of some higher goal. Thus morality always involves a choice, and that choice is not always between a clear-cut good line of action and a clear-cut bad line. It may be between two or more good lines of action, and there may also be many wrong ways that involve different degrees of evil.

Since knowledge of the factors involved in any decision seldom results in a judgment that this or that action is best without qualification, it might seem that a rational decision is impossible. But knowledge or intellect is not the only factor involved in a decision of conscience; there is also will supported by feeling. Our decision is ethically good only if we have a good will (supported, if possible, by healthy emotions) that inclines us to follow our best information and ethical insight, even if they are not conclusive. An informed conscience needs knowledge of the facts and of the law, but it also requires a disciplined or virtuous affection for what will truly satisfy our needs in an integral manner. This element of affection is unappreciated by many contemporary ethicists who seek to turn ethical decisions into rational balancing acts, without consideration of the virtues or character which make good ethical reasoning sure and easy.

Certitude in Ethical Decisions - not on exam

Health care professionals today know only too well that ethical decisions may involve a real agony of conscience. People may be faced with the realization (1) that, although they have tried to get adequate information, they still do not have all the facts or the clear understanding of values that they really need to make an objectively correct decision; and (2) that even when they have acquired the best knowledge available, the best alternative may remain unclear, because every alternative has advantages and disadvantages. Such uncertainty causes many to think that in practical matters an ethical decision is finally nothing but a leap in the dark.

This is not the case. To act ethically, we need to have practical, not speculative, certitude. There may and usually does remain a speculative or objective doubt as to whether what we decide will actually work out for the best, but there must be no practical doubt. A person's conscience must be certain that for him or her, here and now, on the basis of the best information practically available, the best thing to do is A rather than B. Otherwise, the person would be acting blindly rather than on the basis of good will applied to the best information available.

When in doubt about whether a course of action is ethical, people should give the benefit of the doubt to existing custom, to established and well-known laws, or to their usual way of acting, and they should accept what has already been done as if it were well done. For example, procedures and policies well accepted in the medical profession should be used as norms of ethical behavior unless the contrary can be reasonably established. This conservative presumption is based on the fact that in human life what is customary and established at least has the merit of long experience, reflection, and survival. The world cannot be changed every day. On the other hand, people may also make the liberal presumption that they are free to do what seems most attractive and subjectively better, provided there is no clear law or reason against it or the rights of others to consider. For Catholics this freedom supposes loyalty to the living tradition of the Christian community in its authoritative expression by the popes and bishops.

Catholics and an Informed Conscience - not on exam

If we are to follow our informed conscience, how does a Christian go about informing his or her conscience? Since Christians believe that the ultimate ethical principles are to be found in the life and teaching of Jesus Christ, this means going beyond merely philosophical ethics to the Bible, in which we have an inspired record of that life and teaching. Yet the Bible has been interpreted and applied in many different ways. How are we to know which is right? Catholics believe that Jesus himself provided an answer to this question by choosing twelve apostles to instruct the people and promising them the guidance of the Holy Spirit until the end of time (Jn 16:7-16). Moreover, Jesus appointed St. Peter the head of this college of the apostles to maintain the unity of their teaching (Mt 16:17-19); Lk 22:30-34; Jn 21:15-19). This teaching authority (technically called *Magisterium*) continues in the bishop of Rome or the Pope. Although there are disagreements among Christians about how to interpret even these texts of the Bible, it is difficult to deny that in the course of history the Roman Catholic Church has been able to maintain a unity and consistency of teaching difficult to find in the many Protestant denominations or the many national Orthodox Churches.

Consequently the Second Vatican Council declares:

> Bishops who teach in communion with the Bishop of Rome are to be revered by all as witnesses of divine and Catholic truth; the faithful, for their part, are obliged to submit to their bishop's decision, made in the name of Christ, in matters of faith and morals, and to adhere to it with a ready and respectful allegiance of mind. This loyal submission of the will and intellect must be given, in a special way, to the authentic teaching authority of the Bishop of Rome, even when he does not speak *ex cathedra* (with full authority) in such wise, indeed, that his supreme teaching authority be acknowledged with respect, and sincere assent be given to decisions made by him, conformably with his manifest mind and intention, which is made known principally either by the character of the documents in question, or by the frequency with which a certain doctrine is proposed, or by the manner in which the doctrine is formulated.[2]

Therefore a Catholic seeking to inform his or her conscience about some ethical question will first of all inquire if there is a papal teaching on the subject and then whether the local bishop, or that bishop along with the national conference of bishops, has given instruction on the question, and what type of instruction this is. If he finds that an ecumenical council under the leadership of the Pope, or the Pope in his own right, has declared that a teaching is contained in the Word of God and is to be believed by all the faithful (seldom the case as regards moral questions), then such a teaching is to be considered definitive and certain ("infallible") and not subject to revision. Such decisions by the Magisterium leave no room for further discussion, except for explanation, clarification, or further detail. Because these definitions a. rare, they are called the use of the *extraordinary* Magisterium.

Most documents of the Church that instruct us in how to form our consciences, however, are only exercises of the *ordinary* Magisterium and have a wide range of certitude, from the documents of Vatican II (which deliberately made no definitive declarations) to the Sunday sermon of a priest or deacon. Obviously these are not all of equal value in settling ethical questions, and some may contain serious mistakes. Consequently it is erroneous to quote Church documents to settle ethical questions without carefully examining their precise authority, even when these documents issue from the Vatican or are signed by the Pope himself.

Nevertheless, it is an even more serious error to disregard anything but the infallibly defined teachings of the Church and follow one's own opinions in other matters. Those who think that nothing but defined teaching is binding on all Catholics forget that the Magisterium could not define a doctrine infallibly (extraordinary teaching) unless it was already contained in the Church's ordinary teaching, since the Magisterium has no authority to add to Revelation, but only to interpret and explicate it. Thus the ordinary teaching of the Church contains a great deal of infallible teaching, although it has not yet been explicitly declared such by the Church. Infallible ordinary teaching can be recognized by signs, such as that it has been taught universally in the Church in a continuous way as revealed and forms an element of liturgical worship and sacramental practice.[3]

Since Catholics in the process of informing their consciences want the best guidance they can get (just as we want the best medical advice we can get for our health's sake), it seems clear that they ought to respect the moral guidance of the Magisterium even when it is not certain that a teaching is either defined or definable. But what are they to do if they find that theologians disagree about some point of morals, or even dissent from the magisterial teaching? The fact that most theologians agree on a point is a sign that this point is correct, but when theologians, no matter how numerous and distinguished, disagree with the Magisterium, it does not make their opinion of equal weight or safe to follow.

The only situation in which a Catholic might in practice form his or her conscience in dissent from the Magisterium would be when after study and prayer it seems clear that from the nature of the documents or their inconsistency with more certain Church teachings, or the certainly known facts, that the official teaching is in error.[4] For example, a scientist might know that a teaching which is not defined, or clearly infallible from other signs, rests on a scientific error; or a biblical scholar might know that a teaching which is not defined, or clearly infallible by other signs, rests on a mistranslation of a Biblical text, in which case dissent would be justified.

It should be obvious that in moral questions which are complex and in which the arguments, both pro and con, are seldom totally convincing, that it would be rare for an individual to have sufficient certitude of this sort to override the well-considered teaching of the Magisterium, and especially of the Pope. Many people who maintain the teaching of the Church to be in error (as in regard to contraception, adultery, or abortion) seem to proceed from a dualistic concept of the human person or a secular value system.

Thus when a Catholic considers the teaching of the Church in medical matters, he or she should not seek merely to obey that teaching but to understand it, and above all to assimilate the values that give rise to the teaching. In regard to abortion, for example, one must learn to distinguish between direct and indirect abortion, but also one must seek to assimilate the value that each person is sacred, no matter what qualities and characteristics the person possesses or does not possess.

Concrete Application of Moral Norms

Catholic health care professionals need not feel in medical matters that they are sinking into a theological morass when applying Church teaching to medical issues. They need only keep in mind that there are two different levels of moral certitude: (1) the theoretical level of principles and value priorities and (2) the practical level of concrete application of these principles to particular problems of moral decision. At the theoretical level of principles and values, Jesus Christ has given Christians ample guidance on "the weightier matters of the law, justice and mercy, and good faith" (Mt 23:23); and they are clearly expressed in the ordinary teaching of the Church.

The practical level of concrete application of ethical principles is a complex and difficult area where official Church teaching can be of great help, but where perfect clarity or undebatable certitude would not be expected. At this practical level one can only say, "I am as sure of my decision as I can be, but I realize that I could be wrong" (moral certitude). Health care professionals are well aware that the clarity and high probability of scientific laws are not to be expected in the application of these laws to particular medical decisions. For example, it may be difficult to determine whether tube feeding for a particular patient is a comfort measure or a life prolonging measure. It is painful to have to make a life-and-death medical decision without being sure how the principles in the medical textbook fit the particular case; yet such decisions have to be made every day. In the same way, moral decisions cannot be made simply by referring to theological textbooks or to official Church documents.

The fact that the pastoral guidance of the Church at the level of concrete application leaves considerable room for individual and institutional judgment makes it obvious that the effort of Christians to acquire and act on a well-formed conscience involves no little risk and conflict. Hence a vital factor in such efforts is self-criticism or maturity of moral judgment. People have to be aware of their own biases, narrowness of experience and outlook, and half-conscious motivation. Consciences have their own psychological and spiritual pathologies—as do emotions—and they have often been weakened or distorted by defective ethical education.

In light of the foregoing, the material on well-formed conscience may be summarized as follows. When making a decision about health care, each person has the responsibility:

1. To inform themselves as fully as practically possible on both the facts and the ethical norms

2. To form a morally certain practical judgment of conscience on the basis of this information

3. To act according to this well-formed conscience

4. To accept responsibility for their actions

3.5 Patients' Rights

Since each person has the primary obligation of caring for his or her own health, each also has the obligation to seek and choose professional people to help advise them concerning health care. Yet this does not mean that persons can surrender to others the responsibility of making decisions about their health. Professionals are helpers, not keepers.

No one is a good judge in his or her own case; precisely because health is so personal a value, it is something about which it is hard to be objective. People tend to delude themselves both as to how well they are and as to how sick they are. Thus to be whole and healthy, each person must be humble enough to seek help from others more expert, or at least more objective about their problems.

Not only humility, but also courage and hope are required. Fear, apathy, shame, and self-punishment are important psychological and moral factors that prevent people from getting the health care they need. The most dangerous aspect of any disease condition is that it may make the victim despair of health or be afraid to seek help to obtain health. At the psychological level, neurotics and alcoholics notoriously deny their problems and resist therapy. Physically sick people also seem to have an almost instinctive dread of recognizing their illness and facing the pain of its cure. Even hypochondriacs, who seem only too eager to claim sickness, use the illusion of one disease to hide from themselves some other sickness—perhaps at the psychological, ethical, or spiritual level—which would be even more painful to face. They crowd the physician's office in unconscious avoidance of the psychotherapist or some moral or spiritual counselor.

Perhaps the reason people resist the truth about themselves is because they are organisms who tend, once an acute crisis has passed, to adapt to a chronic disease by integrating it into their way of life. Once such a distorted integration has become fixed, they sense real peril in returning to the acutely painful crisis that might be provoked by a new effort to become really well. Hence they dread physicians and avoid them as long as possible. Thus both psychological and physiological diseases are allowed to escalate dramatically before people can submit themselves to treatment. The same principle holds at the ethical and spiritual levels, so that most profound moral and spiritual conversions are brought about only after a deep conviction of sin. Jesus noted that it was the publicans and prostitutes who were most likely to enter the Kingdom of God (Mt 21:31).

Choosing a Physician

Even when people have the humility and courage to seek a physician, they are faced with very serious ethical problems in choosing a good one. For example, their choice may be very much restricted by the complex organization of modern medical care and the maldistribution of its services. Or, the patient may not be able to judge accurately the professional ability of the physician.

Certainly it is true that in every age many, perhaps most, people have been quite irresponsible in selecting their medical guides. The very fears that prevent people from seeking help also cause them often to prefer the quack (medical, psychological, ethical, or spiritual) to the competent guide whom they suspect may make them face a painful reality. The quack knows how to exploit these fears, this flight from real diagnosis and cure, to gain control over the patient. Not all quacks are incompetents, since very able guides can easily be tempted to use their own gifts to gain power for themselves, as the history of illicit medical experimentation evidences.

To escape enslavement to the incompetent or exploitative professional, people need to be conscious of the rights that correlate to their responsibility to choose professional help prudently. In 1973 the American Hospital Association formulated a document entitled *Patient's Rights* (see Appendix). Although it was never adopted universally by hospitals, it does give a good summary of what a patient should be aware of when evaluating his or her rights in regard to a physician or health care facility. They can be summed up as follows:

1. The right to the whole truth
2. The right to privacy and personal dignity
3. The right to refuse any test, procedure, or treatment
4. The right to read and copy medical records

The rights proposed above all rest on the fundamental concept of informed consent, which is discussed in Chapter 6. If the patient is to give free consent, then he or she must also be able to refuse any test, procedure, or treatment. The right to privacy and personal dignity implies the right of patients to refuse to be involved in any professional procedures that make them objects to be examined or discussed for the benefit or convenience of professionals or students rather than for the patient's own therapy.

If this consent is to be not only free, but also informed, then the patient has the right to the whole truth, including access to read and copy medical records. Many professionals deny these rights on the grounds that the patient is not able to understand the technical information known to the physician and may be harmed by it. Such difficulties do not disprove patients' rights to know so that their consent may be fully informed, but only establishes the professional's duty to communicate this information in ways that are helpful, not harmful, to patients.

Thus the underlying ethical issue of trust between patient and health care professional arises. Is competency the primary consideration in choosing a physician? Certainly it is the specific qualification most people seek in any professional, including their physicians. If physicians are not also trustworthy, however, in the sense that they are sincerely dedicated to helping the patient get well, then their medical competency is dangerous—as in the case of the brilliantly competent surgeon eager only for more bodies on which to demonstrate his skill.

Patients have an obligation toward their physicians as well. People should not, therefore, lightly accept the idea that personal responsibility for their own health is satisfied merely by assuming a critical attitude toward physicians and demanding their rights from them. Such a responsibility also includes willingness to trust physicians once they have been prudently chosen, to make good use of their advice, and to cooperate with their healing efforts. While people should never be afraid to protect their rights and to insist that physicians give patients all the information they need to give informed consent to treatment, they should also give them a deserved respect. Trustworthy and competent health care professionals do people a very precious service, for which they deserve profound gratitude, good reputation, and fair and prompt payment.

3.6 Conclusions

The primary responsibility for one's health care rests with each individual. Each in his or her commitment to life must practice a stewardship of the body and mind God has given them by making ethical decisions of health based on an informed conscience. To properly inform their conscience, they need both to obtain the best medical advice available and the teaching of the Church. This implies a careful choice of the health care professionals who serve them and an insistence on their rights as patients.

Footnotes

1. Austin Flannery, editor, "Church in the Modern World," N.16, *Documents of Vatican II* (Collegeville: Liturgical Press, 1975).

2. *Ibid.*, N.25.

3. *Ibid.*

4. "Human Life in Our Day," *Pastoral Letter of the American Hierarchy*, (Washington, DC: United States Catholic Conference, 1968), p. 18.

Study Questions

1. The philosopher, Nietzsche, contended that Christianity is a "life-negating" religion, because Jesus was a celibate who allowed himself to be crucified without defending himself and who proclaimed an other-worldly Kingdom of God instead of affirming the maximum enjoyment of this life. What do you think of this understanding of Christianity?

2. Design a life plan promoting optimal health for a man or woman whose life work is that of a busy physician (or a business executive). What habits are to be avoided and what encouraged?

3. How could the physicians of a small city be involved in the city's problems of environmental pollution and stewardship of local resources of water, green space, fauna, and flora?

4. List and describe the resources available to Catholic medical professionals faced with making conscientious decisions to difficult ethical problems.

5. Prepare a "Bill of Patient's Rights and Responsibilities."

Cases

1. Bill, a 35-year-old cocaine user, has a high-paying job and no family responsibilities. He is told by his physician that recent studies have shown that cocaine presents a serious cardiac risk to middle-age persons because it releases large amounts of adrenaline into the system. Bill, however, figures that he can afford financially to continue the habit and that we all have to go some day, and is willing to take his chances. Does Bill have any moral responsibility to give up cocaine? Why?

2. In Ibsen's famous play, *An Enemy of the People*, a physician attempts to awaken the townspeople to the danger arising from pollution of the water system. They don't want to hear his warnings because his information hurts some people's reputations and his proposals for a remedy tread on the other people's toes.

   Can you think of current situations where there is resistance by vested interests or by the public to problems of stewardship and preventive medicine? What could medical professionals do to overcome this? Does the medical profession itself sometimes support such resistance?

3. A number of Catholic theologians have supported the concept of "freedom of choice of abortion" despite the declarations against abortion by the Vatican and the American bishops. They have argued: (1) it is not always necessary or helpful to support morality by law; (2) there is no national consensus on the question; (3) a law against abortion could not be enforced; (4) it might lead to an increase of illegal abortions; (5) in some cases, such as rape or danger to the mother's health, abortion seems medically justified. What would be the proper process to inform one's conscience on this issue?

4. Several modes of treatment are possible for breast cancer: radical surgery to remove the whole breast and adjacent areas; surgery to remove only the tumor; chemotherapy and radiation therapy without surgery. Mary has a small malignant tumor without evidence of metastasis (spread to other organs). Her physician, Dr. D, is convinced on the basis of his personal experience that the risks are lower if radical surgery is performed at an early stage of the pathology. He knows Mary is very upset with the diagnosis and to spare her further confusion he tells her his judgment without explaining that other physicians disagree as to the proper treatment in such cases or what the alternative treatments are.

   Have Mary's rights been violated? Would she have a case for a malpractice suit if she is dissatisfied with the result of the operation which has disfigured her, even if the radical surgery saved her life?

5. Rudolfo is admitted to a city hospital for observation. Because he is such a difficult patient, he has to be physically tied down to his bed. The restraints are improperly fastened, however, and he is nearly strangled one evening when an orderly raises his bed. As a result of the accident, he suffers severe brain damage and is left permanently unconscious. The hospital wants to

remove all life support, but Rudolfo's attorney believes that the hospital should continue to care for him. What are the ethical responsibilities of the hospital in this case?

Chapter 4

Responsibility of Health Care Professionals

Though each of us is primarily responsible for his or her own health and health care, the communal nature of the human personality makes it clear that we need the help of others in our endeavors to maintain or restore health. Thus we need the help of health care professionals and society.

4.1 What is a Profession?

Because health care is only one among several professions basic to the culture of any advanced community, to delineate the ethical responsibilities of this profession it is necessary first to consider the nature of the professions in general, then to define the specific role of the health care profession, and finally to identify its relationships with other professions.

The older medieval professions were divinity (theology), physic (medicine), and law. They were "person professions" centered on a counselor-client relationship. They did not produce goods for sale or works of art for enjoyment, but worked to heal, guide, or protect some person in a life crisis. Industrial society has greatly fostered the professions, but it has also depersonalized them. No longer are they centered on conviviality of persons but on the productivity of an impersonal system. They no longer deal with better interpersonal communication, but with more efficient exchange of power.

This slow depersonalizing transformation of the professions is reaching its completion today just as industrial society itself seems about to yield to a new postindustrial society. Neither progressive capitalism nor revolutionary Marxism has been able to fulfill the promises of scientific technology to produce a society of abundance and freedom. This promise seems illusory in view of the ecological doomsday predicted by some authorities.

In postindustrial society the source of power will no longer be economic ownership (whether capitalist or socialist) but rather knowledge and its communication. Such power means a still greater role for the professions. This knowledge can be used to bring about greater social conformism and dependency on the professionals, or it can be used to open the system to wider and more genuine social participation by all. In either case, the profession would be radically reconstructed.

Will professionals become technocrats whose technological mastery must extend itself to behavior control? Or will they become the persons who help others to transcend the depersonalization of technological systems? If professionals choose the latter alternative, then the professions must again be personalized. They must be reconstructed so as to eliminate the threefold depersonalization that they have suffered in the epoch of industrial society: that of the client, the profession, and the client-professional relationship.

Clients have been depersonalized by the proliferation of specialism. They are no longer thought of as complex organisms but as collections of organs.

The parts are healed, not the person, such that the very meaning of healing, that is, to make whole, has been lost.

Professions themselves have been depersonalized by a loss of clear identity. This loss is notoriously true for the ministry and is now evident in law, teaching, and medicine. A recent study showed that psychiatrists, psychoanalysts, and psychiatric social workers all do much the same thing, yet are considered members of three different professions. What is even more confusing is that many ministers, lawyers, and physicians counsel clients in ways not easily distinguishable from those of psychotherapists.

Contributing to this confusion of identity today is the tension within the profession between the goals of research and the goals of practice. How then can a professional make that kind of personal commitment always regarded as a mark of a profession if it is not clear to what he or she is professed?

Third, the validity of the professional-client relationship is being questioned. Professionalism seems to imply an elitism that is ultimately socially destructive. Ivan Illich, studying the problems of underdeveloped countries, has launched an all-out attack on schooling and the concept of the teaching profession and has extended the same criticism to medicine.[1] He contends that the industrial model for organizing the professions has progressively restricted access to knowledge and skill, placing them in the hands of elites, on whom the public is more and more dependent, but from whom the public receives less and less adequate service. He argues that both capitalist and Marxist politics are based on the same invalid professional ideal, and that the Third World is desperately striving to make the same mistake.

Personalistic Concept of a Profession

Today the term *profession* is used for almost any prestigious occupation because it has the aura of an ideal. It is a symbol rather than a reality. Nevertheless, the sociologists have devoted much time to developing a good empirical definition of a profession. Robert Merton explains the social value of a profession very succinctly:

> First, the value placed upon systematic knowledge and intellect: *knowing*.
> Second, the value placed upon technical skill and trained capacity: *doing*.
> And third, the value placed upon putting this conjoint knowledge and skill to work in the service of others: *helping*.[2]

Moore and Rosenblum use a scale to define professionalism. Professionals must rate high on the following six operational attributes:

1. Professionals practice *full-time occupations*.

2. They are committed to a *calling*, that is, they treat their occupation "as an enduring set of normative and behavioral expectations."

3. They are distinguished from the laity by various signs and symbols and identified with their peers—often in formalized *organizations*.

4. They have esoteric but useful knowledge and skills through specialized *education*, which is lengthy and difficult.

5. They are expected to have a *service orientation* so as to perceive the needs of a client relevant to their competency.

6. They have *autonomy* of judgment and authority restrained by responsibility in using their knowledge and skill.[3]

The problem with contemporary definitions of a profession (which fundamentally come down to Merton's "knowing-doing-helping") is that they fail to distinguish clearly the original group of person professions from other highly developed occupations to which the term has been extended but which do not deal directly with persons. Today accounting, engineering, architecture and the other arts, and business are considered professions, since they also involve knowing, doing, and helping. Yet their immediate objective is not personal but productive. Obliterating the distinction between the person professions and productive occupations is characteristic of industrial society and its depersonalization of the professions. If professions are to be repersonalized, the distinction between profession and productive occupation must be drawn once more.

To call the technologies and the arts (engineering, business, fine arts) professions is confusing and dangerous because this designation disguises the fact that they produce things and do not directly help persons. Certainly the technologies should educate their practitioners to be more sensitive to the human uses to which their product will be put, but this humanization of technology will be hindered if industrial society persists in its tendency to lump the technologies and the person professions together under one name and to judge them all in terms of productivity.

A true profession therefore is rooted in theory but aimed at practice—a practice that does not produce things external to persons, but a service directly to persons themselves. Furthermore, this service is not applied to persons who receive it passively but facilitates those persons' own activity. It aims at healing them, at making them whole, at freeing them to act on their own. Person professionals should not act on clients nor dominate them, but enable them to become fully, autonomously themselves. Thus a true profession cannot properly be elitist. It communicates power rather than enforces dependency.

Finally, professional help in the full sense is concerned precisely with those problems which are deeply personal, or are matters of life and death. Such help engages both professional and client in a profound responsibility both to each other and to the larger community. This personalistic concept of a profession can reconstruct the professions and professional education for the future.

The proper task of the medical professional then is to deal with problems at the biological and psychological levels of human functioning. Obviously, at the psychological level counseling of a certain type plays a major therapeutic role. At the biological level, however, it is not so obvious that the physician's role is still primarily that of a counselor. Yet if the thesis put forth in Chapter 3 is correct—that all persons have primary responsibility for their own health— then the physician's primary responsibility is to help patients make good health decisions (not make such decisions for them), which requires a counseling process. People cannot make a good decision about how to care for their health unless they have the required information. In more complicated cases this information can be obtained only by consulting a physician. To some extent the physician is playing the role of a teacher in giving this information; but more is involved than that, since the information required is not abstract biological truth but a concrete assessment of personal health and the possible ways of dealing with the problems it presents. This kind of guidance is required from a physician, and it engages the physician in a special type of counseling.

4.2 Ideals of the Medical Profession

To make sure that the personalistic concept of the health care professions is not a mere ideal but rather is put into practice requires a brief look at the crosscurrents of purpose at work in the historical development of the medical professions. The health care profession comprises others besides physicians. But physicians are the leaders of the health care team and we are able to understand the other health care professions only if we grasp the history and ideals of the medical profession. For this reason we concentrate on physicians in the rest of this section, but much of the content applies to other health care professions as well.

The history of medicine shows that physicians have been considered both priests and scientists. This duality, upon closer examination, reflects the mind-body or psychosomatic duality of the human being who is sick. In Greece (where modern Western medicine originated) the first father of medicine was Asclepius, who was the "mild god." Asclepius' priests presided over shrines (the first clinics) where the sick came to worship, to sleep, and to have their dreams interpreted. The symbol of the medical profession today is still a staff with entwined serpents because the serpent, symbol of wisdom and the healing power of Mother Earth (that is, Nature), was the cult animal at these shrines.

This Greek myth of the god of healing manifests a basic truth about the medical profession: the physician to this day retains something of a priestly ministry in the service of the healing forces of nature. Something similar is true of every profession because all professions deal with the sacred dignity of the human person and rest on the sacred covenant of trust between client and professional. This priestly ministry is especially true of the medical profession because its direct relation to life and death gives it a sacred character. A person's trust in the physician is almost like trust in one's mother, a primordial confidence in life support. While this trust can be abused and exploited, it is valuable when it is authentic. No one can be healed without trust. Thus the most significant distinction in understanding the history of medicine is not between scientific and nonscientific medicine, but between authentic medicine and quackery. Authentic medicine has both priestly and scientific dimensions.

Why did it take until the nineteenth century for the rapid development of the scientific side of medicine to begin? Perhaps the development of scientific medicine was somewhat retarded by its priestly aspects. It is not inevitable, however, that these two aspects should hinder rather than complement each other. Others have pointed out that scientific medicine could not get far until the development of chemistry and biology. But why were these sciences also so slow to develop? Greek thinkers clearly recognized the method and value of empirical sciences, but it seems they were discouraged from engaging in experimentation in sciences and clinical practice in medicine by a social system based on the sharp division between the liberally educated freemen who despised manual work and the slaves or serfs who performed it. This barrier between theory and practice, between the spiritual realm and the realm of matter, seems to have been the major obstacle to the development of science and scientific medicine.

Nevertheless, the Christian concern for the poor and respect for the human body as the temple of the Holy Spirit began to break through this Greek contempt. Christianity has been the religion most concerned with organized health care because of its belief in personal charity and of the integral relation of the body to the human person. In spite of practical efforts to realize this Christian ideal, however, the state of scientific knowledge and the level of social organization were so low that until the end of the Middle Ages the chief efforts were directed more to caring for the sick and dying than to healing them.

The Christian Physician

The current debates about the humanization of medicine reflect the resurgence of the priestly aspect of the medical tradition that has never died and that will always be part of medicine. Therefore the charismatic character of the physician, which arises from the priestly side of medicine but is also enhanced by the miraculous powers of scientific technology, should be respected. The charismatic atmosphere is an important element of the professional relationship and is essential to the healing process. This atmosphere makes it possible for the patient, often distrustful, to place the necessary trust in professional help. It also gives medical professionals a sense of personal dignity, dedication, and responsibility that immeasurably contributes to their satisfaction and persistence in a difficult vocation. Moreover, self-respect is a guard of other ethical values. Nothing is so likely to keep medical professionals from abusing their position for financial or other gains as this sense of self-respect. Increasing commercialization of medicine will be disastrous, and the medical profession will become an anonymous functionary in an industrial or a government bureaucracy unless self-respect of health care professionals prevails.

On the negative side, however, as with the clergyman, overemphasis on the special status of the physician is open to great abuses. The physician can become an unquestioned, dogmatic authority in medicine and in all other matters as well. The medical profession often jealously defends its authority and its prerogatives, refuses to discipline members of the profession, and claims the right to settle ethical and social questions that affect the profession on the grounds that lay persons have no right to opinions in such matters.

Therefore, the physician who wants to develop a sound ethical judgment must (1) have a profound respect for the medical profession as a vocation that has both scientific and priestly aspects and (2) have a clear understanding of the limits of this profession and of its interrelation to and dependence on other professions that also deal with the human person.

The Christian Perspective

Christian health care professionals are called by their faith to understand this vocation in a special way, just as professionals of other religions or philosophies of life are called by theirs. Christians think of life as a gift of God and the body as a marvelous work of divine creation to be reverenced as a temple of God (1 Co 6:19; 2 Co 6:16). They also think of the human person not only as a living body, but also as a body living with spiritual life open to a share in the eternal life of God. Consequently, the Christian health care professional thinks of sickness as an evil desecrator of the temple. Even when sickness cannot be overcome, the struggle against it can be lived through as an experience that can further moral and spiritual growth. Thus the Christian physician or nurse is truly a minister of God, cooperating with him in helping suffering human beings overcome their suffering in order to live more fully.

The Christian medical professional finds a model in Jesus Christ, the Healer. While physicians do not have supernatural or miraculous powers, they do have medical skill, which is also a gift of God, and can imitate Jesus' compassion for the patient and his reaching out to the most neglected, even the lepers. This Christian attitude cannot be a matter of mere pious words; rather it is a profound dependence on God, who gives the physician and nurse the inspiration, insight, and courage to carry out their work as professionally and as skillfully as possible.

Moreover, one should not make the mistake of thinking that the ethical aspect of medicine pertains only to its personal, priestly side, since it also penetrates its scientific aspect. The scientific approach to disease is built on the devotion to objective truth and the courageous, persevering effort to advance this truth through research and criticism. Dedication to objective truth and scientific integrity is an ethical value of the highest order. Nothing is gained if the effort to humanize or personalize medicine interjects an unhealthy sentimentalism or occultism into its practice. Sound ethical judgment can be based only on critical scientific knowledge.

On the negative side, however, the scientific method as now understood and practiced often tends to reductionism, that is, the assertion that the scientific method is the exclusive road to truth. Since the scientific method deals only with the limited aspects of reality that can be measured and experimented on, such a reductionist attitude can compel physicians to ignore and deny facts and experiences outside those rather narrow limits. When reductionism is rigidly applied, the patient is treated as a soulless machine. In the history of medicine, this mechanistic approach has been profitable to the degree that is has used the scientific method intensively, but it has ultimately limited the advance of medicine. Again and again, biologists and physicians sensitive to the holistic character of living organisms and the human person have revolted against reductionism and opened new, broader, and more fruitful lines of research.

Thus sound ethical judgment must completely respect scientifically established medical facts, but it cannot rest on these facts alone. It must be open to all humanistic approaches to understanding and evaluating the human condition.

4.3 Personalizing the Health Care Profession

At the heart of every profession there is a counseling relationship between persons, and this relationship takes on a special mode in health care. Ethical decisions about health matters depend first of all on a cooperative effort of patients and professionals without which patients lack the information they need for an informed conscience. Ethical decisions also depend on peer relationships between members of the health team who must pool their information and expertise. Such cooperation between patients and professionals and between professionals and colleagues demands trust and effective communication, which are rooted in sound personal relationships. Therefore, unless mutually beneficial relationships are established and maintained in the health care facility, there is little hope of ethical, humanistic health care.

Although there are many models of counseling relationships that may be applied to the professional-patient interaction, the most significant models from an ethical perspective are the psychoanalytical model and the medical model. We consider each model in order to indicate the mutual ethical responsibilities of patient and physician.

The Psychoanalytical Model

In the psychoanalytical model the client comes to the therapist because of painful anxieties that make normal life difficult or impossible, with the goal of trying to resolve emotional conflicts whose unconscious origin is unknown to the client. The therapist's responsibility is not to diagnose the illness by labeling it, but to help the client come to an understanding of the causes of his or her problems and to cope with them more effectively. To achieve this, the therapist must gradually win the client's trust and help the client step by step to interpret the symbolism of the symptoms. The therapist must grant the client the right to have his or her behavior interpreted as symbolic rather than judged morally and to have the client's sufferings counted worthy of sympathy. The therapist must help the client not to act out symptoms, but to discover their underlying meaning and thus to come to a deep and realistic self-understanding. Finally, the therapist must help the client acquire new skills in coping with the problems of life and terminate dependence on the therapist. To do this, the therapist must personally arrive at self-understanding through the same process.

The client must come to trust the therapist, speaking more and more freely, cooperating by undertaking the task of working through symptoms, rejecting escape from the process by suicide or even by a flight into health. The client's will to get well and become independent of the therapist must also be reinforced. This process depends on an intense one-to-one relationship in which the patient withdraws from the familial and social situation in which he has become ill. It also demands toleration by family and society of the patient's temporary withdrawal from ordinary relationships and responsibilities.

The dependence of the client on the therapist is essentially a recapitulation of the parental relationship, but a healthy one rather than the unhealthy one from which the client has suffered. The therapist is a good mother in taking on the attitude of what Carl Rogers called "unconditional benign acceptance" and also a good father in the increasing role of interpretation and confrontation with reality. The libidinal, erotic elements of the transference of the client to the therapist are gradually turned toward the real love objects of the client's independent life. By no means is it easy for clients to come to such total trust in their therapists, since they have learned to distrust any mother or father. Clients must accept the tasks (1) of trusting the therapist and (2) of trying to recover health and normal independence.

On their part, therapists undertake the moral burden of being faithful to this trust reposed in them by their clients. Therapists must listen, not judge, and (to a degree) must sympathize. Therapists must set limits on "acting out" by clients and must insist on "working through." They must approve and reinforce the client's progressive achievement of insight and gradually confront them more and more with the demands of reality. For therapists to be ethically true to this trust, they must be personally aware of any tendency toward countertransference (that is, the development of a relationship in which the therapist begins to use the patient to meet the therapist's own emotional needs) and must strive to keep this human tendency within limits.

Today these mutual duties, which clearly involve considerable virtue on the part of therapists and a desire for virtue and willingness to grow through suffering on the part of clients, are often formalized in a contract made at the beginning of therapy. In this contract therapists make sure clients understand and accept the goals and limits of therapy and are aware that they can hold a therapist liable for the therapist's half of the contract. Thus therapists are unethical when they fail to make such a clear contract (which is an aspect of informed consent) or fail to adhere strictly to it. Therapists should not assume moral obligations beyond the limits of this contract.

Such limitations raise certain difficulties, however, the chief ones being: (1) What if the patient is contemplating suicide? (2) What if the patient is contemplating some act injurious to another party, for example, physical attack, theft, adultery, or divorce? (3) What if the patient proposes sexual relations with the therapist? (4) What if the patient refuses to work seriously at the therapy or needlessly delays its termination? These problems are discussed at greater length in Chapter 12. Here we need only point out that these actions constitute a breach (perhaps not culpable) of the contract on the part of the client. They relieve the therapist from his contract, but they leave him obliged (not as a professional, but simply as a citizen) to prevent harm to a third party or to prevent an insane person from harming himself.

Medical Model

In strong contrast to the psychoanalytical model is the medical model, yet it too gives rise to many ethical issues. In the medical model the professional goal is to treat a physical illness so as to restore normal physical functioning to the degree possible. The physician first seeks to diagnose the disease, then to prescribe a course of treatment (in which the physician is assisted by nurses and others) through medicine, surgery, nursing, or change of regimen. The physician must also make a prognosis and if possible offer the patient hope. The patient, on the other hand, is relieved from blame for his or her condition and from ordinary responsibilities to work and family, but is expected to be cooperative with the professional staff. Families and society are expected to support the patient psychologically and to contribute to the expenses.

Patient passivity raises the main ethical issue characteristic of this model. If the health care profession is only a servant to the patient because primary responsibility for the patient's health remains the patient's, then it follows that the professional has no rights over the patient, except those given by the patient's informed consent. Hence, ethically speaking, an implicit or explicit contract must regulate all that goes on in the medical model.

What are the essential features of this medical contract? First, the contract limits the obligations assumed. In the medical model a physician does not assume the role of a psychotherapist or of an ethical or spiritual counselor. Efforts to repersonalize medicine should not demand that the medical doctor assume all the roles proper to a complete health team. Of course, physicians need to be aware of nonphysical factors that may be affecting the patient's health in order to seek the help of other members of the health team in dealing with such factors.

The implied contract between a patient and the primary care physician, however, obligates the physician to undertake a serious effort to help the patient discover the nature of the problem and the type of help that is appropriate to it, medical or otherwise. The patient who does not feel well comes to a physician as a first, obvious step in an effort to determine the source of the discomfort. If the possibility of a physical cause can be eliminated, the patient then has the information necessary to take the next step—seeing another type of counselor or other action. But if the physician fails to listen or to make an adequate examination or sends the patient away confused or with a placebo or tranquilizer, the patient still lacks the necessary information for rational decisions. A well-known study of hospital care showed that a high percentage of patients were incorrectly diagnosed because of the failure of physicians to listen carefully to patients' complaints and to recognize nonmedical factors in their conditions.

Second, the medical model, like other professional relationships, is based on trust. The physician, therefore, must establish trustworthiness within the limits of the contract. As it relates to trust, the contract should have three elements.

1. *Concern.* Fundamental to the contract is the physician's concern for the patient's well-being. Trust will never exist if the patient believes that the physician is concerned only about the fee or is acting out of mere routine like a machine or a bureaucratic functionary. The physician must communicate interest in the patient as a person, not as a kidney or a heart, and a willingness to do for the patient whatever is professionally possible, not limited by mere self-interested motives. For this reason, Paul Ramsey has rightly emphasized that the professional contract is something more than a contract; it is a covenant in the theological sense.[4] Thus the professional contract also implies the promise to continue the care of the patient even when the patient is no longer able to insist on its fulfillment.

This concept of covenant, however, should not be exaggerated. God himself insists on the responsibility of his people to respond to their own obligations under the covenant. Hence the physician also has the right to demand cooperation from the patient. Moreover, the physician's contract is not universal, but limited by his own competence, so that the physician is not obligated to do more than inform the patient when a problem exceeds his competence and refer him or her to another specialist or another type of nonmedical counselor.

2. *Knowledge and skill in medicine.* Health care professionals have the fundamental responsibility, within their specialties, to be expert in both the science and the art of health care, up-to-date in knowledge, experienced, of good judgment, and skilled in procedures. Personal warmth does not substitute for

medical expertise. Professionals communicate such expertise to patients by evidence of their education and licensure, by reputation, and also by the care and thoroughness with which they deal with patients.

3. *Communication.* Since patients retain fundamental rights over their own bodies, and the fundamental knowledge of how they feel not only at this minute, but also throughout the day and in varied situations, physicians cannot hope to make a proper diagnosis, carry on successful treatment, or make an accurate prognosis without adequate communication with patients.

Health Care Fees

To these basic ethical obligations of the medical doctor, a fourth can be added that applies also to the psychotherapeutic models: to set or refuse an appropriate fee. In a capitalist society it is assumed that a professional should be paid as any other worker is paid according to the laws of supply and demand. It is assumed that a service is just as much a commodity for exchange with a value measured in monetary terms as is any other product. Consequently, some persons argue that there is nothing ethically wrong with organizing the medical profession on the basis of profit like any other industry and they actually speak of "the health industry"! They believe that the stimulus of the profit motive has been the chief cause of the rapid technological development of American medicine.

Furthermore, some argue that the fee is actually a part of therapy, since it causes the average person to refrain from asking for unnecessary services which might overload the system and deprive others in real need from getting proper attention. Moreover, the fee promotes a cooperative attitude on the part of the patient and thus shortens the time of treatment.

Yet the question can also be raised as to whether this capitalistic assumption is a realistic and practical fact. At no time in the history of medicine has the market system operated fully in the professions because there have always been people who desperately needed professional help but who could not pay for it. Either the professional had to provide free services or payment had to be made by a third party. In fact, since the rise of health insurance, Medicare, and Medicaid, most health care *is* paid by a third party, the insurer or the government, who determines standard fees.

If our account of the nature of a profession is correct, it should be clear why profit cannot be the primary basis of any profession, but must be considered a secondary and highly variable feature. The medical profession, like any true profession, must rest not on bargaining but on trust; and it provides a service that is concerned with life and death, matters so precious as to be priceless. No monetary value can be set on the spiritual light given by a priest, the defense of human rights provided by a lawyer, the risk of his own life provided by a soldier, or the search for truth shared by a teacher. Nor is there any price for the service of a physician in the battle to live.

Unfortunately, recent developments in the organization of health care endanger and erode its professional goals. The growth of for-profit and investor-owned health care facilities have made profit and not personal service to those in need the overriding purpose of many facilities and the people employed therein. As Paul Starr declares in *The Social Transformation of American Medicine*:

The emergence of corporate enterprise in health services is part of two broad currents in the political economy of contemporary societies. The older of these two movements is the steady expansion of the corporation into sectors of the economy traditionally occupied by self-employed small businessmen or family enterprises. In this respect, the growth of corporate medical care is similar to the growth of corporate agriculture. The second and more recent movement is the transfer of public services to the administrative control or ownership of private corporations—the reprivatization of the public household.[5]

Hence professional fees are not payments measured by the value of the service provided (which is truly priceless), but a *stipend* to be measured only by what professionals need to live and work without distraction. The ability-to-pay principle is not unjust as long as it remains within the bounds of the more fundamental principle that professionals are public servants who have no right to expect in return for services anything more than a standard of living that will make it possible for them to perform those services with liberty of mind and health of body and to adequately fulfill family and social obligations.

A Christian health care professional can only conclude that a professional living is essentially a modest one in which simplicity of life style and freedom to be available to serve others is the only honorable measure of remuneration. Nor can the popular argument be accepted that physicians, since they spend years in difficult study, work long hours, and assume great responsibility, deserve to make money. The rewards of any profession are to be found not in some extraneous gain, but in the satisfactions of knowledge and of interesting, satisfying and absorbing work. Such an ideal is not easy to realize, nor is it often realized in its purest form; but even when imperfectly realized it is what has given the medical profession its own vitality and health.

4.4 Professional Communication

In health care, as in all professional relationships, adequate communication between professional and client is a fundamental ethical requirement. In the medical model opportunities for such communication may be rather sharply restricted, but they are still crucial. Within these limits, what are the duties of physicians and nurses?

The first obligation is to listen to the patient. Yet often, while professionals concentrate on filtering out medically significant information, patients are attempting to express a rhapsody of symptoms, fears, fantasies, evasions, cries for attention, and so forth. The work-pressured professional cannot afford to sit and hear a long and rambling discourse from a self-pitying patient. But the health care professional needs to remember that "the medium is the message," that is, the way patients are (or are not) communicating may be the most significant symptom.

Therefore, no matter how busy they may be, health care professionals have the responsibility to acquire the art of medical dialogue by which they can help patients say what needs to be said. The first rule of this art is for the professional to repeat back to the patient what the professional has heard that seems significant and to ask whether it is what the patient meant. This feedback not only reassures the patient, but can also gradually train the patient to give relevant information. A second rule is to obtain the patient's cooperation by explaining the purpose of questions, since unexpected and cryptic questions are often threatening and confusing.

Of course, professionals also have the right to require honesty and frankness from clients. When they suspect deliberate deceit, they should deal with the situation explicitly and directly as a breach of the patient's contract with the professional. In most illnesses, however, psychological factors may cause communication to be distorted by unconscious elements of self-deceit, denial, confusion, or panic. Psychotherapists in particular have to deal with this perplexing inability of some patients to communicate openly, but therapists also experience in themselves something of the same ambiguity.

Health care professionals cannot expect truth from their patients unless they are equally truthful with them. Lack of frankness by professionals is usually excused as concern to spare the patient, but is just as often the result of unconscious fear on the part of the professional. Chapter 11 discusses the problem of telling the truth to the incurable or dying patient. Here it suffices to say that the fundamental principle in all such situations is that the patient has the right to the truth, however difficult it may be for the professional to communicate it.

Confidentiality

Patients have the right to the truth about their health because they have the primary responsibility for their health. They also have the right to privacy about those aspects of life which do not directly affect others. Human community is based on free communication, which is impossible if confidences cannot be shared. Hence health care professionals have a serious obligation to maintain such confidences that protect the patient's right to confidentiality.

How is a professional to act when questioned by others about a patient's condition? All Catholic moralists agree that it is always wrong to lie, even to protect confidentiality, but not all agree on how to define lying. The meaning of any human statement must always be determined from the context in which communication occurs. Consequently, when persons ask questions which they have no right to ask, the context renders any answer given essentially meaningless, so that it is ethically inconsequential whether that answer in a normal context would be true or false. Thus health care professionals who are questioned about confidential matters may without lying or even falsehood reply in any way that protects confidentiality. This fact, however, cannot excuse a physician from frankly answering questions put by a patient or the patient's guardians, because these persons have the right to know. Thus, whether one has the obligation to reply to a question with unambiguous and accurate information then depends on the questioner's right to such information.

It is not easy to draw the line between what individuals have the right to keep private and what they may have the duty to make public. Hence, the contract between professional and patient should determine this as exactly as possible. If professionals are convinced that to do the best for a patient they need to discuss the case with consultants or before other members of a team or the professional staff, the professionals must obtain the informed consent of the patient. Most patients (or, when they are incompetent, their guardians) readily permit the therapeutic use of information, but they should have the opportunity to restrict the use of this information when entering into contractual relationships with the professional. One of the most difficult problems, however, is the need of researchers to have access to records, especially when doing epidemiological studies; yet even here it should be possible to guard the privacy of individuals from public knowledge.

Nevertheless, the right of confidentiality, sacred as it is, is limited by the rights of other persons and by the individual's own limited rights of self-disposal. Patients may behave in ways which directly injure themselves and indirectly or directly injure others. In all these cases the family or society has an obligation to prevent harm both to the patient and to the public because all are members of a community that exists for the good of each of its members in relation to all others.

Hence, generally speaking, professionals have not only the right but also the duty to communicate information necessary to prevent serious harm to the patient or to others, even when it is given to them in confidence, to those who may be able to prevent this injury. When what is revealed is an intention to commit a crime (including suicide), the professional has the obligation to reveal to appropriate persons whatever information is necessary to prevent such a crime. When no crime is contemplated, but there is probably danger of harm which can be prevented, the professional should discreetly do what is likely to be helpful in preventing such harm. Ordinarily this should not be done without first warning the patient of exposure if the patient refuses to desist.

Serious problems about confidentiality have been raised recently by the computerization of health records and also by the requirement of private and government health insurance plans that physicians report the nature of a patient's illness as a condition of receiving payment. It is clear enough that a physician does not have the right to give information of this sort without the patient's permission. This, however, leaves the larger question of how patients are to obtain the benefits to which they are entitled without giving such permission. The insurance or public agency has the right to ask proof from patients that they have used funds for a legitimate medical purpose, but the agency also has the duty to design adequate controls that do not require detailed information which might be embarrassing or injurious to the patient. Computerization of health records should always require the patient's permission, and even when permission is given, care must be taken to limit the availability of these records to a few authorized persons.

So to fulfill their obligations to serve the patient's health, health care professionals have the responsibility:

1. To strive to establish and preserve trust at both the emotional and rational levels

2. To share the information they possess with those who legitimately need it in order to have an informed conscience

3. To refrain from lying or giving misinformation

4. To keep secret information which is not legitimately needed by others, but which if revealed might either harm the patient or others or destroy trust.

4.5 Peer Relationships

Health care professionals need good personal relationships not only with those they serve, but also with their colleagues on the health team. Problems of leadership and accountability, of common decision making and cooperation in carrying out decisions, of adequate communication and mutual support not only have psychological importance, but also are profoundly ethical.

In health care the problem of mutual responsibility is crucial. If health care professionals do not care enough about each other and their common enterprise to accept the painful task of maintaining group standards in a fraternal and humane way, they cannot hope to personalize health care.

The need for improved peer relationships and professional communication is evidenced in medical malpractice suits. A federal commission concluded that malpractice suits frequently result (1) from poor communication between physicians and patients and hence from inadequately informed consent on the patient's part; (2) from patients' frustration because physicians seem unresponsive to their complaints; (3) from patients' misinformed, unrealistic expectations about the benefits of treatment; and (4) from growing public conviction that consumers need to defend themselves against arrogant, self-serving professionals. It is noteworthy that the first three of these factors (and perhaps in large part the fourth) reduce to a failure in communication, a skill in which physicians are often not well trained.

Two opposite remedies have been proposed for the malpractice problem. One answer is *peer review*. It is argued, plausibly enough, that in a field so highly technical as medicine no one is competent to evaluate professional performance except peers in the profession or even in the same medical specialty.

On the other hand, some observers argue that peer discipline has never been successful in protecting the patient or even in maintaining high standards of medical competence. A profession, they contend, is too concerned with its own autonomy to be very diligent in disciplining its members. Consequently, these critics believe that disciplining a profession must first of all concern those who suffer from malpractice or neglect. Health care consumers must know and defend their own rights by all available economic, legal, and political means. Since the primary responsibility for health must remain with each person to whom the professional is only a servant, the ultimate right to call the medical profession to account must be in the hands of those the profession exists to serve. This is why the users of health services have the fundamental right to the final word in regulating the profession through public law.

In this matter it seems that the physician and the lawyer are in a somewhat different position than the minister, teacher, and scientist. These latter professionals deal with objective truth as such, and the public has no right to silence the voice of truth. But the lawyer is an officer of the court, that is, he or she is subordinated to the legislative and judicial officers of the government who represent the people in determining the law. The medical professional also does not stand for truth as such, as a scientist must, but is providing a service to human physical or mental health, a service which must ultimately be judged in terms of its practical enhancement of human well-being. Consequently, the medical profession must accept a public, practical evaluation of its services. Of course, health care professionals in their secondary role as scientists have a right and an obligation to speak out for objective truth about biological and medical matters, but this does not give them complete autonomy in the realm of medical practice.

4.6 Conclusion

The medical profession and every learned profession must have a genuine but limited autonomy. As health care users become more knowledgeable about what is and what is not good medical care, they will become increasingly able to detect serious incompetence or negligence in the service they receive. But at last, this awareness will only raise questions; it will not be sufficient in most cases to pass judgment. People may have doubts that an operation recommended by their surgeons is really necessary, but all they can do to find out is either to ask for more convincing answers to their questions or to consult another professional.

It would seem, therefore, that a satisfactory system of discipline for the medical profession must be a combination of both peer discipline and consumer discipline. A medical review board must include both professional peers with requisite technical knowledge and experience and also health care users (along with legal advisers) to ensure that the medical professionals are more concerned for the served than for their own self-interest as the servants. At the same time, it is essential that medical information be made more easily available to all users so that each can know and defend his or her own rights and interests.

The real remedy for malpractice and unjustified malpractice litigation is a more personalized practice of medicine which will reduce misunderstanding between professional and patient and will correct human failure by professionals through mutual cooperation and discipline within the health team itself. The notion of fraternal correction is part of the Christian ethos (Mt 18:15-18). Applied to a profession, it means that the members do not simply ignore or hide the defects of colleagues out of indifference or self-interest, but are seriously concerned to help them overcome these defects and repair the consequences. It also implies that even those workers in subordinate positions have a right and an obligation to correct superiors and that the superiors have an obligation to listen to such corrections.

If such mutual support and discipline are to be possible in a health team, it must rest on a profound mutual trust and respect which can be built up only by persistent effort. One of the marks of a Christian health care facility, therefore, should be this striving to establish the personal relationships within the staff and administration that will be the basis for such professional cooperation.

Footnotes

1. Ivan D. Illich, *Medical Nemesis: The Expropriation of Health* (New York: Pantheon, 1976), p. 9.

2. Robert Merton, "Some Thoughts in the Professions in American Society," address, Brown University, 1960.

3. W. Hunt Moore and Gerald Rosenblum, *The Professions: Roles and Rules* (New York: Russell Sage Foundation, 1970), pp. 51-65.

4. Paul Ramsey, *The Patient as Person* (New Haven: Yale University Press, 1970), p. 14.

5. Paul Starr, *The Social Transformation of American Medicine* (New York: Basic Books, 1982), p. 445.

Study Questions

1. What distinguishes the classical professions from other useful occupations? Why is the maintenance of high ethical standards in these professions so important for society as a whole?

2. Write a modern version of the "Hippocratic Oath" which expresses what you believe to be the principal ethical values of the medical profession.

3. Write a verbatim report of a dialogue between a physician and his or her patient showing how the physician can establish rapport and trust and good communication and how he or she might fail to do this.

4. Are there any situations in which a medical professional is justified in revealing embarrassing or damaging information about a patient to a third party? Name and explain.

5. If you were a physician who wanted to set up a team approach to care for patients in an intensive care unit, what possible difficulties would you anticipate? How would you avoid them? Do these factors involve questions of fairness (justice)?

Cases

1. Mr. Wagner is chief executive officer of a 500-bed general hospital. Financial pressures for earlier release of patients have arisen from new Medicare regulations. During a meeting to formulate policies to meet these pressures, Wagner gets into a heated argument with Dr. Critch, chief of the medical staff. Finally, Dr. Critch says, "I am a medical professional. You are a businessman. Who are you to interfere with my professional judgment?" To which Wagner angrily replies, "But I also am a member of the medical profession. I have a degree in hospital administration." Was Wagner right? Where would you draw the line?

2. Two physicians, Dr. A and Dr. B, were medical school classmates but ten years later they have developed very different "professional manners." Dr. A dresses very conservatively, always wears his white coat in his office, impresses his patients with a very crisp, authoritative manner, and always appears to be very busy. On the other hand, Dr. B dresses informally, does not "look like a doctor," and cultivates a rather folksy manner with his patients. Dr. A's patients are afraid to ask him questions but have great confidence in his skill. Dr. B who does not have as great a reputation wonders if he ought to imitate Dr. A. Is Dr. B making a mistake? If so, what should he do about it? Or is Dr. A mistaken? How could he improve communication with his patients without losing their confidence?

3. On January 17, 1985, a convicted criminal was executed in Texas by lethal injection because he had been an accomplice in the murder of a narcotics agent. He was executed by a physician. What are the ethical issues involved in physicians assuming such a role?

4. Jane is 14 years old and pregnant as a result of incest with her father. On a routine visit to the family physician, Dr. Y, she explains what has happened and he confirms the pregnancy. She begs him not to tell her parents, because then her mother will discover what has happened. She is convinced that her mother will blame her, rather than her father, because her relations with her mother are very bad. Dr. Y, a Catholic, tells her he never performs abortions so Jane asks him to refer her to some physician who does. Dr. Y wonders whether professional confidentiality and perhaps even legal complications forbid him from informing the mother and trying to stop the abortion and the continuation of the incestuous relationship. But he is also worried that Jane will go to a disreputable and unsafe abortionist. What principles will help him solve his problem?

5. Nurse R has a low opinion of the professional conduct of Dr. Q. The latest example involved a comatose patient. She agreed with Dr. Q that the patient's family should be encouraged to give consent to disconnecting the respirator. After several days of discussion the family called the doctor and gave their consent. That evening he phoned Nurse R and ordered her to remove the respirator as soon as the family got there to be with the dying patient. She did not protest that this unpleasant task had been delegated to her, because she knew any protest would anger Dr. Q. With the family at the bedside, she

removed the respirator and to her and their horror the patient went into convulsions before dying. The family now blames her. What can Nurse R do to prevent such situations in the future?

Chapter 5

Social Responsibility for Health Care

Since individuals are mainly responsible for their own health and the health care profession has a responsibility to be of service in this pursuit of health, does society have the responsibility to individuals and the health care profession in the pursuit of health? What are the ethical responsibilities of local, state, and federal governments? And what are the bases for these responsibilities? American culture and political thought are paradoxical in its prevailing attitude toward these questions. Long ago the principle was accepted that government should promote and regulate universal free education for all children at least through high school, but for some reason Americans have hesitated to accept wholeheartedly the principle that government should promote and regulate universal free basic health care. Only since World War II have local and federal governments become involved in the issue of comprehensive health care.

Although there have been efforts by local, state, and federal governments to extend health care to the elderly and poor through programs such as Medicare and Medicaid, we believe these programs follow a model of providing health care that is seriously flawed. In this chapter we discuss the models of health care used in the United States and offer a different model founded on Catholic social teaching.

5.1 Models of Health Care

Among health care professions there is a tendency to discuss all social issues in terms of two opposing models: free enterprise versus socialism. Actually, three models of the social organization of health care are being debated in the United States.

Pluralist Model

The pluralist system actually exists, but some people regard it as no system at all. Its regulatory principle is the market in which persons with health needs compete for the services of health care professionals, principally on a fee-for-service basis, and professionals compete to sell their services. Today, however, these professional health care providers no longer act merely as individuals, but are organized in a spectrum of health care institutions, of which the hospital is chief.

Each of these health care facilities requires the cooperation of many medical specialists assisted not only by nurses but also by many different kinds of technicians and auxiliaries. Furthermore, an increasing number of physicians are organized in group practice of various types, such as health maintenance organizations (HMOs) and preferred provider organizations (PPOs). In some of these organizations physicians are prepaid by patients a fixed salary or a fee based on the number of patients served (capitation). Thus in a pluralist system there is no single organizational structure but a plurality of health providers, some acting individually, but most acting through some institutional group.

The difficulties with this present system have become very apparent in recent years. It is an inefficient system because it does not provide for long-range planning and it wastes resources in overlapping services and duplication of expensive plants and equipment. There are no national priorities for health care, so we have inconsistent actions: the federal government limits the funds for Medicare and neonatal care programs while funding transplants from living donors. More serious still, the present system has not provided access to adequate medical care for many socially and geographically disadvantaged groups. Nor has it demonstrably raised the general level of health in recent years. Finally, it seems subject to ever-mounting costs, which at present absorb at least 10 percent of the gross national product.

Other defenders of pluralism look for ways in which free-market mechanisms can be brought into play to afford better cost control and greater effectiveness in meeting real rather than artificial needs. While some doubt professional monopoly is really the major factor in raising health costs, others assert this and call for restrictions on monopolistic practices on the part of medical societies such as the use of ethics codes to prevent advertising and limit access to information by which consumers might be able to make competitive choices. Other economists believe some degree of government regulation is inevitable, but advise that it should not emphasize planning so much as provide economic motivation for hospitals to control costs (for example, by budgetary measures), limits on new hospital construction, and encouragement to shift to more outpatient care.

Centralized Model

Because of such difficulties with the present pluralist model, a second centralized (or regional) model has been widely proposed and defended. In this model the United States would be divided into regions, each to have all health care organized in a unified system. At the bottom of the pyramid would be a large number of primary care physicians with their auxiliaries who would care for the great majority of health problems requiring only a minimum of specialized knowledge and equipment. For cases exceeding such care, there would be a second level of hospitals or other facilities with complete staffs of specialists and advanced equipment. Finally, for cases of still greater difficulty, there would be a third or even fourth level of institutions equipped to give the most advanced care in which medical education and research would be located. In such a system, long-range planning would be possible, and this system could move the focus of health care from its present emphasis on the cure of disease toward emphasis on prevention so that each region would become an HMO.

To think of the pluralist model as free enterprise and the centralized model as socialism is a serious mistake. Because of the monopolistic control by the medical profession, the pluralist model is in fact a free enterprise system only in a very limited degree. In such a model, health consumers are seldom in a position to make intelligent choices between competitive alternatives either because they lack information or because these alternatives are very limited.

On the other hand, the centralized model is by no means incompatible with a free enterprise system as it now operates in the United States. The American way of life has moved toward a high degree of rationalization and monopoly in industry as well as in government. Such centralization has not changed the class structure of American society in any radical way. It would be perfectly possible to set up a centralized model in such a way as to leave a considerable choice to both the consumer and the provider. It could even include voluntary health insurance and fee-for-service features. What is essential to such a system is that it be centralized on a regional basis and bureaucratically planned.

Participatory Model

The participatory model is based on the view that there must be planning (as in the centralized model), but this is not the same as advocating a planned society. In a planned society, whether it be governed by a democratic bureaucratic elite or by a Marxist bureaucratic elite, individuals have their health cared for but lose any real control over how it is to be done. In a market system, individuals have scarcely more control because they lack the information or alternatives to choose from. What is needed therefore, according to those who seek a third model, is a system in which consumers play a real role in the planning process. The great problem in adopting the participatory model is the resistance of health care professionals. They have been educated to believe that the maintenance of high-quality health care demands professional autonomy and forbids interference by lay persons.

The essential steps to developing a participatory model are (1) assumption of responsibility by each person for his or her own health, (2) restoration of a sound professional-client relationship, and (3) education of medical professionals to be able to work in this relationship.

Christian Social Thought

For Christian health care professionals, the first step in seeking a better organization of health care in the United States and in the world must be to free themselves from the ideology that leads Americans to analyze every social issue in terms of the American free enterprise system and the tyranny of socialism and communism. Unfortunately, most American Christians identify Christian social teaching with the American way of life. Such identification of any human culture with the Gospel is certain to be misleading, since the Gospel stands as a prophetic criticism of every culture, approving some of its features but correcting others.

The authentic social teaching of the Catholic Church, for example, contains some strong criticisms of Marxist socialism and communism, chiefly on three grounds—(1) its atheistic materialism, (2) its denial of the right of private property, and (3) its tendency to totalitarian government. This teaching also contains a vigorous criticism of capitalism on the grounds of (1) its deterministic reliance on economic laws, the so-called magic of the market; (2) its advocacy of unregulated competition and the profit motive, and (3) its neglect of the Christian advocacy of the poor. Recent Church documents have pointed out that capitalism and communism alike have become colonializing powers either politically or economically and are thus largely responsible for the wars and poverty that oppress the great majority of humankind. Christian health care professionals, therefore, should base their thinking about the social organization of health care on the principles of the Gospel and not on the principles of the free enterprise system any more than on those of socialism.

Apart from ideological bias, no one economic system anymore than any one political system is simply natural, right, or Christian. Such systems are human inventions, each with some advantages and some disadvantages, to be selected according to particular historical circumstances. These merits need to be evaluated both from a theoretical point of view and from a practical, experiential point of view. In judging them ethically, we must consider both their congruity with fundamental moral and Gospel principles and their pragmatic results in a given situation.

To design a fundamental revision for providing health requires radical thinking, and it is here that Catholic social thought can make an important contribution to finding new solutions. These solutions must rest on three principles that have been previously expounded on in this book: (1) every human being has a fundamental right to health, as acknowledged in the *Universal Declaration of Human Rights*, article 25, because human rights are based on essential human needs; (2) individual persons have the primary responsibility to promote their own health; and (3) as social beings people also have the right to seek the help of others when necessary to fulfill this responsibility and reciprocally have the duty to give the same help to others as far as they are able. These concepts are better understood in the context and analysis of the concepts of common good and subsidiarity.

5.2 Common Good and Subsidiarity

Common Good

Most social evils and injustices are the result of exclusion of some persons from the common good in which they have a right to share. The ancient evil of slavery was precisely such an unjust institution wherein the slaves contributed to the common good but were not permitted to share fully in it, not only in regard to economic goods, but also in regard to spiritual goods such as education, freedom, political participation, respect, and even the right to worship the gods of the city. Thus the distribution of the common good is a fundamental demand of social justice.

Jesus, moreover, taught an ethics that clearly went beyond even this demand for distributive justice based on merit (that is, each receives in proportion as he contributes). Jesus proclaimed the coming of the Kingdom of God (Mk 1:15), which was not merely a heavenly kingdom but was also the fulfillment of the Old Testament prophecies of the Reign of God on the earth. When Jesus said to Pilate, "My kingship is not of this world" (Jn 18:36), he did not mean by "world," the earth, but the present sinful order of power struggle. He was saying to Pilate, "I am not competing with you power brokers. I am building a kingdom built on a different principle; on service, not on dominion." He taught his followers to pray, "Your Kingdom come, your will be done, on earth as it is in heaven" (Mt 6:10).

The Beatitudes (Lk 6:20-22; Mt 5:3-11) in their original form were the joyful announcement to the poor (that is, those excluded from the common good) that at last they were to be included in that common good, not only economically, but spiritually ("the poor have the good news preached to them") (Lk 7:22). Consequently, the principle of the early Church was "from each according to his ability, to each according to his needs," a principle Marx borrowed from the Acts of the Apostles (32:35). Thus the common good requires love and mercy and the distribution of good according to need. The mark of all Jesus' work was his concern for the neglected, the outcast, the leper, the prostitute, the Samaritan heretic, and the pagan unbeliever.

A Christian ethics of health care distribution must be based not on merit, and certainly not on the ability to pay, but on need, because the needy are the most neglected. Moreover, social oppression is the chief cause of their illness—an oppression from which the more affluent members of society profit. Hence those who are helpless by reason of poverty, disease, defect, or age (the unborn or the senile) should be the first consideration of any health plan.

Yet all persons should contribute to the plan according to their *ability*. Thus the social responsibility for health care falls first on those who have the ability to heal, the health care professionals, and second on those who have the ability to pay, that is, those who have financially profited the most from society. For such affluent individuals to claim that they have made their wealth simply by their own efforts is an absurdity. They may have worked hard, but their wealth would not have been possible without the cooperation of the society of which they are a part. Consequently, their debt to the common good is in proportion to the wealth they have received from it.

Subsidiarity

From this notion of the common good, the notion of subsidiarity follows logically. Subsidiarity implies that the first responsibility in meeting human needs rests with the free and competent individual, then with the local group. Higher and higher levels of the community must assume this responsibility (1) when the lower unit cannot assume it and (2) when the lower unit neglects to assume it. The higher level should never be content merely to take over responsibility, but it must work to return responsibility to a lower level. *The main objection to many social reforms has been that they have not provided for this progressive decentralization.* For example, the welfare system in the United States has perpetuated poverty rather than helped the dependent to become independent.

Therefore, the kind of health care program that Christians can consistently support must aim at preventive medicine, at achieving a healthier people who can care for themselves, rather than an ever-increasing dependence on technical medical care and professional help. As Plato observed, "A society that is always going to the doctor is a sick society" (Republic III, 405A). To achieve this fundamental objective, society must seek the sound political and economic organization of society.

Before secular humanism became the dominant philosophy of modern society, Christian thinking was able to advance the notion that a society is not simply a two-level structure of government and citizenry, but an organic community containing many mutually interdependent functions. Hence the power to make social decisions ought to be kept as close as possible to those who experience those problems and are most strongly affected by the decisions concerning them. Only in this way can the dignity of the least members of a community be acknowledged and their interests effectively served by the greater members. A paternalism that decides everything for those it claims to serve is really nothing but a form of domination and tends to become self-serving.

Subsidiarity requires us to share decision-making power not only at various vertical levels of local, state, and federal government, but also among horizontal sectors representing various functional bodies. Each person in a society is related to as many such functional bodies as he or she has basic needs. The role of government is to coordinate and encourage the full development of these different organs of society, not to deprive them of their decision-making capacity.

This application of subsidiarity to the organization of society on the basis of social functions, rather than on the basis of a struggle between isolated individuals defending their rights and a centralized government having all the powers of social decision, we call functionalism.

5.3 Functionalism

Functionalism is opposed on the one hand to communism and national socialism because they are totalitarian, concentrating all decision-making power in the hands of the state and the military. On the other hand, it is opposed to the competitive individualism of unregulated capitalism or free enterprise, with its hidden tendency to monopoly resulting in concentration of decision-making power in the hands of an interlocking power elite. Functionalism is not a mere theory, since it has a powerful influence, through Catholic statesmen, on the formation of the European common market and of codetermination by management and labor in West Germany, Yugoslavia, Japan and other countries.

Politically it might seem that functionalism would have little chance in the United States. Certain features of some institutions, however, are in fact functionalist. For example, higher education in the United States, in contrast to the statism of the lower school system, remains largely functionalist. Decisions about educational policies in our colleges and universities are for the most part still made independently of government by faculties and accrediting agencies and by the right of students to choose their own schools. On the other hand, the increasing control of the government over schools by reason of their economic dependency is working strongly to destroy their functionalist character.

Similarly, the growth of labor unions in the United States once seemed to promise the eventual development of functionalism in the economic sphere. Unfortunately, the unions have largely neglected the social aspects of their original purpose and have been co-opted by the capitalist market system in which they are becoming just another monopoly. Fortunately, this trend toward monopoly shows some signs of a reversal in the growth of consumerism, participatory democracy, and social ecology, as well as in the increasing dissatisfaction with poorly designed liberal reforms, so many of which have served only to enlarge the power of government bureaucracy. Health care reforms need to take advantage of this growing criticism of the so-called American way of life to propose a more personalistic and functionalist conception of society.

In view of Christian goals, we should be aware of lessons learned by the United States in regard to health care. The first of these is that the pluralist system did not adequately care for the poor, nor did it do much about positive health improvement. It tended to an exaggerated professional elitism, to place strong emphasis on monopolization and the profit motive, and it never produced a system of medical education that was personalistic. On the other hand, the pluralist system should be credited with promoting very rapid technological and scientific progress and with developing a great number of health care facilities equipped to give high-quality care. It must be noted, however, that this progress has led rather to greater expenditure of resources on the sophisticated treatment of relatively rare ailments than to better care for the health of the majority.

The contemporary trend is to create a "market-oriented" centralized system aimed at correcting some of the defects of the former system, although not in a very radical manner. Such a new system will greatly increase the bureaucratization which, as evidenced by the welfare system, DRGs (Diagnosis Related Groups) and other federal controls, can cost a great deal and accomplish very little. A centralized system will provide more health care, but there is no certainty it will promote better health. Nor is a bureaucracy likely to personalize the health care it gives.

It seems, therefore, that while some form of national health care program is the only practical way available to extend care to the neglected of society, Christians should not have any illusions about the adequacy of such programs, but should critically support the new schemes for national comprehensive health care, stressing the need to incorporate into these plans as many functionalist features as possible. For example:

1. Comprehensive health care should aim primarily at the promotion of positive health, not merely at the cure of acute disease or the prolongation of life through sophisticated techniques. Therefore, it should work for (a) removal of the environmental and social causes of ill health, including the commercial exploitation of unhealthy patterns of living, and (b) provision of preventive health education, which will give persons control over their own health.

2. Priority should be given to the problems of the most powerless, poorly informed, and least able to pay. These persons should not be cared for paternalistically, but should be admitted at once to participate in the power of decision about their own health needs.

3. Decision-making power should not be confined to a government bureaucracy nor to autonomous professionals, but should be shared by all concerned in mutual interdependence.

4. Planning should proceed in such a way as to avoid tendencies to increase dependence on higher levels and to promote a gradually increasing decentralization both in control and funding. This decentralization, however, should not be used as an excuse for the government to neglect the monitoring of health care and the supplementation and correction of defects at lower levels of organization.

5. Planning must be a continuous process of decision making that adapts to experience and new needs, rather than a fixed plan based on projections that may be mistaken.

The concepts underlying all such efforts to organize society, including its health care institutions, in such a way as to counteract tendencies to totalitarian bureaucratism on the one hand, and competitive individualism on the other, can be summarily formulated.[1]

Human communities exist only to promote and share the common good among all their members "from each according to ability, to each according to need" in such a way that (1) decision making rests *vertically* first with the person, then with the lower social levels, and *horizontally* with functional social units; and (2) the higher social units intervene only to supply the lower units what they cannot achieve by themselves, while at the same time working to make it easier in the future for lower units and individuals to satisfy these needs by their own efforts.

5.4 The Health Care Facility as Community

Considerable sociological effort has been devoted to understanding the modern health care facility. It seems to be a curious mixture of several types of organization.

1. It retains something of its original character as a hotel or temporary residence, with the primary function of care and custody. Thus some facilities for incurables become permanent or long-term residences approaching a total institution of the sort studied in Erving Goffman's well-known work *Asylums*.[2]

2. It is also a place of cure in which the medical staff provides diagnosis and treatment for patients. Acute care is usually offered in a hospital or in a clinic offering minor surgical procedures.

3. Finally, it may also be a school in which there are teachers and researchers (overlapping roles, as in any modern university) with their students and research staffs. The students are engaged both in class work and in supervised clinical practice, and some are interns and residents in actual full-time practice.

Especially interesting is the fact that the nurses are at the point of intersection of all these functions. They are often themselves students in training, but they also provide care, that is, they are the persons who actually carry out the host function of the hospital. At the same time, nurses are an essential part of the medical staff engaged in cure, since it is they who execute many of the treatment procedures and cooperate closely with physicians in observing patients and monitoring treatments.

Today the organizational complexity of the health care facilities is further intensified by the fact that they are becoming governmental agencies for the administration of public funds for health care. As such they are also staffed with social workers who help patients return to a wider community. Thus the health care facility today becomes one of the principal formative institutions of society, providing a model community that is bound to have a profound effect on the average American's understanding of social and personal interrelationships.

If the modern health care facility is to perform these varied functions effectively, it has to solve a number of basic ethical questions. In discussing total institutions, Goffman has shown that a prison, a small village, or a monastery can never be really complete because it lacks the resources to satisfy all human needs. If a health care facility is not to foster regressive behavior in its inmates, it must find ways to be open to wider influences.

Hence, hospitals or nursing homes in which patients remain for long periods have two special obligations. First, they must constantly seek ways for their patients to retain contact with the life of the outside world and engage in a variety of stimulating and enriching experiences and occupations. Second, they must find ways to involve patients in some genuine participation in making the decisions that affect their own lives. Obviously, senile or mentally disturbed patients may have little capacity for such participation, but too often this incapacity has been fostered by patterns of institutional life, which have given them no opportunity to express their preferences or to take at least some responsibility for themselves and others.

Today, largely because of the inflation of health costs, great efforts are being made in acute care hospitals to reduce the stay for patients, so that now the average stay is less than a week. This is not only less costly, but often also better therapeutically and ethically. The hospital has an ethical responsibility not to disrupt the home life of patients. While the sick have the right to be relieved of many ordinary social obligations, they need to be helped to experience sickness as a part of life, not as an interruption in living.

Consequently, in spite of inconveniences to the staff, better health care facilities no longer discourage visitors, not even small children, but find ways to facilitate continued family contact and opportunities for the family to share in the therapeutic process. Similarly, when their condition or convalescence permits, patients should be encouraged to assist their fellow patients, especially in long-term care. The sense of isolation, abandonment, and helplessness is perhaps the most traumatic aspect of being sick; but sickness can also be an important occasion to draw people together in a shared effort of healing.

Such patient participation also requires that patients have a choice as to when they get up in the morning and retire, what they eat and wear, when they should receive visitors, and who these visitors should be. Hence there must also be a constant, imaginative effort to enlarge the scope of patients' activities which should be measured not by the convenience of the hospital staff, but by therapeutic and human values.

The communal orientation of a health care facility as described here is primarily patient centered, but the patients will not be treated as persons if the professionals who care for them are themselves alienated by feelings that their own needs are neglected or their rights infringed. These professionals invest a great part of their lives and energy in the life of the institution and are rightly convinced that they have special rights based on their dedication, expert knowledge, and experienced judgment.

Professional Freedom

Perhaps the most important of these professional rights is the autonomy of professional judgment. Physicians need to be free to examine their patients and to order the treatment they think best. Nurses need to feel that their responsibility for their patients is just as professional as that of physicians. How can this necessary autonomy be reconciled with the communal character of the health care facility as an institution?

Generally speaking professional freedom in health care institutions, like academic freedom in universities, must be vigilantly protected. The hospital administration's duty is (1) to ascertain the competency of all professionals it admits to its staff and (2) to bring to the attention of a professional's peers any evidence or complaint about unprofessional or unethical behavior. If these peers fail to maintain standards, then the administration has no recourse but to terminate relations with the offender. The procedures to be followed in such cases should be clearly stated in the written policies and contracts of the institution.

The administration not only has such disciplinary responsibilities, but it also has a positive duty to unify the multiple functions of the institution in a manner which permits both the patients and the staff to form a truly human community not merely a "health factory." Faulty communications between physicians, nurses, auxiliaries, and administration and within these subgroups produce an atmosphere of tension very deleterious to the services, which can directly affect the psychosomatic health of the patients, especially in mental health care facilities. Modern administrative and communications theory affords important resources for improving such situations provided that they are used as tools to achieve ethically acceptable goals and not merely to oil an impersonal machine.

Finally, as the inflation of health care costs continues, many ethical questions arise from the economic policies of health care facilities reflecting the severe pressures from which they suffer. Here two important patient rights come into question: the right to emergency care and the right to treatment once the patient is admitted. The courts have generally upheld the legal obligation of hospitals with emergency wards (and even of those not so equipped to the extent of their resources) to care promptly for all persons who come to them in serious need of medical attention and to continue to care for them until they are ambulatory or can safely be transferred to another hospital which is willing to receive them. Recent research indicates that not all hospitals are respecting the rights of patients in this regard and that "dumping" patients without health insurance is becoming a national problem.[3] The courts are also beginning to develop a doctrine on the rights of patients in so-called custodial institutions to treatment as well as to care. Christian and humanist ethics both have accepted the teaching of the parable of the Good Samaritan (Lk 10:25-37), but in public institutions this concern for one's neighbor must be legally enforced.

All these ethical and legal questions, which arise from the ideal of the health care facility as a community of care and cure, faced with the realities of modern depersonalized and competitive society, can be solved only at the price of an unremitting effort to give priority to persons over institutions and properties. Every health care facility suffers from the proliferation of bureaucratic rules intended to protect the institution from exploitation by the crazy or the crafty. This red tape is destructive to patients and staff. The chief remedy against this ever-present danger is training the staff to deal with borderline situations in a flexible and prudent manner and to provide a variety of methods by which self-criticism can be promoted and criticism from outside can be heard. To achieve this interplay, it is necessary to develop the staff not merely as a hierarchical structure of command responsibility, but as an interacting health team.

5.5 The Health Care Team

Because of the highly specialized character of modern medicine, health seekers must entrust themselves not to a single physician but to a *health care team*. This section discusses those members of the health care team with whom the patient must deal directly—the physician, the nurse, and the social worker—to determine what reciprocal ethical obligations exist between the patient and these three kinds of professionals. To fulfill these ethical obligations we suggest a new version of relationship between health team members.

Traditionally, the chief decision maker in any health care team is the licensed physician. Consequently, no serious step toward treating the patient can be taken without a physician's permission.

Today the concept of the licensed medical doctor as a general practitioner has been vastly altered by the growth of medical specialization. In 1950 only about 36 percent of physicians in private practice were specialists, while in 1986 about 70 percent are specialists. This rapid decline of the general practitioner as the primary care professional has deprived patients of the advantages of having their health problems evaluated by someone who knows the patient in his or her family context over a long period and who thinks of the patient as a whole person with a continuous biography.

Perhaps the key to this difficulty of knowing the patient personally is to be found in a better understanding of the nurse's proper role. Originally, the nurse was the person most concerned with caring for the patient and in continuous contact with the patient. Therefore patient-centered health care, which this book is advocating, would dictate that the nurse is the central professional figure, not the physician.

Today, however, nurses have been burdened with other tasks. For too long they spent much of their energy in housekeeping chores—making beds, carrying trays, and so forth. Today they have been largely relieved of these tasks by auxiliaries, but they are still much occupied with technical tasks: injections, medications, intravenous feeding.

Under present circumstances, as nursing education has advanced, able nurses have sought administrative and teaching posts as the only way of advancement open to them. They would find nursing itself much more interesting, however, if it became the real focus of health care, so that the role of the nurse, female or male, in direct contact with the patient is seen as primary care and the real source of unity in the health team. Then the nurse assigned to a given patient would become the authority having responsibility for the patient as a person and would help the patient make use of all the resources furnished by the health team.

This personalistic, mediating function today is often performed by the medical or psychiatric social worker. Sociological study of the medical profession has led to the acknowledgment of the great importance of the social dimension in treating disease. Hence, persons trained in social process have been added to healing teams. The social worker interviews patients to discover possible social factors of ethnic culture, economic status, and family structure which may have caused the disease, which may hinder treatment, or which may prevent rehabilitation. Commonly, such workers help patients regarding both their legal rights and their opportunities for public financial assistance and other matters connected with illness. They also act as a liaison with the patient's family and help find ways to assure family stability in the absence of the patient from the home. Finally, social workers undertake the patient's reentry into society.

The social worker is chiefly concerned with patients in their normal life patterns, and the nurse with patients undergoing the actual experience of sickness and healing. Consequently, these two roles are very closely connected and together constitute primary care in the strict sense of direct concern with the patient as a person. The physician's role, on the other hand, is more specialized since it is focused precisely on the diagnosis and treatment of a pathological condition or its future prevention. If this analysis is correct, the physician cannot be the sole decision maker in the health team. Rather, the patient has the ultimate decision and is helped in this decision in the first place by the nurse and social worker who are acquainted with patients in their total personalities and life situations, in the second place by the primary care physician, and in the third place by various specialist physicians.

Recently, some hospitals have begun to recognize the need for pastoral care, not as an occasional intervention of religious ministry from outside the institution by a visiting clergyman, nor only as a convenience for patients who wish religious ministration by a resident chaplain, but as a regular part of patient care, since all patients, religious or secular, have problems of ultimate concern that affect the success of the healing process.

Physicians will not find it easy to reconcile their proper professional autonomy with the requirements of teamwork or to relinquish the idea that they have sole decision-making power in health care while all others are merely their executive assistants. If the health team concept is to have real significance, physicians must come to acknowledge that they need the help of others not only in carrying out decisions, but also in making them if the people entrusted to their care are to be well served.

Commonly, when continuing education programs in ethics are offered to the professional staff of a hospital, the nurses take advantage of these, but the physicians are notable by their absence. Because physicians occupy a leadership role on a health care team, they must be as well-acquainted with the ethical policies of the institution as are other members of the staff; yet they often excuse themselves because of their heavy workload, as if the nurses had it easy! *It would be entirely reasonable for Catholic institutions to specify as a condition of granting hospital privileges to physicians, or for medical staff and residents, attendance at a certain number of hours of continuing education in the ethical policies of the institution.* A hospital administration which puts this issue on a professional, rather than an informal level, will find that physicians will accept this responsibility as they do so many others, and will soon come to view it as a reasonable and necessary part of the continuing education which today is demanded of all health care professionals.

5.6 Health Care, Ethics, and Social Policy

The federal government has made some attempt to give ethical guidelines for social policy in regard to health care. In the late 1960s and early 1970s Congress became uneasy, in fact, disturbed, about the implications of scientific progress. Revolutionary advances in science and technology were predicted, for example, genetic engineering and DNA splicing, and it was feared that these advances might have damaging effects on individuals and society. At the same time, public outrage arose over some scientific research projects that had violated the human rights of some individuals. For example, a study was made public in which aborted fetuses were decapitated in order to perform pharmaceutical tests. Moreover, the Tuskeegee Syphilis Study in which the cure for syphilis was withheld from some poor black men afflicted with this disease was exposed in the press.

Because of general apprehension about revolutionary scientific developments and the sharp public reaction to specific abuses in the area of research, Congress established The Commission for the Protection of Human Subjects of Biomedical and Behavioral Research (CPHS) in July 1974. As its name indicates, the mandate for this commission was to set ethical guidelines for research projects involving human beings, especially those whose rights might be violated. When the life of this commission ceased, the Secretary of the Department of Health, Education and Welfare appointed an Ethics Advisory Board (EAB) in the spring of 1978 to continue the study of ethical issues and public policy. This advisory board was superseded a few months later by another group created by Congress, called The President's Commission for the Study of Ethical Problems in Medicine and Biomedical and Behavioral Research (PCEMR).

Accomplishments

The productivity of these three federal commissions has been impressive. The CPHS published more than 10 studies in its 4-year life on subjects such as research on fetuses, children, prisoners, and the mentally infirm. It also studied psychosurgery, put forth ethical guidelines for delivery of health care by government agencies, and set standards for institutional review boards. In the Belmont Report the CPHS sought to synthesize the ethical principles it had used in its studies. The EAB, because of its short existence, studied only one ethical problem at length, that of in vitro fertilization. The PCEMR was commissioned by Congress to consider many ethical issues, such as brain death, access to health services, withdrawal of life-support systems, and testing in regard to genetic disease. During its existence, the PCEMR published 10 studies on these and other topics.

Evaluation

Although we do not attempt to evaluate any of the documents emanating from these federal commissions, we offer the following general comments.

1. The very fact that Congress recognizes the need for ethical norms in the field of research and therapy is a step forward. For the most part, the norms set forth by the commissions are useful and protect the rights of scientists and physicians as well as subjects and patients.

2. The norms formulated by the commissions are designed with our pluralistic society in mind. Thus they seek to enunciate what most scientists, politicians, and religious thinkers will agree on. Although they do not state it explicitly, it is clear that they avoid controversy, so some of the more difficult and important ethical issues are not considered, such as the value of fetal life, the time when human life begins, and the meaning of health.

3. Although some of the more important norms concerning physician-patient relationships are considered, for example, informed consent and justice in selection of research subjects, there is little consideration of the pressing ethical questions concerning the society-physician-patient relationship, such as: Is there a *right* to equal health care for all? Should all feasible care be financed publicly? What are the goals for our national health programs?

4. The basis on which these ethical statements are formulated is not the nature of the human person, the covenant between physician and patient, the just society, nor religious teaching. Rather, the basis is what is culturally acceptable, that is what norms seem acceptable to the American public. Deciding ethical responsibilities in this manner is dangerous because it justifies whatever is popular. The ethicist should continually question and evaluate what is culturally acceptable, judging it on more fundamental values.

5. The motivation for observing the norms of the federal commissions is mainly monetary. If a person or institution does not observe these norms, the person or institution will not receive federal funding and might be subject to malpractice litigation. Thus, in a certain sense, these "ethical statements" emanating from the federal commissions are legal norms insofar as the motivation for observing them is concerned. Although ethicists may differ in detail as to the proper motivation for ethical activity, avoiding legal sanctions is not considered by any ethicist to be the ultimate justification for ethical action.

In sum, the deliberations of the federal commissions have been worthwhile in that they have brought to our attention the need for ethical norms in the field of research and therapy. But, because the agencies avoid some of the more important questions as they concentrate on expressing consensus and because the norms are based on a weak foundation, it is clear that more rigorous thinking must be applied to the modern ethical issues in medicine, research, and health care.

5.7 The Catholic Health Care Facility

Originally, Catholic health care facilities were founded principally by religious orders of sisters and brothers to give health care to the neglected and, especially in areas where Catholicism was not the chief religion, as a means to witness to the ethical and spiritual aspects of health care in accordance with Catholic values. Today in the United States, the dominance of secular humanism as a philosophy of life has so influenced and pressured the operation of such

Catholic health care facilities that many wonder whether these institutions are any longer Catholic in any significant respect.

What characterizes a Catholic health care facility? In the United States such a facility has several obvious characteristics.

1. It has a Christian and Catholic ministry and therefore receives apostolic direction from the ordinary of the diocese. Under his guidance and interpretation it follows the *Ethical and Religious Directives for Catholic Health Facilities* approved by the United States Catholic Conference (USCC), which outline the proper spiritual care patients should receive, the duties of the hospital as a representative of the Catholic Church, and the medical procedures prohibited in Catholic health care facilities. Many of the ethical problems presented in this book are treated in the *Directives*, but not some of the more recent issues, such as transsexual surgery and behavior control. The *Directives* were last revised in 1975, and suggestions for future revisions may be sent to the USCC through the bishop of the diocese.

2. A Catholic hospital is usually sponsored by a religious community of sisters or brothers who have basic financial ownership and responsibility for policy. In the future they may be sponsored by the laity yet because they are publicly presented as Catholic be responsible to the Church.

3. It is not a for-profit institution but has as its principal goal the service of the right to health of all persons, and especially the neglected. Thus it has made what Pope John Paul II and the United States bishops call "the option for the poor." Although investor-owned corporations are not evil in themselves, they are out of place in the health care setting because their goal is making a profit for investors.[4]

4. It has a pastoral care program that involves sacramental as well as a counseling ministry staffed by priests, religious, and lay persons. In larger health care facilities there may be full-time ministers representing religious communities other than Catholic.

5. Such institutions usually are marked by various Catholic symbols, such as statues, religious pictures, and crucifixes in the rooms.

All of these characteristics (even the last) are more than superficial. They express the character of the hospital as a ministry of the Catholic Church, based on the interrelations of the whole person in all the biological, psychological, ethical, and spiritual dimensions dealt with in this book.

There is something deeper, however. Catholics essentially conceive of the healing ministry as an extension of the ministry of Christ. Jesus was prophet or teacher, king or shepherd, priest or sanctifier. The Second Vatican Council has taught that this threefold ministry should be reflected in all the works of the Church and in every member. Healing is part of the shepherding function of the Christian community, since building this community entails concern for each weak member who needs restoration to vital life and participation.

Jesus healed people radically by penetrating to the spiritual core of the human personality and liberating the person from original or social sin and also from individual, personal sin, with the more superficial but real effect of healing them also psychologically and physically. A Christian hospital, therefore, is also concerned with the radical healing of those for whom it cares. The experience of sickness and healing in such a hospital should be also an experience of personal spiritual growth through suffering and redemption.

What should make a Catholic hospital a special kind of community and a model for other healing communities is that its members, both professionals and patients, are clearly aware of the presence of Christ the Healer in the midst of the community making use of his ministers—physicians, nurses, technicians, administrators, and patients in relation to each other—in his work of healing. This presence of Christ should also be celebrated ritually through the sacraments and proclaimed through the word of Scripture and of preaching, with Christ's promise of renewed life more powerful than death.

Such a religious conception of a health care institution need not weaken but should enhance its competence in all the arts and sciences of modern medicine. Without that religious commitment, a hospital or long-term care facility becomes a depersonalized machine that hurts as much as it heals. In the same way, unless a Catholic health care facility gets its vitality from its own religious faith and system of values, it will become more hurtful than healing, a scandal rather than a witness of Christ's presence in a suffering world.[5]

A significant development in Catholic health care is the recent formation of health care corporations in which a number of hospitals under the sponsorship of the same religious order or different religious orders are united in a single corporation. This enables the corporation to provide the individual hospitals with much needed research and education and a more effective public voice in influencing public health care policy. It is essential that such large corporations give as much attention to the Christian values to which they are dedicated as to economic and administrative problems. Otherwise, they become a business and do not promote the values that should characterize health care. As Paul Starr wrote:

> The organizational culture of medicine used to be dominated by the ideals of professionalism and voluntarism, which softened the underlying acquisitive activity. The restraint exercised by those ideals now grows weaker. The "health center" of one year is the "profit center" of the next.[6]

5.8 Conclusion

Perhaps the greatest ethical issue in health care in the United States is the issue of social responsibility. The health care system in the United States is advanced and sophisticated insofar as research, knowledge, and therapy are concerned, but it is poorly designed insofar as provision of care is concerned. Too many people, especially those without health care insurance or without adequate coverage, are unable to receive the health care they need. The poor and frail elderly are especially deprived in this regard.[7] There are no easy answers to the problem. But some solution to the problem of providing adequate access to health care for all must be found in the immediate future. The federal government must cooperate to overcome the injustices that are present in our provision of health care. Neither the federal government nor health care professionals and corporations will act, however, unless private citizens express their displeasure with the shocking lack of health care for many people.

Footnotes

1. Pope John Paul II, "Rich in Mercy," *Origins* 10 (26) December 11, 1980.

2. Erving Goffman, *Asylums: Essays on the Social Situation of Mental Patients and Other Inmates* (Chicago: Aldine, 1982).

3. Robert Schmitt, MD, *et. al.*, "Transfers to a Public Hospital," *New England Journal of Marketing*, 314 N.9 (February 27, 1986) pp. 552-557.

4. Kevin O'Rourke, "An Ethical Perspective on Investor-Owned Medical Care Corporations," *Frontiers* 1 (1), September, 1984.

5. Kevin O'Rourke, *Reasons for Hope* (St. Louis: Catholic Health Association, 1983), p. 53.

6. Paul Starr, *The Social Transformation of American Medicine* (New York: Basic Books, 1982), p. 448.

7. G. J. Bazzoli, *Health Care for the Indigent* (Chicago: American Hospital Association, 1985).

Study Questions

1. The free market system of capitalism seems to have produced a higher standard of living and higher levels of technological progress and productivity than has centralized planning in socialist countries. Should we not, therefore, promote the highest possible degree of competition in the delivery of health care? Please explain your answers.

2. If a national or even a regional system of universal health care is developed in this country, what policies should be built into it that will maintain subsidiarity and limit the growth of a cumbersome and oppressive bureaucracy?

3. According to the concept of functionalism, health care is an autonomous sector of our national society whose concerns should have easy access to government power without resorting to covert lobbying. In what respect is this the case in the United States at the present time, and in what respect is it not?

4. Many TV dramas have hospitals as their settings and health care professionals as their characters. In what ways do they and do they not realistically portray health care facilities as human communities?

5. What do you think of the proposal in this chapter to assign the nurse rather than the physician to the key role in a health care team? Is the notion of a health care *team* itself realistic?

6. Report on the most recent developments in the federal government's regulation of and provision for universal health care.

7. What changes would you make in the Catholic health care facility best known to you to make it more authentically Catholic?

Cases

1. In a city of 60,000 population there are two not-for-profit hospitals, one Catholic and one nondenominational which compete with each other. Neither is usually filled to capacity. A group of physicians build a for-profit hospital in the city and compete with both. They have a financial advantage in that they refuse charity patients beyond the minimal percentage required by government regulations, while the Catholic hospital has always gone beyond this minimum, and the nondenominational institution has followed the same practice in order not to fall behind the Catholic institution in public support. The for-profit hospital uses its advantage in part to bring advanced equipment into the city and thus to attract those able to pay. Discuss the pros and cons of for-profit hospitals.

2. Dr. N moves from Canada to the United States because he resents the government regulation involved in the national health care system of Canada. He says in his experience these regulations make it more difficult for a conscientious physician to follow his own best judgment in fulfilling his obligation to his patients. He finds, however, that, in the U.S., Medicare requires a great deal of paperwork and so he decides to refuse Medicare patients. He then finds that his own income has fallen. To increase it he is tempted to recommend more surgery than he might otherwise have done. What are the ethical questions which Dr. N must ask himself?

3. Dr. S, a surgeon, has been reported to the chief of staff, Dr. P, by Dr. T, an anesthesiologist, who has observed several rather strange incidents in the operating room. He suspects that Dr. S is either an alcoholic or using drugs. Dr. P assures Dr. T that he will speak to Dr. S about the matter. Dr. S admits that he has a problem but promises to be more careful in the future. Nothing more is said about the matter until a malpractice suit is brought against Dr. S and the hospital because of an operation in which he removed a healthy ovary instead of the pathological one, thus rendering the woman permanently sterile. At the trial neither Dr. P nor Dr. T mention the matter of the drug dependency because they are not asked the question directly by the attorneys. When it comes to light through one of the nurses, they answer truthfully but claim that they had done what they could about the matter and were unaware that Dr. S had continued his misconduct. What is the responsibility of these physicians with regard to policing their own profession prior to court action?

4. Hospital C specializes in the rehabilitation of patients with disabilities. In order to encourage the patients to a more positive attitude toward their disabilities, they have a policy of employing as many persons on the staff who are themselves handicapped yet function effectively. A new administrator, however, prefers a staff chosen simply on the basis of its competence. How do these two models relate to the conception of a health care facility as a community?

5. Dr. C is responsible for setting up a staff for the intensive care unit. What should be the criteria for selecting the physicians, nurses, and auxiliaries for

such a staff from the viewpoint of personal relations? What ethical problems may arise in making such a team effective?

6. In a city public hospital, tax revenues set severe budgetary limits. This hospital is the recipient of many minority patients with low incomes who are rejected by other local hospitals for lack of insurance. It is purposed to begin heart transplants at this hospital because Dr. M of the staff, an excellent cardiac surgeon is very interested in the procedure. Objections are raised that becoming involved in something so sophisticated and expensive in this type of hospital is a poor use of resources. Dr. M points out that charity patients have even more heart disease than the average population. Don't they have a right to full care? What would be your position?

7. St. Ann's General Hospital is sponsored by a congregation of Catholic sisters. Because of declining vocations they have only a few sisters on the staff; none of them are actually engaged in nursing. The medical staff is only about 30 percent Catholic and the nurses are of many religious affiliations or none. The congregation, however, retains ownership of the corporation and influential positions on the board. What should be their objectives in policy decisions if the hospital is to remain Catholic in more than name? What relation should the hospital have to the local Catholic bishop?

Chapter 6

Norms of Christian Decisions in Bioethics

6.1 Ethical Methods

Need for an Objective Method

Some philosophers today deny that there is any objective method of arriving at ethical decisions. They argue that, although it is possible to decide between conflicting views in the sciences by checking the *facts*, in disputes over ethics it is not facts that are in question but *values*, and values are simply a matter of individual preference. Thus the statement, "Abortion is wrong" is not a statement of fact such as "The earth is round," but simply means, "I don't like abortion," or "Abortion is ugly." Such a theory of ethical decision is called *emotivism* because it reduces ethical judgments to statements of emotional reactions.

Emotivism as an ethical method was best defended in modern times by the philosopher Jean Jacques Rousseau, who argued that most people have naturally good emotional instincts, when these have not been distorted by bad education. His views have greatly influenced American culture. When politicians appeal to the "wisdom of the American people," they probably mean "the emotional reactions of the majority must be right." In debates about medical ethics, it is not uncommon to meet physicians who think that attention to the instincts of decent doctors is the best way to settle any ethical question. The difficulty with this approach is that it provides no method of public, objective discussion but leaves problems to rhetoric and passion. Whose instincts are sound? After all, some people feel that all blacks and Jews should be wiped out. Consequently, it is important that we try to find an objective and logical method of settling what is right and wrong, even though this method may not be fool-proof.

Deontological Methodologies

Probably the most common ethical methodology rests on the principle that an action is right when it conforms to laws or rules laid down by legitimate authority and wrong when it violates these laws. Such a method is called *legalism* because the ultimate standard of right and wrong is the law. It is also called *voluntarism* because it considers that a law obliges because it is the *will* (Latin *voluntas*) of the legitimate lawgiver. Finally, it is called *deontologism* (Greek *deontos*, duty), because it conceives ethical behavior as dutiful, obedient, and law-abiding.

There are, of course, various kinds of lawgivers and various kinds of law. If we believe that the ultimate appeal is to the authority of the state (or of our peer group), this is *legal positivism*. For example, many people considered abortion wrong when it was still forbidden by state laws but right after the Supreme Court voided these laws. The total inadequacy of such a view is evident from the fact that Hitler was careful to act legally, but it was he who made the laws! It would never be possible to argue for the abolition of a law as unjust, unless there were some higher standard than the law of the state.

Consequently, throughout history people have appealed to a "higher law," namely, divine or eternal law, the will of God, since God is the supreme authority whose will is always righteous. How are we to know God's will? One way is through revelation, which Jews believe is embodied in the Hebrew Torah and oral tradition based on it. Christians believe it is in the Bible, and Muslims believe it is in the Quran. An appeal to these scriptures (which in ethical matters have much in common) involves problems of interpretation. Protestants, for example, rely on a personal, sometimes very literal, interpretation of the Bible; Catholics believe the Bible must be interpreted authentically by the living tradition of the Roman Catholic Church under its pope and bishops. Another way, accepted by Catholics, of knowing God's will is to begin with the divine law revealed in the Bible, but to supplement this by using natural law (i.e., human reason and experience used to determine what actions best serve true human welfare) to apply the biblical law to many detailed questions, such as those arising in modern medical practice, and also as the basis of objective discussion with non-Christians for whom the Bible lacks authority.

In the eighteenth century another form of deontological ethics arose among the so-called Enlightenment philosophers, who rejected Christian revelation but were not inclined to adopt Rousseau's subjective emotivism. The chief thinker of this school, who is still influential in medical ethics, was Immanuel Kant, who proposed a kind of deontological method known as *formalism*. According to this our emotional preferences, which provide us with values, must be checked against certain rational standards of a purely formal kind. The principle standard is the *categorical imperative*, namely, that any choices we make must be such that we would be willing for everyone else to make the same choices (*universality*). For example, if I were to choose to lie for my own benefit, would I really be willing that others lie to me? Since I would prefer they not lie to me, I must not lie to them. Kant thought that this method was advantageous because it made no appeal to any standard except the individual's own conscience (that is it was an *autonomous* ethics not a *heteronomous* one depending on the authority of another). Nevertheless, it is open to serious criticism because it is purely formal and has to rely on emotivism to establish any concrete values or practical rules.

Because of the weakness of this formalism, a number of recent ethicists have tried to modify Kant's system by postulating a number of general rules, such as the principles of fairness and beneficence. These are proposed as needing no other justification than that they help us settle ethical questions in a consistent way. Such a method, however, still is open to the objections that (1) it does not provide concrete rules and (2) consistent behavior does not always mean consistently good behavior. There are consistent liars and crooks.

Teleological Methodologies

The weakness of any deontological system is that it does not give any ultimate reason why the will of the authority itself is right or wrong. We ought to question whether we ourselves are righteous. Often the state is obviously unjust in the laws it makes. Even God, as Job complained, sometimes seems to be unfair. Laws are useful and necessary guides for our ethical decisions, but still we cannot help questioning whether some laws are just. Teleological methodologies seek to answer this question.

The word *teleology* has as its root the Greek *telos*, or goal. A teleological method in ethics seeks to justify or reject an action by determining whether it is an effective or a self-defeating means to the goal of *true* human fulfillment in the community. Some persons choose as their goal in life some kind of illusory self-fulfillment which, even if it is achieved, leaves them miserable, such as the man who devotes all his energies to financial success only to discover he is rich, lonely, and afraid of death.

Utilitarianism

Teleologists are divided into two very different schools of thought whose debates are responsible for many of the hottest controversies in medical ethics today. One of these schools is so popular that many identify the term teleology with it, supposing there is no other kind. This is *utilitarianism* (or consequentialism). Utilitarians believe that the goal of human life is maximum satisfaction or, in other terms, one which produces more satisfactory consequences than unsatisfactory ones.

Some utilitarians are *act* utilitarians, who say that there are no universal ethical rules but that every action must be judged in its unique context. Some Christian ethicists call themselves situationists or contexualists and adopt act utilitarianism. The pioneer medical ethicist Joseph Fletcher argued that there is only one general ethical rule: "Do what is most loving in the circumstances." He was never able to define what "most loving" means in practice. Most utilitarians, however, favor *rule* utilitarianism, which accepts general ethical rules such as "Thou shalt not kill" as *prima facie* rules that are generally obliging but admit exceptions in some circumstances. Also, to avoid reducing their system to the subjective preferences of emotivism, they contend that the supreme principle of ethics is not merely *my* maximum satisfaction in life, but the greatest good for the greatest number.

The weakness of utilitarianism is that it can be used to justify almost any action because it provides no objective way of measuring the good and bad consequences of an action. Jeremy Bentham, the English philosopher famous for his defense of this system, believed it possible to establish a "unit of satisfaction" and thus measure satisfactions much as we weigh economic values in units of dollars and cents. But how can we find a common quantitative unit of measurement for the very qualitatively different kinds of "satisfactions" that make up a truly fulfilled life? Can I weigh the price of friendship, success in my work, and good health one against another? Can we sacrifice the life of one innocent person to save the lives of 10 others?

Proportionalism

Another form of teleological ethics which has been put forward by a number of Catholic moralists and which is to be found in a good deal of current writing can be called *proportionalism* because it seeks to reduce ethical decisions to a single fundamental principle of proportion, which can be stated as follows:

> An action is morally good if the premoral values that it promotes outweigh the premoral disvalues it promotes; otherwise it is morally evil.

Premoral values are physical, psychological, or social values considered prior to their moral evaluation. For example, nutritious food is a human value, yet morally considered it is a disvalue for a person who needs to diet. Proportionalists admit that there are some abstract moral norms, such as "Do good and avoid evil" and "Love your enemy" which are absolute; that is, admit no exceptions for any purpose or in any circumstances. They also concede that we can state concrete moral norms, such as "Do not murder" and "Do not fornicate," which also are absolute. The very terms in which they are formulated imply a moral judgment, since "murder" and "fornicate" imply that such an action is ethically unjustifiable.

They do not admit that concrete norms stated in value-free terms such as "Thou shalt not kill" and "Thou shalt not engage in sex outside marriage" can be absolute, but maintain that all such concrete norms stated in value-free terms admit, at least in theory, of exceptions in certain circumstances. Thus the norm "Thou shalt not kill" is *prima facie* (generally speaking) valid, but in certain circumstances and for certain purposes it does not hold: one can kill to defend oneself, or as punishment for a capital crime.

How, then, do we know when we can ethically make an exception to a generally valid concrete moral norm? For example, when can we make an exception to the general norm that to kill an unborn child is wrong? Proportionalists argue that the criterion in making such legitimate exceptions is the principle of proportion. If the values achieved by the act outweigh the disvalues or harm caused, then the act is moral, even if it violates the generally valid concrete norm. Thus it is not murder to kill an enemy in self-defense because the value of my life outweighs that of my attacker, since I am innocent and he is a criminal. Similarly, the interests of a woman who has been raped may outweigh the value of the life of her unborn child.

Proportionalism is a popular theory even among Catholics because it seems both to maintain the *prima facie* validity of traditional Christian norms, such as those which forbid homicide, abortion, extramarital sex, and lying, and at the same time to permit exceptions in difficult cases where the insistence on such norms seems to be inhumane. Nevertheless, proportionalism as a methodology is open to serious theoretical and practical objections and seems very difficult to reconcile with the Bible or the teachings of the Catholic Church.[1] It is sufficient here to point out two of its weaknesses.

First, we must ask proportionalists how they are going to measure or weigh the relative values or disvalues of a human action? Caiaphas used a proportionalist argument in arguing for the death of Jesus: "Can you not see that it is better for you to have one man die than to have the whole nation destroyed?" (Jn 1:49). But how do we weigh the value of one human life against another? Or how can we decide that the happiness of one individual is of more or less value than the life of another? Proportionalists have not been able to give any practical, objective answer to how this proportion is to be determined fairly without simply lapsing into utilitarianism or situationism.

Second, if we are to weigh values and disvalues, there must be some values that are nonnegotiable or absolute against which other values are weighed, such as the right of an innocent person to life. To violate such nonnegotiable values is to do something intrinsically evil that cannot be justified by any circumstance or good intention. That is why in our justice system we recognize the right of a person to be considered innocent until proved guilty. Therefore to deny there are any exceptionless concrete moral norms amounts to saying that it is sometimes permissible to do evil for the sake of good, or that the end justifies the means, views which have always been rejected by Christians.

Proportionalists attempt to answer this last objection by saying that they do not maintain that it is permissible to do moral evil for the sake of good, but only to do premoral (or ontic) harm when the good achieved is greater than the premoral harm caused. This answer, however, revives the first difficulty already discussed. To say that a value is premoral means that it is unrelated to the good of human persons, since any value which is a human, personal value has a moral character, as has been shown in Chapter 1. Thus the command, "Thou shalt not kill" in the Bible does not mean that killing, in the abstract, is wrong; but it does mean that to kill an innocent, nonagressive human person is always wrong. If killing a human person in self-defense can be justified, it is not because the premoral benefits of killing outweigh the premoral harm done, but because the aggressor has by his own harmful actions forfeited the absolute moral right to life, which innocent persons possess in all circumstances.

Prudential Personalism

Another form of teleological methodology that avoids these difficulties and is more consistent with the teaching of the Catholic Church is adopted in this book. Prudential personalism is based not on the principle of proportion but on that of moral discrimination, which will be explained later. (See p. 88.) Prudential personalism agrees with proportionalism that in every moral decision we must take into account not only *prima facie* concrete moral norms but also the circumstances and the purposes of the actors; but contrary to proportionalism it maintains that some basic human values, corresponding to the basic needs of the human person discussed in Chapter 1, are nonnegotiable, that is, they do can never be violated.

Thus some (but by no means all) concrete moral norms are valid in all circumstances and for any purpose. For example, it is always wrong to kill innocent human beings, it is always wrong to commit incest or rape, and it is always wrong to perjure oneself. Such actions strike at the nonnegotiable values of human life on which all human society is based, and they are contradictory to our love of neighbor and therefore our love of God. This methodology, therefore, is *prudential* because it takes full account of the circumstances and purposes of human actions, but it is a *personalism* because it protects the dignity and basic rights of the person against violation by anyone or by society.

6.2 Christian Principles of Ethical Action

How do Christians reach decisions concerning specific concrete issues? They apply Christian principles to particular cases. By a principle we do not mean *a priori* rules that are deduced from more abstract value statements, which in turn have been deduced from broad, metaphysical axioms. Nor do we mean mere postulates or assumptions accepted for the sake of consistency in behavior. Rather, we mean practical generalizations derived from human experience of our basic human needs and confirmed by the Gospel.

Adultery is not wrong merely because it violates some ideal model of marriage, but because human experience tells us adultery involves a serious breach of trust which destroys or weakens marital love that is a basic human need. This experience was confirmed by Jesus in the Sermon on the Mount (Mt 5:27-30). Thus moral decisions are not automatically deduced from general principles because actual decisions depend on wide and rich experience, good will, and sensitive, normal, and disciplined emotions as well as good logic. To make good moral decisions we must be good persons who have a realistic understanding of what it is to be fully human.

Christians realize that because of the widespread wars, poverty, ignorance, hatred, cruelty, and waste of human talents, what it is to be truly human is not always clearly evident. In all times and cultures people have been able to see the difference between those who are "human" and decent and those who are "inhuman" and evil. Nevertheless, what some people admire appears contemptible to others.

It is only in Jesus Christ that Christians see the true and complete picture of what it is to be truly a normal human being: truthful, courageous, compassionate, wise, unselfish, forgiving, and faithful. Consequently, it is to his example that we look to define moral principles in their precise meaning. At the same time we know that his example can be appreciated not only by Christians who declare themselves his followers, but by people of all faiths who have learned about his life. Thus Gandhi, a Hindu, kept the New Testament on his bedside table because he recognized in Jesus a supreme model of human goodness.

Christians, however, believe that Jesus is much more than a model. Because he is truly the Son of God, he is the source of the power of grace by which it becomes possible for us all to grow in likeness to him. This following of Jesus is not merely something individual; we need to live it as members of the community he founded and in which he continues to live spiritually—the Christian Church, whose visible unity is to be found in the headship of the successor of St. Peter, the Pope. This Church is made up of both saints and sinners, but they work together that all might become more like Jesus. Through the Bible, which the Church has preserved, and the living tradition by which the Church correctly interprets the Bible, as well as by the support and example of fellow Christians, we members of this community are helped to keep the life and teachings of Jesus clearly before our eyes. When controversies and disagreements arise about what is the Christlike thing to do, we can arrive at a clear and sound decision of conscience through the guidance of this community, the Church.

The great disciple of Jesus, St. Paul, taught us that the actions by which we follow Christ must be motivated by faith, hope, and love (1 Co 13). Faith, hope, and love work toward the satisfaction of our deepest human need, the need to live in the community of persons centered in the three-personed God. Our unison with God and neighbor through Christ is Christian love. Christian hope is the dynamic movement toward the realization of this community that is God's kingdom, even here on earth. And the conviction that God has called us to this kingdom and is willing to give us the power of the Holy Spirit by which we can attain it is Christian faith. Christian prudence is faith in its practical aspects as it enables us to be open to the guidance of Christ's Spirit, who alone knows the way to God through the many illusions and dead ends of life in a sinful world.

Thus faith, hope, and love, because they make us Christlike and thus fulfill our deepest human needs, are the ultimate principles of Christian ethics. Prudence (in the sense we are using here) does not signify mere caution or compromise as it often does in common parlance. Rather it means the ability to assess the circumstances of an action and determine the best way to reach the goal to which God has called us in Christ. Thus prudence often involves daring and courage and always requires a practical wisdom that gets the job done.

Non-Christians who seek to develop ethical norms may agree that faith, hope, and love are important human values, but they may differ in the emphasis they give those values and they may not understand them in a Christocentric manner. Thus faith, hope, and love are common to many value systems, but in an analogical way. This does not imply that non-Christians never experience the realities to which the terms faith, hope, and love refer. Catholic theology admits that non-Christians may be living by grace, but when they experience these realities they do not name or understand them in the same way as Christians. Christians claim no monopoly in the true God or his grace, but only that the gracious God has made himself fully, explicitly, and intimately known to humanity in Jesus Christ. Thus these three Pauline terms of faith, hope, and love serve as a way of classifying a set of ethical principles that are explicitly but not exclusively Christian and that can be applied to bioethical issues. In the remainder of this chapter, we will formulate and briefly explain 12 such principles which play the major role in bioethical decision.

6.3 Principles of Christian Faith

Christian faith, which enables us to understand not only our natural needs but, more important, our deeper needs awakened by God's grace, is a kind of knowing, a light that guides our way in life. Hence the principles of faith instruct us how to form a prudent conscience, because forming a prudent conscience is fundamentally (but not totally) a process of knowing and a strengthening and deepening of human insight and reason. Christians are aware that in forming their consciences they depend on the Holy Spirit to overcome the prejudice and blindess of sin (Rom 1:18-20). With this assistance and the light of faith we are guided in making prudent decisions by six principles. If our faith is to be practical, we must take care to inform our own conscience (*principle of well-formed conscience*) and enable others to do the same (*principle of free and informed consent*). We must then apply this information to our actual decisions (*principle of moral discernment*), taking special care when our actions, although good in themselves, may involve bad side effects (*principle of double effect*) or involve us in cooperation with others who do something we would prevent if we could (*principle of legitimate cooperation*). In particular, as professionals we must respect the right of others to privacy when they confide their own moral problems to us (*principle of professional communication*).

1. Principle of a Well-Formed Conscience

This principle has already been discussed in Chapter 3 in connection with personal resonsibility for health (see page 25).

To attain the true goals of human life by responsible actions, in every free decision involving an ethical question, people are morally obliged to do the following:

    a. Inform themselves as fully as practically possible about the facts and the ethical norms.

    b. Form a morally certain judgment of conscience on the basis of this information.

    c. Act according to this well-formed conscience.

    d. Accept responsibility for their actions.

2. Principle of Free and Informed Consent

To protect the basic need of every human person for health care and the person's primary responsibility for his or her own health, no physical or psychological therapy may be administered without the free and informed consent of the patient, or, if the patient is incompetent, of the person's legitimate guardian acting for the patient's benefit and, as far as possible, in accordance with the patient's known and reasonable wishes.

The principle of free and informed consent is unquestionably one of the most important in medical ethics because it is at the heart of the physician-patient relationship discussed in Chapter 4. It is a corollary of the principle of well-formed conscience. If I have an obligation to inform my own conscience, I must also enable those who request my professional advice to do the same. Responsible consent to therapy must be informed consent, that is, the patient must be told the nature of the proposed therapy, its probable benefits, its possible risks, and other possible treatment choices. Moreover, consent must be free, that is, the patient must be permitted to make decisions without undue pressure of time, emotional upset, confusion, persuasion, or threat.

The information must be given in terms understood by the patient and preferably with feedback from the patient to make sure that he or she has understood correctly. The professional should not feel excused from this principle merely because the patient seems uncooperative, ignorant, or unable to speak English well; he or she is obliged to do what is possible to communicate the information adequately. It is true, of course, that such communication is often difficult and in emergencies may not be perfectly achievable, but a serious effort must be made.

For so-called proxy consent the legitimate guardian should always act not for the guardian's interests but for the patient's benefit and should respect the patient's known or probable wishes, provided these are reasonable. If the professional has good reason to think that the guardian is not acting in this responsible way, an effort to protect the rights of the patient must be made, by legal action if necessary.

3. Principle of Moral Discernment

This principle, which distinguishes prudential personalism from other forms of theological ethics (see page 85), maintains that,

To make a conscientious ethical decision, one must do the following:

    a. Proceed on the basis of a fundamental commitment to God and the authentic dignity of human persons, including oneself.

b. Among possible actions that might seem to be means of fulfilling that commitment, exclude any which are in fact intrinsically contradictory to that commitment.

c. Also consider how one's own motives and other circumstances may contribute to or nullify the effectiveness of the other possible actions as means to fulfill one's fundamental commitment.

d. Among the possible means not excluded or nullified, select one most likely to fulfill that commitment, and act upon it.

For example, a surgeon faced with a problem of recommending a high-risk surgery to a patient will (1) guide his decision by his overriding sense of responsibility before God for the welfare of his patient; (2) consider possible ways of treating the patient's condition with or without surgery, and exclude those which are so risky, experimental, or ineffective as to be contradictory to the patient's nonnegotiable right to life or other such basic needs; (3) also consider whether his judgment may be prejudiced by financial considerations or ambition to make a name for himself, and whether in the circumstances of the patient's life and the available medical facilities, the possible value of the surgery may be nullified; (4) among the remaining possibilities choose and act on one that will most likely benefit the patient and reflect a real concern on the surgeon's part for the patient as a person.

The first of these points of commitment to God and the dignity of the human person is the underlying motivation of the Christian life, which should be part of all the helping professions. It connects this principle with the principle of love, to be explained later in this chapter. The second point is the difference between prudential personalism as a methodology and proportionalism, since the latter denies that there are any concrete moral norms that, apart from circumstances and intention, can absolutely exclude any type of action as intrinsically evil. The third point is the prudential aspect of prudential personalism, which takes into account not only the intrinsic nature of an action but also all its circumstances. Finally, point four shows why this principle belongs to teleological ethics: according to it, moral decisions depend on the judgment of the relation of the action as a *means* to the goal or commitment (point one).

4. Principle of Double Effect

To form a good conscience when an act is foreseen to have both ethically beneficial and physically harmful effects, the following conditions should be met:

a. The directly intended object of the act must not be intrinsically contradictory to one's fundamental commitment to God and neighbor (including oneself).

b. The intention of the agent must be to achieve the beneficial effects and as far as possible to avoid the harmful effects (that is, must only indirectly intend the harm).

c. The foreseen beneficial effects must be equal to or greater than the foreseen harmful effects.

d. The beneficial effects must follow from the action at least as immediately as do the harmful effects.

Developing a well-formed conscience with prudent moral discernment also demands care in the possible harmful side effects we foresee resulting from our good actions. Since it is not possible to avoid all such side effects and at the same time to fulfill our obligations to do the good from which they result, we need a principle to guide us in such dilemmas. For example, to save someone's life, a physician may perform an amputation. Although the crippling effect of the surgery is foreseen, it is not desired or chosen as such. The handicap is an undesirable side effect. Because the handicap is not what is chosen, it is not a moral effect, but only a physical effect, since morality always pertains to free choices. Thus the two "effects" referred to in the title of this principle are not both moral or ethical effects. Rather, the effect that is freely (directly) chosen is morally good and the other effect is physically harmful, but it is not freely chosen (it is indirectly chosen).

Proportionalists eliminate the first, third, and fourth of these conditions and accept only the second, because they do not admit that it is possible to state any concrete moral norms that are exceptionless; that is, they do not admit that any kind of concrete action can be judged to be intrinsically wrong (contradictory to a fundamental commitment to God and neighbor) unless at the same time we consider the circumstances in which it is performed. We have explained the inadequacy of such a methodology. It is impractical and arbitrary because there is no precise way to weigh the complex positive and negative values involved in human actions.

Proportionalists retort that, if this is so, how can the third of the above conditions be fulfilled? Our reply is that in a prudential personalist methodology the first condition is the essential one, and the other three merely suggest tests by which it can better be determined if the first condition is actually being fulfilled. Consequently, all that the third condition demands is not the precise, determinative weighing of values on which the entire methodology of proportionalism depends, but merely that an action, already determined to be intrinsically moral (first condition), is not vitiated by circumstances that result in obviously greater evils than the good intended. The second and fourth conditions are required for the same reason, to ensure that the agent directly intends only the intrinsically good effect.

An example of the application of this principle is an operation to remove the cancerous uterus of a pregnant woman, which will also kill her unborn child. The physician rightly decides that this is ethical because his direct intention is morally good (to save the woman's life from the cancer), thus fulfilling the first condition; and he knows that he is being honest in his decision because (1) he would save the child's life if he could (second condition), (2) the value of the mother's life is equivalent to that of the child's (the third condition), and (3) the removal of the cancer is what saves the woman's life, not the child's death (fourth condition).

5. Principle of Legitimate Cooperation

To achieve a well-formed conscience, one should always judge it unethical to cooperate formally with an immoral act (that is, directly to intend the evil act itself), but one may sometimes judge it to be an ethical duty to cooperate materially with an immoral act (that is, only indirectly intend its harmful consequences) when only in this way can a greater harm be prevented, provided (a) that the cooperation is not immediate and (b) that the degree of cooperation and the danger of scandal are taken into account.

To carry out our responsibilities we usually have to cooperate with others. We frequently foresee that this may involve us in conduct on their part which we believe to be objectively wrong, although we realize that those with whom we cooperate may not in their own consciences perceive it as evil. When possible we should inform them and try to dissuade them, but often we know this will have no effect and may even injure them or ourselves. Must we, therefore, refuse to cooperate with them?

We must refuse to cooperate if we would involve ourselves in *formal* cooperation, that is, agreeing with, advising, counseling, promoting, or condoning the objectively evil action of another, because formal cooperation demands that we directly intend the evil action itself, which is morally equivalent to doing it ourselves. If, however, the cooperation is merely *material*; that is, our cooperation is with the good that is being done and only indirectly with evil, which we would prevent if we could, then such cooperation is permissible and even obligatory if (1) the refusal to cooperate would result in a greater evil than if we cooperate and (2) if the cooperation is not immediate and is more remote the greater the evil involved. The main reason for these conditions is to verify that one truly avoids formal cooperation. The closer the cooperation and the greater the evil the more it requires a serious justifying cause. In judging the evil involved, even in material cooperation, an important additional consideration is the scandal that may be caused or the bad example given to others.

For example, a physician who thinks abortion is wrong, yet performs one because his patient demands it or even merely refers her to another physician cooperates formally. A nurse who disapproves yet takes an active part in the procedure, cooperates immediately, and her action is not justified. Yet a nurse who cares for the patient after the abortion cooperates only materially and remotely. Such cooperation might be justified if her refusal would imperil her ability to continue in her profession and scandal can be avoided. This would not justify, however, working in a facility devoted exclusively to abortions, since this would certainly give scandal.

6. Principle of Professional Communications

To fulfill their obligations to serve patients, health care professionals have the responsibility to do the following:

a. To strive to establish and preserve trust at both the emotional and rational levels.

b. To share such information as they possess which is legitimately needed by others in order to have an informed conscience.

c. To refrain from lying or giving misinformation.

d. To keep secret information which is not legitimately needed by others and that if revealed might harm the patient or others or destroy trust.

It is obvious that, if professionals are not truthful to patients, there cannot be free and informed consent. Hence good communication is needed between professional and patient, which is impossible without (1) trust, (2) contact among people who have the needed information, (3) clear formulation and expression of this information, and continuous feedback by which failures in communication can be corrected. Modern communication theory has shown that this work of communicating depends first on good emotional relationships among the communicators, since emotional conflict is a powerful barrier to communication and brings into play all sorts of uncontrollable, unconscious factors.

The duty to tell the patient the truth does not, of course, dispense one from the responsibility to do it in a sensitive, compassionate, and tactful manner and in the proper circumstances. Moreover, professional secrecy has some limits. Although a Catholic priest is absolutely bound by the secrecy of the confessional, the medical professional may in some rare situations reveal confidential matters, namely, when the patient is considering suicide, is involved in a serious crime or serious injustice to a third party, or is seriously incompetent.

Why Are These Christian Principles?

The foregoing six principles are not exclusively Christian, since anyone who is convinced that human beings have inalienable rights should agree with them. Nevertheless, Christian faith makes these principles clearer and more certain and uses them in a practical way as guides to prudent decisions. Christian faith convinces us that all human persons are created in God's image as intelligent, free, and morally responsible. Consequently, they must strive to base their free decisions on correct information, and must truthfully share this information with each other, at the same time respecting the consciences and privacy of others. In using this information they must discern what actions are always wrong because they contradict commitment to God and neighbor and the fulfillment of basic human needs, but they must also take into consideration the concrete situations in which they act and the possible side effects of their actions, even when these are essentially good.

In the Sermon on the Mount (Mt 5-7) Jesus taught us that if we are to keep his Father's commandments it is necessary not only to do good but to do it from the right motives. This is why it is essential that the direct intention of all our actions, no matter how complex or ambiguous the situation in which we have to act, should be ethical. St. Paul (Rm 3:8) rejects the notion that we can do evil so that good may come from it. If we are to achieve the happiness for ourselves and others that God wants us to have, it can only be by means that are themselves good, because evil means can yield good results only in the short run and even then they injure the integrity of the agent. In the long run they are always counterproductive.

6.4 Principles of Christian Love

We have just considered the norms that guide our thinking as we strive to make intelligent realistic moral decisions. These norms are rooted in one of our basic human needs, the need for truth. Another basic human need is the need for society. Our fundamental motivation is the drive to self-fulfillment, but human self-fulfillment is possible only through relationships with other human beings, and above all with the three divine persons, Father, Son, and Holy Spirit. The ethical norms that govern these relationships can rightly be called norms of love.

Love is not only a kind of feeling, but also the practical *will* that leads one person to be concerned about another and that person's true needs. Furthermore, love motivates people to help others fulfill these needs by sharing with another the values they themselves enjoy. In any Christian ethics the fundamental truth is that there is a Triune God and that "God is love" (Jn 4:8). God loves us not because he has first needed our love, but because his love for us has made us lovable.

> God's love was revealed in our midst in this way: he sent his only son to the world that we might have life through him. Love, then, consists in this: not that we have loved God, but that he has loved us and has sent his son as an offering for our sins. If we love one another, God dwells in us and his love is brought to perfection in us (1 Jn 4:9-10, 12).

Three particular norms help to define the content of Christian love: (1) every person must be valued as a unique, irreplaceable member of the human community (*principle of human dignity*); (2) every person must be encouraged to play a role in the common life and fully share its fruits (*principle of common good, subsidiarity, and functionalism*); and (3) all persons must be helped to realize their full potential (*principle of the totality of the human person*).

7. Principle of Human Dignity

All ethical decisions (including those involved in health care) must aim at human dignity, that is, the maximum, integrated satisfaction of the innate and cultural needs of every human person, including his or her biological, psychological, social, and spiritual needs as a member of the world community and national communities.

Although today the unique value of every being is affirmed by all the world religions and philosophies of life and the inalienable rights of the person are nominally guaranteed by the constitutions of most governments, yet these rights are contradicted by three prevailing trends: (1) persons are swallowed up in totalitarian, bureaucratic institutions; (2) persons who are not needed for the efficient operations of these institutions—women, the very young, the very old, the uneducated, the defective—are treated as nonpersons; (3) even successful persons find their happiness not in sharing their lives with others but in private, individualistic satisfactions.

This principle not only states one basic human need but also includes all the others. In short it sums up the true goal of human life: self-actualization in relation to God and neighbor. Jesus said, "Treat others the way you would have them treat you: this sums up the Law and the Prophets" (Mt 7:12). That is, respect your own human dignity and that of others.

8. Principle of the Common Good, Subsidiarity, and Functionalism

Human communities exist only to promote and share the common good among all their members "from each according to ability, to each according to need" in such a way that:

a. Decision making rests vertically first with the person, then with the lower social levels and horizontally with functional social units.

b. The higher social units intervene only to supply the lower units what they cannot achieve by themselves while at the same time working to make it easier in the future for lower units and individuals to satisfy these needs by their own efforts.

The principle of human dignity requires that various levels of responsibility be established within the community. In Chapter 3 we showed that the primary responsibility for health rests with the individual, and hence the work of health care professionals must be conceived as a cooperative service for individuals in their personal search for health (Chapter 4). At the same time no individual is self-sufficient in this search but can achieve health only with the help of health care professionals and the support of the community (Chapter 5). Consequently, it is important to observe subsidiarity (that is, to keep decision making as close as possible to the persons concerned in the vertical organization of society) and functionalism (to keep decision making widely spread in the horizontal organization of society). At the same time, those who have the highest authority must protect and promote the common good.

This principle is only a way of spelling out the implications of the principle of human dignity by showing the respective roles of the individual, subgroups in the community, and the total community so that by this division of labor the dignity of every member of the community will be fully recognized and actively promoted. It has its source in our basic need to preserve life.

The Christian specification of this principle is given by St. Paul in 1 Co 12-13. He shows that the Christian understanding of person, based on Jesus' concern for the "little ones" and the "least brethren" (Mk 9:33-37), must be the principle that governs the Church, conceived as the Body of Christ, ensouled by the Holy Spirit, and the model for the coming kingdom of God. The conception of social authority as service rather than domination is at the heart of the Gospel (Mk 10:41-45).

9. Principle of the Totality of the Human Person

To promote human dignity in community, every person must develop, use, care for, and preserve all of his or her natural physical and psychic functions in such a way that:

a. Lower functions are never sacrificed except for the better functioning of the whole person and even then with an effort to compensate for this sacrifice.

b. The basic capacities that define human personhood are never sacrificed unless this is necessary to preserve life.

This principle makes explicit another aspect of the principle of human dignity by requiring self-respect as well as respect for others. Unless a person respects his or her own integrity, which includes one's natural bodily and psychic integrity, and seeks to preserve and perfect one's own gifts, that person cannot expect the community's respect. This principle and the principle of the common good maintain that the community and the person are complex systems of mutual interdependence of parts of a whole. Person and community differ radically, however, because a person is a natural, primary unit whose parts depend completely on the whole and exist for its sake. On the contrary, the community is a system made up of primary units—persons—and so exist for their sake, not merely as isolated individuals, but as sharers in a common, profoundly interrelated life. To claim that the community ought to function like one person results in totalitarianism, which sacrifices the person to the collective state.

Human wholeness consists in the interdependence of higher and lower spiritual and bodily functions. Consequently, the lower functions cannot without qualification be sacrificed to the higher functions. This sacrifice might be to the advantage of the higher function but will not be to the good of the whole person, since that good is essentially complex, irreducible to the good of one part, even if that part is the highest.

To be a complete human being, therefore, is not merely to have the higher level of functions but to have all the basic human functions in harmonious order. This order requires the subordination of the lower functions to the higher functions but also forbids their total sacrifice. Nor can this dependence be simply supplied by some means external to the person. For example, the ability to produce babies in test tubes does not of itself justify the elimination of the reproductive power of humans. Nor does the possibility of intravenous feeding justify the elimination of the human alimentary system. Human perfection requires that people reproduce and eat in a human manner. Substitutions of external means of life may be justified temporarily out of necessity, but they do not improve on human nature.

Human body functions contribute to higher functions not merely by supplying what is needed for physiological brain functions; they also supply part of the human experience that is essential to human intelligence and freedom. Bodily feelings (movement, eating, sexuality, manipulation of the environment) develop one's self-awareness and relation to the community. Thus, if a child were conceived in a test tube and gestated in an artificial womb and then raised in a laboratory, it is doubtful that he or she would have essential human experiences. The following norms pertain to human integrity:

1. Primarily, human health is not merely a matter of organs but of capacities to function humanly.

2. Generally speaking, any particular human functional capacity can be diminished when necessary for the good of the whole person; that is, so that the person can better exercise all other human functions.

3. Secondary functions can always be sacrificed for more basic ones. For example, a finger can be removed to save the use of the hand because the capacity of action given by one finger is secondary in relation to the capacity given by the hand as a whole.

4. Primary or basic functional capacities, however, cannot be destroyed to promote even more important capacities except when it is the only way to preserve the life of the whole person. For example, the capacity for emotional feeling must not be sacrificed to the power of scientific thinking. The capacity to think humanly cannot be sacrificed in order to think more technically.

Why then is it sometimes permissible to sacrifice one of these basic human capacities to preserve life? Because in this case it is not a question of sacrificing one basic capacity for another, nor for the better functioning of all other human capacities, but of sacrificing one function so that the whole person should continue to function at all. Only in such extreme necessity does basic integrity yield to the good of the totality.

The great importance of this principle for medical ethics is that it establishes a norm for setting priorities when one human value must be subordinated to another. In Chapter 1 we discussed this hierarchy of values in terms of the biological, psychological, social, and spiritual dimensions of human personality. The spiritual and social values have higher priority than the psychological and biological values, but such priority must not be understood dualistically as if the lower can simply be sacrificed to the higher values.

The specific character of this principle arises from the Incarnation in which the Word of God became flesh as Jesus of Nazareth, lived a bodily life, died, and was resurrected in the body transformed in glory. Consequently, Christian anthropology, while admitting a certain polarity in the person because of a commonality with the animal and earthly world and a spiritual intelligence, freedom, and openness to God, yet opposes any kind of dualism that would deny the dignity of Christ's body, human resurrection, and that persons are the "temples of the Holy Spirit" (1 Co 3:16). This principle is well expressed by the writer of Ephesians (5:21-33) when he makes the analogy between Christ's love for the human race, a man's love for his wife, and one's love for one's own body.

6.5 Principles of Christian Hope

After discussing the norms of faith and love, let us now consider what theologians call the eschatological aspect of ethics (looking to the final coming of Jesus Christ in the fully realized kingdom of God). The person and the community are not structures of static relations but are dynamic—loving, growing, developing, and evolving. This is why we have opted for a teleological, goal-directed, means-ends ethics. Furthermore, human goals are not always clearly envisioned in advance. The kingdom of God, on which Jesus centered his preaching, is a goal so mysterious that he could express it only in terms of parables.

Recently, Christian theologians have developed theologies of hope and theologies of liberation to bring out the many ways in which the Gospel is not merely a declaration that heaven is better than earth, but a call to transform the earth as we journey heavenward. In this way they are finding areas of agreement with humanism and Marxism which teach that to be human is to work for the future. In health care this sense of hope is the source of all healing, so that to be a health care professional is constantly to affirm the possibility of turning suffering into a victory over disease and death.

Three ethical norms relate in a particular way to Christian hope. Our hope enables us not only to endure the sufferings of life courageously, but to grow as persons through this experience (*principle of growth through suffering*). Hope also enables Christians to entrust themselves to another in the lifelong commitment of marriage and to look forward to sharing this gift of life and love with a family and the future (*principle of personalized sexuality*). Moreover, not only do we have hopes for our families but for the whole of human society and the good earth which is its home (*principle of creative stewardship*).

10. Principle of Growth Through Suffering

As bodily pleasure should be sought only as the fruit of the satisfaction of some basic need of the total human person, so suffering and even bodily death when endured with courage can and should be used to promote personal growth in both private and communal living.

In any teleological ethics the ultimate criterion of morality is true happiness. An action is morally good because it leads to happiness for persons. People sometimes fail to take into account, however, that in the actual conditions of human existence not all that appears to be happiness is really so. The only authentic happiness is one which satisfies the whole person in his or her deepest and most ultimate needs and does so permanently. Thus it is quite possible for persons to think they are happy because they have achieved goals that are partial, superficial, and unstable. On television we witness the extravagant joy of winners in giveaway contests, knowing that in fact such happiness will quickly fade and prove to have been utterly fake.

It is also possible for persons to have really achieved goals that are encompassing, profound, and lasting and yet to be in a state of great suffering because circumstances do not yet permit the full experience of satisfaction. A great writer who has completed a masterpiece or a scientist who has achieved the discovery of a lifetime or a statesman who has successfully carried through a great reform may feel for a time exhausted, torn by inner conflict, and depressed. Yet such persons are to be envied because ultimately they will realize they have reached the goal of their whole lives.

Thus, from an ethical point of view, it is essential to understand that true human happiness cannot be measured merely by pleasure, comfort, or freedom from anxiety, tension, and guilt. Normally pleasure, comfort, and peace are the consequences and the signs of the achievement of authentic human goals and the fulfillment of the true human needs, and hence they are good and desirable. But they are secondary signs and not the proof or measure of real human achievement.

Relevant to ethical questions, therefore, people need to look at the deeper and more total need and not to measure good and bad merely in terms of pleasure and pain. Short-range goals, that is, immediate satisfactions, have to yield ethically to long-range goals. Yet we cannot live without some short-range, moderate pleasures, and strains and pains cannot be endured too long. A work ethic by which life is simply striving for a far-off, never-attained goal is a bad ethic. Authentic fulfillment, however, is not to be found by the maximization of sensual pleasure (as hedonism insists), but rather by intensifying deeper spiritual pleasures along with moderate bodily pleasures and by realizing that one is able to develop as a person through suffering.

The Christian faith, then, looks upon suffering and death in two different ways. On the one hand, death is evil because it is the result of sin. On the other hand, it is a liberating and grace-filled experience, if the proper motivation is present. These two views are not contradictory; rather they are complementary. Suffering and death, joined to the suffering and death of Jesus, the Lord of life, represent not dissolution but growth, not punishment but fulfillment, not sadness but joy. God allows suffering and death to enable us to live with

Christ now and forever. This principle, supremely exemplified in the Cross of Christ, is rooted in the basic human need to preserve life, since people suffer only in order to achieve a renewed, purified, and enriched life. In Chapter 11 this principle of growth through suffering and its applications to health care are discussed in more detail.

11. Principle of Personalized Sexuality

The gift of sexuality must be used in keeping with its intrinsic, indivisible, specifically human teleology. It must be a loving, bodily, pleasurable expression of the complementary, permanent self-giving of a man and a woman to each other which is open to fruition in the perpetuation and expansion of this personal communion through the family they responsibly beget and educate.

This principle concerns personalized sexuality because it is based on an understanding of sexuality as one of the basic aspects of a person that must be developed (personalized) in ways consistent with an enhancing of human dignity.[2] Because human sexual life is not merely a matter of animal instinct but requires free decisions, it sometimes raises serious ethical dilemmas. These problems might well be considered under norms of love, but more properly they belong to the norms of hope because sexual love in a very special way looks toward the future. The survival of the human community, as well as the maturation and fulfillment of the individual, depends in a notable way on the right use of the gift of sex.

Sexuality is a complex of many values that are generally recognized in every ethical theory, but whose interrelation and priority are the subject of much disagreement. These generally recognized values can be summarized in four chief categories:

1. Sex is a search for sensual pleasure and satisfaction, releasing physical and psychic tensions.

2. More profoundly and personally, sex is a search for the completion of the human person through an intimate personal union of love expressed by bodily union. Ordinarily, it is also conceived as the complementation of the male and female by one another so that each achieves a more complete humanity.

3. More broadly, sex is a social necessity for the procreation of children and their education in the family so as to expand the human community and guarantee its future beyond the death of individual members.

4. Ultimately, sex is a symbolic (sacramental) mystery, somehow revealing the cosmic order.

These values are commonly recognized in all the great religions and philosophies of life and are protected and developed in every viable human culture.

In our modern culture, dominated by secular humanism, these values are generally thought to be combined in sexuality by sheer accident through the purposeless process of biological evolution. Consequently, many today argue that we are free to combine or separate these different values according to our own purposes and preferences. Thus for secular humanists it seems entirely reasonable sometimes to use sex purely for the sake of pleasure apart from any relation to love or family; sometimes to use it to reproduce (making babies in a test-tube) without any reference to pleasure or love; sometimes as an expression of unselfish love, but without any relation to marriage or family.

For secular humanists, moreover, if sex is a symbolic mystery, it is because love and sexual ecstasy are often considered the highest happiness in life, without which no one can be complete as a person. Consequently, for many secular humanists sexual morality can be reduced to two fundamental norms: (1) laws or social attitudes that hinder human freedom to achieve these sexual values in ways the individual desires are unjust and oppressive, and (2) sexual behavior, at least among consenting adults, is entirely a private matter to be determined by personal choice, free from any moral guilt.

The Christian attitude to sex agrees with that of secular humanism in recognizing these same four values of sexuality but differs in its conviction that sexuality is a gift of the Creator, who in his wisdom and love for humanity created in his image has so intertwined these values that we cannot separate them without injury to that same image. The Catholic Church has often been accused of a negative attitude toward sexuality. It is true that in the course of her long history, the expression of her teaching on sexuality has sometimes been colored by the secular culture in which she has lived. Consequently, the pagan philosophy of Plato, who taught that sex is a result of the fall of the human soul into the tomb of the body, and of the Stoics, who rejected physical pleasure and erotic love as unworthy of a philosopher and saw no value in sex except procreation, as well as current secular humanism, have sometimes distorted the ways Christians have thought and spoken about sex.

Nevertheless, genuine Christian teaching on sexuality is clear enough in the Scriptures and was given a rich and accurate expression by Vatican II and Paul VI's encyclicals, *Humanae Vitae*, and John Paul II's *Familaris Consortio* based on the Council.[3] Genesis 1-3 teaches that God created persons as male and female and blessed their sexuality as a great and good gift. Jesus confirmed this teaching, and perfected it by affirming that men must be as faithful in marriage as women (Mk 10:2-21; 1 Co 7:10). Nevertheless, Jesus also taught that although sexuality is a great gift, its use in marriage is only a relative value, which can be freely sacrificed for the sake of higher values. Thus, for the Christian, the celibate or single life with its freedom from domestic cares to be of service to others, can be even more personally maturing and fulfilling than married life. St. Paul (1 Co 7:25-35) also emphasizes the value of the single life, but teaches that marriage is a sacrament in that the love of husband and wife is a symbol that shows us the love of Christ for his people (Ep 5:22-23).

From this Biblical teaching it is clear why Vatican II and the papal encyclicals teach that sexuality was given to us to help us love one another whether we freely choose to marry or to live the single life of service to society. Any use of sex outside marriage is ethically wrong, because (1) it is a selfish pursuit of pleasure apart from love, as in masturbation, prostitution, or casual or promiscuous relations; or (2) it expresses love, but not a committed love involving true self-giving, as in adultery or premarital sex; and (3) it is committed, but practiced in a way contradictory to its natural fulfillment in the family, as in contraception or the relations of committed homosexuals. The reason such actions are ethically wrong is not some repressive rule of the Church, but because they are contradictory to the intrinsic value and meaning of sexuality as designed by the Creator and blessed by him. Human culture and customs have undergone many revolutions, but such changes cannot alter the basic structure of human nature without destroying humanity itself. The medical-ethical problems that the application of this principle raises are discussed in detail in Chapter 8.

12. Principle of Stewardship and Creativity

The gifts of multidimensional human nature and its natural environment should be used with profound respect for their intrinsic teleology, and especially the gift of human creativity should be used to cultivate nature and environment with a care set by the limits of actual knowledge and the risk of destroying these gifts.

The hope that leads human beings to endure the inevitable pain of human existence and to overcome human mortality by the perpetuation of the human community also leads us to struggle with the environment. The author of Genesis 3 profoundly symbolizes the evil of sin by the expulsion from the Garden, the burden of sexism for Eve, and the burden of struggle with the environment for Adam. These are the fundamental realities of the human situation, yet Scripture says they are not what God wanted for humanity. God has given persons the power of intelligence, restored by grace in Christ, the new Adam, by which they can deal with these problems. Yet, although they may deal with these evils well or badly, they cannot escape the struggle and still remain human.

This principle requires us to appreciate the two great gifts that a wise and loving God has given us: the earth, with all its natural resources, and our own human nature ("embodied intelligent freedom"), with its biological, psychological, ethical, and spiritual capacities. Recently, we have come to recognize that our earthly environment is a marvelously balanced ecological system without which human life could never have evolved. Although we certainly have a need and a right to cultivate and perfect our earthly home, to till and irrigate its soil, to build cities, and to use its raw materials for the wonderful devices of modern technology, we should not do this ruthlessly but must take the utmost care to conserve our ecological system unpolluted and unravished, and to cycle its raw materials and its energy supplies. We have already discovered how much damage the thoughtless exploitation of natural resources can do to our own lives.

Similarly our own human nature, our bodies, and our minds are wonderfully constructed. We have the need and right to improve our bodies and to develop medical technologies that prevent and remedy the defects to which they are liable. But we must do so with the greatest respect for what we already are as human beings. Our bodily and mental functions have natural teleologies, which cannot be eliminated or misdirected without injury to our humanness.

Consequently, a technology based on the false principle that "If it can be done, it should be done" is a misuse of our creative intelligence. Rather we should ask ourselves, "Should it be done?", and only if the answer is "yes" develop and use the technology to do it. Thus the God-given gifts of our environment and our humanity are ours in stewardship, but because the greatest of our natural gifts are our intelligence and freedom, the stewardship should be creative. Our creativity should be used as a co-creativity with the Creator, not a reckless wasting of his gifts.

This principle is rooted in the basic human need for truth, since it is God-given human intelligence, the capacity for truth, which makes persons co-creators with God. Its specifically Christian character derives from the fact that the risen Christ is the pledge that the Kingdom of God will eventually be built, and the coming of his Holy Spirit gives persons the power to share in this building of the Kingdom, the house built not on the sand of pride but on the rock of faith (Mt 7:24-29). The Gospel does not encourage Christians simply to wait until the Lord returns, indifferent to the world's fate as Marxists and humanists charge. Rather, Christians are called to play a historical role in the liberation of the human race from poverty, disease, and oppression with the assistance of the power of God, with a special "option for the poor."

6.6. Coordination of the Principles

Why have we chosen to list 12 principles rather than a few broad ones? The main reason is that in the actual process of bioethical decision making, each of these 12 plays an important role. In fact, these could be still further multiplied by additional corollaries. Our list, however, can be coordinated and simplified by showing how it flows from the four basic needs of human persons enumerated by Aquinas (see page 9):

1. The need to preserve life: the principles of totality and growth through suffering.

2. The need to procreate: the principle of personalized sexuality and moral discrimination.

3. The need to know the truth: the principles of well-formed conscience along with the rules for resolving conflict cases (principles of double effect and legitimate cooperation), and finally the principles of informed consent and professional communication, which provide the conditions for a prudent conscience.

4. The need to live in society: the principles of human dignity and of the common good and subsidiarity along with the principle of stewardship, which relate human society to the environment and to the use of all gifts for the common good.

6.7 Summary

To sum up this discussion of the principles that govern bioethical decisions from a Christian point of view:

1. Faith requires persons to act with an informed conscience, which requires the intellectual effort of moral discrimination between right and wrong, even in complex cases wherein moral actions involve evil side effects or material cooperation. It also requires a relation of trust between persons (especially between professional and client) in which there is an honest exchange of the information necessary for an informed conscience.

2. Hope requires persons to accept growth through suffering, to continue the human community through the institution of the family, and to fulfill in a creative manner their stewardship of their own nature and the world God has given them.

3. Love requires a profound respect for human dignity, no matter what the condition of the person. It also requires a proper love of one's self and a responsibility for one's own health. Finally, it requires persons to work for and share in the common good.

Footnotes

1. John Connery, "The Theology of Proportionate Reason," *Theological Studies* 44 n.3, (Sept. 1983) p. 489-498; G. Grisez, *The Way of the Lord Jesus*, (Chicago: Franciscan Press, 1984), Chapters 4, 8, 35, 36.

2. Karol Wojtylo (Pope John Paul II), "Human Sexuality," in *Towards a Theology of Praxis*, Alfred Bloch and G.T. Czuckza, editors, (New York: Crossroads, 1982), pp. 57-104.

3. Pope John Paul II, "The Christian Family in the Modern World," (Nov. 22, 1981), in Austin Flannery, *Post Conciliar Documents* (North Port, NY: Costello Publishing, 1982), p. 815-898.

Study Questions

1. How might (a) an emotivist, (b) a religious deontologist, (c) a legal posivist, (d) a Kantian formalist, (e) a situationist, (f) a utilitarian or consequentialist, (g) a proportionalist, and (h) a prudential personalist justify (with or without exception) the proposition: "It is wrong for a physician to lie to a patient"?

2. What is the difference between an ethical *principle* and an ethical *decision?* How are they related?

3. If ethics is based on sound reasoning based on historical personal and social behavior that promotes or harms human well-being and happiness, what do the teachings of Jesus add to this?

4. Give health care examples of problems that exemplify each of the 12 principles mentioned in this chapter.

5. How does one internalize an ethical principle? Is internalization of a principle the same as obeying a command?

Cases

1. Mary T is a moderately retarded girl aged 16. She is able to work in a laundry which is a great assistance to her mother who works in an office and cannot stay at home with her. Her father is dead. Her mother, Mrs. T, discovers that some of the men who work in the laundry are trying to date Mary, probably with sexual intentions. She consults Dr. P, a conscientious Catholic, about having Mary sterilized. The mother, also a Catholic, knows that sterilization is not approved by the Church, but she argues that in this case it is justified as the lesser evil, since Mary may get pregnant which would be a heavy burden, while it is not so important if she becomes sterile, since she is too retarded to marry. What should Dr. P do? What should he say to Mrs. T? To Mary T?

2. Dr. Q is called in to operate on Mr. R who has been wounded in a gang war. He knows that Mr. R is a notorious criminal who, if he lives, may very well be tried and sentenced to death for the torture and murder of the daughter of one of the rival gang leaders. It occurs to him that he could easily let this man die on the operating table without the attending anesthetist or nurses realizing what he is doing. It would save the government a lot of expense. What ethical principles should he consider in making his decision?

3. Nurse M is told in confidence by Dr. X of a difficult decision he is making. Mrs. S has carcinoma of the womb. He has told her of this and she is deeply depressed. He has not told her that she is also pregnant. She does not suspect the fact since she attributes the cessation of her menstrual periods and her swelling to the tumor. He has decided to go ahead and operate to remove the womb (thus also killing the child) without telling her of the pregnancy lest it depress her further. Can Nurse M keep this information from Mrs. S and assist the physician in the operating room? How do the six principles of Christian faith apply to Nurse M's decision?

4. Hemophilia is a dangerous genetic disease transmitted through the mother. It is life-threatening, often very painful, and requires expensive transfusion therapy. Dr. G proposes to gradually eliminate it from the population by passing a law requiring all hemophiliac women to have their Fallopian tubes ligated. He argues that this is for the common good and that the government has the responsibility to correct problems that are not corrected at a lower level. Since the parents of girls carrying this defective gene do not have their daughters sterilized, the government must order it done. Furthermore, it is for the good of the girls themselves to sacrifice their fertility to avoid the burden of caring for a hemophiliac son. Discuss these arguments in light of the three principles of Christian love.

5. Sigmund Freud suffered from cancer for some years yet refused to take painkillers because they dulled his thinking and interfered with his research on the healing of mental illnesses which he believed were rooted in sexual repression. Yet he also believed that sexual repression is necessary for the progress of civilization which, therefore, necessarily causes mental illness and great personal suffering. In view of the three principles of Christian hope, what would you say to Sigmund Freud about the paradoxes which so troubled him?

Chapter 7

Human Research and Triage

In this and the remaining chapters we apply the 12 principles of ethical decisions explained in Chapter 6 to the chief ethical issues debated today in health care. First we consider issues involved in medical research and in the allocation of scarce medical resources (triage) because these are general issues affecting all aspects of health care. Then we cover more specific topics. The principles applied in this chapter are chiefly informed consent, decisions of conscience, totality of the person, and double effect.

7.1 Human Research

> When science takes man as its subject, tensions arise between two values basic to Western society: freedom of scientific inquiry and protection of individual inviolability.[1]

These words introduce another major study by Jay Katz and others concerning the legal and ethical issues of human research. That research on human beings is often useful and often necessary for the common good is undeniable. Many beneficial vaccines and other therapies, such as open heart surgery and successful treatment of certain birth defects, have required human research, but it has often been abused. The world should never forget the horrors of the experiments carried out on innocent human beings in the name of scientific progress in the Nazi concentration camps. Aside from such atrocities, other egregious violations of human rights have occurred in the United States, such as the withholding of newly discovered penicillin from patients in the Tuskeegee syphilis study, the Willowbrook experiments in which retarded children were used as subjects, and the injection of live cancer cells into unknowing subjects in the Chronic Disease Hospital case.[2] Psychological research has also given rise to serious debate about behavior control. Such abuses often are not the product of demented or perverted minds but result from lack of care and ethical sensitivity on the part of well-motivated researchers who overlook the rights of human beings in an effort to ensure scientific progress.

Today, in an effort to obviate excesses and facilitate progress, the federal government requires that every institution that carries on research projects with public funds establish an institutional review board (IRB).[3] An IRB monitors the research protocols mainly by analyzing the risk-benefit ratio for the patient, by evaluating the informed consent process, and by examining the scientific procedures insofar as they might affect the safety of the human subject. Because there is risk to the human subject involved does not mean a research protocol would be rejected by the IRB, but does require that the risk be proportionate to patient benefit, that free and informed consent on the part of the subject be assured, and that the protocol of the scientific investigation be as safe as possible. If not, the research project must be rejected by the IRB. In the U.S., most research is carried on by the National Institutes of Health and in medical schools. Funds for this research are provided by the federal government and the pharmaceutical corporations.

In research using human subjects several categories of persons may be involved: (1) normal healthy adults, including the investigator, and elderly persons; (2) sick adults, including the acutely and terminally ill; (3) people living in highly controlled situations, such as, prisoners, soldiers, and students; (4) children, both healthy and ill; (5) mentally incompetent persons, whether adults or children; and (6) unborn fetuses or still-living aborted fetuses. Each of these categories presents special problems as indicated by the studies of two commissions appointed by the federal government to set ethical norms for human research:[4]

Human research is either therapeutic or nontherapeutic. Therapeutic research allows one to accept greater risk of harm than nontherapeutic research. Therapeutic research studies the effects of using diagnostic, prophylactic, or therapeutic methods that depart from standard medical practice but hold out a reasonable expectation of success for improving the condition of the subject. Nontherapeutic research, on the other hand, is not designed to improve the health of the research subjects; rather it seeks to gain knowledge or develop techniques that may benefit people other than the subject.

The proper manner of conducting these kinds of research on the various categories of human subjects has become one of the most discussed bioethical questions of recent years. Through seminars and studies on the subject, some ethical principles have been developed to serve as a guide for researchers and for those who support research.[5] As a result of such studies by legal, medical, and ethical groups throughout the world, especially in the generation after World War II, some principles for human research have become widely accepted, even though there may be disagreement concerning their applications in particular cases. These norms produced by medical and legal experts, such as the Nuremberg and Helsinki statements on research with human subjects, are largely in harmony with Christian teaching on human dignity.[6]

7.2 Norms of Research on Human Subjects

We list nine norms for ethical research that involves human subjects. Some of these norms are pertinent to psychological research; some to medical research. Some of the norms are self-evident, but some need explanation for their ethical implications to be clear.

Norm 1. The knowledge sought through research must be important and obtainable by no other means, and the research must be carried out by qualified people.

Norm 2. Appropriate experimentation on animals and cadavers must precede human experimentation.

Norm 3. The risk of suffering or injury must be proportionate to the good to be gained.

Because the principle of double effect[7] is used to justify the possible ill-effects of human experimentation, the proportion between risk and potential benefit is an essential criterion, the benefit being the good effect and the risk being the foreseen but undesired bad effect. Of course, predicting the degree of risk with certitude is seldom possible. Moreover, sometimes, as in the case of the poliomyelitis inoculation in 1954, when the use of some poorly prepared live vaccine resulted in the death of children, or in the swine flu inoculation disaster in the late 1970s, the risks may be greater than predicted. Hence, absolute certainty concerning the nature and degree of the risk cannot be required. To demand such certitude would paralyze all scientific research and would very often be detrimental to the patient. Care must be taken, however, to predict as accurately as possible the nature and magnitude of risk from any particular human experiment, and the bias of enthusiastic researchers in favor of the promise of some new procedure must be subject to review by an IRB. When discussing risk, it is important to distinguish between the frequency and the gravity of a risk. Thus a researcher may state that a risk is light if it happens in only 3 or 4 percent of cases. But if the risk in question is death or serious impairment, then it is a very grave risk for which the probable benefit must be of at least equal value.

When determining the degree of risk that a person might undergo, one must always bear in mind this difference between therapeutic and non-therapeutic research. If the research project is therapeutic, then persons may undergo greater risk because one is seeking to avoid death. The principle of totality is thus involved in therapeutic research.

The same principle of totality cannot be invoked in the case of non-therapeutic research because one person is not related to another person or to a group of persons (the society) as part of the whole. Although a relationship of extrinsic finality exists among different people, a relationship of intrinsic finality or form does not. One person does not exist for the other, nor is one person directed to another person as a means to an end. Each individual person is an end or being in himself or herself and cannot be sacrificed for another. This is the basic reason the public authority has no right to sacrifice individuals for the interest of the state or for scientific progress. Experiments carried out for the good of the state or for scientific progress may provide new knowledge or medical techniques and thus seem beneficial, but if they do so at the expense of human rights and human dignity, they are immoral. In research directed to the common good and not to the individual good of the research subject, the matter of free and informed consent becomes paramount. One may risk one's life for others but the level of risk must be assessed and the action must be freely performed in order for it to be ethical.

Double-Blind Protocols

A special ethical issue arises in double-blind research. The objectivity of scientific research depends largely on the use of controlled experimentation in which a group of subjects is divided into two subgroups, one of which receives the experimental therapy while the other, the control group, receives the standard therapy or a placebo. Sometimes three groups are used, one group receiving the experimental therapy, one receiving a placebo, and one receiving standard therapy or no treatment at all. This sometimes is called a randomized clinical trial. To ensure even greater objectivity double-blind control may be used: not only are subjects not informed as to which kind of treatment they are receiving, but even those researchers who evaluate the effects of the treatments do not know which subjects have received which therapy. Only the double-blind technique can eliminate the placebo effect, that is, the improvement frequently experienced by patients who expect it and the effect of bias on the part of scientists. This raises ethical questions however, since it seems (1) that those patients who do not receive the new therapy are at a therapeutic disadvantage and (2) that none of the patients in the double-blind experiment could have given informed consent to a specific treatment.

Hence, in double-blind experiments the subjects should be informed that, if they consent to the experiment, some will receive the new treatment and others will not, but that none of the subjects will know. The potential subjects will then be free to consent to these experimental conditions or to refuse to participate. If the clinical trial involves a placebo for the control group and the project aims at finding an agent that will mitigate or cure a lethal or disabling disease, then a special ethical issue arises, because the control group may not be receiving adequate therapy for their illness or disease. This is especially true if there is some justification for thinking that the new therapy might be much more effective than older ones. Thus the same protocol may be therapeutic for some and nontherapeutic for others. IRBs and researchers then must be doubly cautious when a double-blind placebo protocol is being designed or reviewed. If the new therapy proves to be effective, then the protocol must be modified and the new therapy made available to all. Of course, a rush to judgment concerning the efficacy of a new therapy must be avoided.

Norm 4. Subjects should be selected so that risks and benefits will not fall unequally on one group in society.

Justice demands that the burdens associated with human progress be shared equitably. In recent years the poor of the world, especially in the United States, have borne an unequal burden insofar as medical research is concerned. Research protocols must be designed to offset this imbalance and to ensure that when the poor take part in an experiment their human rights are respected and they are given the freedom their human dignity demands.

Norm 5. To protect personal integrity, free and informed (voluntary) consent must be obtained.

If it is impossible to obtain consent because the human subject is unable to give it, then proxy consent is required as a substitute.

Requiring informed consent is perhaps the most important and the most debated of the principles involved in human experimentation. All agree that the requirements for informed consent may be summed up in the words knowledge, understanding, and freedom. Thus, the subject must not only know the process or procedure in question but he or she should be able to comprehend it because it is explained in understandable language. Freedom does not imply that one is free from the natural coercion of the need for therapy that might accompany an illness, but it does mean that there is no deception or external coercion involved. However, how consent should be obtained and how knowledge must be communicated to subjects is debated extensively. Moreover, the debate increases as impaired or imprisoned human subjects or children are considered for research protocols.

The most puzzling problems in research occur when one person gives consent for another for whom he or she is morally responsible. Such consent is commonly called proxy consent. This is an unfortunate term, since, properly speaking, a proxy is an agent acting on behalf of another *with* the other's consent, which is precisely the element lacking in these cases. It would be better to call it vicarious consent, since a vicar fulfills a duty for another irrespective of whether the other has authorized it. As such, proxy consent simply means that one person who represents the interests of another by some legitimate title gives consent for the experiment in place of the subject because that subject is incompetent. Decisions of proxy consent must be made in view of the good of the individual, not for society's good or a class good or the good of another person. Otherwise, the person is manipulated and treated as a thing. If the research is therapeutic, there is reason for the proxy to allow risk in proportion to the good that might accrue to the individual in question, since that would be acting in the person's best interest. If nontherapeutic experimentation is involved, however, then the decision is more difficult.

Proxy Consent for Nontherapeutic Therapy

As stated, nontherapeutic research results in knowledge that will be beneficial to others but does not directly benefit the subject of the research. Children, the retarded, the dying, fetuses, and newborns are considered by some to be fitting subjects for nontherapeutic research. They argue that this is ethical because it gives subjects an opportunity to contribute to the common good, something they should desire. Others maintain, however, that a guardian has no right to expose a ward to any risk. The justification for this position is that a proxy should make a decision in accord with the subject's best interests. But since it is not clearly evident how nontherapeutic experimentation is in the subject's interests, and, since the subject does not have the capacity to make a free choice about a free matter, the proxy (guardian) has no right to presume or say anything on the ward's behalf.[8]

Others would allow exposing children and others who cannot consent for themselves to "minimal risk." They maintain that there are some things a child as a human being should do for others, for example, take part in experiments where there is hope of general benefit and only minimal risk. The United States Commission for the Protection of Human Subjects, when determining the norms for fetal experimentation and for children, followed the minimal risk theory when considering nonbeneficial research. Indeed, the Commission would even allow more serious risk of harm if a national committee recommended it.[9]

We follow the more protective opinion, maintaining that proxy consent is not licit in nontherapeutic experimentation, even when the risk is minimal. Two considerations convince us of this. First, because of the principle of human dignity, guardians have responsibility for wards who cannot care for themselves. This principle affirms that no person can achieve fulfillment without sharing in the common good and contributing to it. Hence, when a guardian or proxy consents to subjecting a ward to research, the proxy has the right to do so not on the basis of the presumed consent of the ward, which is merely hypothetical, but on the basis of the ward's actual need for care. Thus theories of presumed consent based on what the ward should do if the ward could consent are weak.

Second, it may be granted that if a guardian in a given case is sure that the ward will suffer only minimal risk and therefore gives proxy consent, the guardian does not fail in his or her responsibility to care for the ward, since "little counts for nothing," as the traditional saying of moralists goes. Such cases, however, cannot be erected into a guideline for general action, since such a rule would open the way for an extensive interpretation under which objectively serious risks come to be subjectively regarded as minimal, as has happened with the proliferation of some unnecessary surgery. Thus, a guardian should be an advocate, jealous of the ward's rights, not ready to yield these rights for the sake of others who cannot act for themselves or for the hypothetical rights of future generations of other children.

Norm 6. At any time during the course of research, the subject (or the guardian who has given proxy consent) must be free to terminate the subject's participation in the experiment.

The reason for this principle is that the consenting subject or proxy may not have been able correctly to anticipate the subjective factors involved, the amount of suffering, anxiety, or depression until they begin to be actually experienced; or the subject or proxy may even discover that the information given was inadequate or deceptive or imperfectly communicated, or the subject or proxy may have second thoughts about his or her own understanding or freedom when the consent was given.

Psychological Research

Special problems are involved in psychological experiments. To discuss these problems more fully, we defer the topic to Chapter 9, after the nature of psychotherapy and its distinctions from medical therapy are more thoroughly explained. At this point, however, we can state that in such experimentation all the precautions necessary in medical experiments must be preserved, especially informed consent, careful calculation of risks and benefits, and precautions against the bias of researchers in favor of their own freedom. We must also add the following special rules.

Norm 7. In psychological experimentations, which shade imperceptibly into social research, the researcher should work with rather than on the human subject.

That is, the researcher must gain the subject's cooperation in the experiment so that the subject will participate with the purpose of gaining greater insight into himself or herself as a person in order to become freer and more realistic in coping with life's problems and also with the purpose of sharing this knowledge and freedom with others.

This principle is based on the fact that psychological experiments with a human subject are also psychological *experiences* for the subject, which can be healthy and psychologically therapeutic or traumatizing reinforcements of maladaptive behavior patterns. In very few cases can such experiences be neutral. Even the experience of filling out a questionnaire can be educational or terrifying. Any experience in which the patient is treated as a passive object rather than as a person cannot be beneficial.

Norm 8. The researcher must avoid breaking down human trust by lying or manipulation, although subjects can give free and informed consent to experiments in which they must learn to interpret ambiguous communications or meet puzzling situations.

In many psychological experiments the researcher does not seem to have any qualms about lying to subjects. Not only is lying intrinsically wrong and contrary to professional ethics, it is also psychologically harmful to the subject because it breaks down the social trust on which human relations are built. Common sense proof of this is supplied by the fact that those who have been subjected to such manipulation often react indignantly when they discover the deception and feel they have been treated unfairly.

This is especially true when dealing with mentally disturbed patients, since elements of distrust, withdrawal, and paranoia present in most forms of emotional disturbance can only be reinforced by deception on the part of professionals who claim to be especially trustworthy and authoritative.

This rule against lying, however, does not prohibit experiments in which previous warning is given that the experiment may involve games in which ambiguous clues are given and embarrassment and defeat possibly experienced. These are risks of the experiment to which the subject must have a chance to give free and informed consent or refusal. Deception in such a case is not a lie, since traditional moral theology has always insisted that it is permissible to use ambiguous clues or language in situations where others are forewarned either explicitly or by the very nature of the situation.

Such games do not usually break down trust if the researcher sticks to the rules. Moreover, they may be highly educational for the participant, since through them the subject gains insight as to how important it is to base one's interpretation of reality on solid evidence rather than on ambiguous evidence or subjective feelings.

Norm 9. Researchers must not take serious risks of reducing the subjects' ability to perceive reality as it is or to make free choices except as a temporary experience through which the subjects can learn to cope with distortions of truth and attacks on their freedom.

This rule states more exactly the special risks involved in psychological experimentation. It excludes permission for any more than temporary damage to patients' ability to remain or become free in managing their own lives. Thus, an experiment would be forbidden if it might cause organic brain damage or induce drug addiction. Similarly, experiments must be avoided that might make the subject unduly liable to hypnotic control or to compulsive patterns of behavior (as might take place in some forms of behavior modification) or that create recurrent hallucinations. A special case of psychological research that may involve risks to freedom is research in dealing with human sexuality. This issue is discussed in Chapter 8 in connection with therapy of inadequate or perverted sexual behavior.

7.3 Triage and Unlimited Resources

What are health care professionals to do when they are unable to give full health care to all those who have a right to it? The issue here is not what to do in long-range planning, because that issue can be settled only by finding ways to provide more health care personnel and equipment, but what to do in the short range when limited resources cannot be immediately augmented. For example, how does a health care system at the present time when donors are rare select patients to receive transplants or use heart machines?

Allocating resources for the short term is often called *triage*, a French word meaning to pick or sort according to quality. The term came into medical usage as a result of wartime experiences and was first explained by Jean Larrey, chief surgeon of Napoleon, in his *Memoirs* as follows:

> Those who are dangerously wounded must be tended first, entirely without regard to rank or distinction. Those less severely injured must wait until the gravely wounded have been operated upon and dressed. The slightly wounded may go to the hospital in the first or second line; especially the officers, since they have horses and therefore have transport.[10]

Recently, however, triage has come to have a wider significance, applying to any situation where patients must be selected for immediate treatment because limited resources dictate that not all can be given equal care.

Ethicists generally agree that triage does not violate justice because it respects the rights of patients as completely as possible in an emergency situation. In applying the principle of triage, two questions must be asked: Who is in greatest need of treatment? and, Who will benefit most from treatment? In the classic cases of wartime or disaster emergencies, as Larrey noted, these two questions yield a threefold division of victims: (1) the dying, whose need is great, but who will benefit least from treatment and who should be made comfortable and left to die; (2) the wounded who will survive without treatment because their need is little and who can be left to care for themselves; and (3) the wounded who will die unless treated, but who will probably survive if treated. Since these last have both the greatest need and can benefit most, they deserve the chief attention.

Today triage problems arise not only in emergency situations but also in situations where no real emergency exists. For example, it may be necessary to select which patients are to be given a new vaccine or drug when a sufficient supply for all is not yet available. The recipients for scarce organs needed for transplantation are also subject to a form of triage. According to recent federal legislation, they are classified by need, and regional centers distribute available organs. Again in such supportive health facilities where patients require almost unlimited attention for chronic, debilitating diseases, similar selective problems are common.

Sometimes, to apply triage, it may also be necessary to use some random principle of selection not based on need or benefit, such as a lottery or the rule of *first come, first served*. Such procedures are not unfair if the need and benefit are approximately the same for all, or if there is no way of discriminating on a need and benefit basis.

The principle of subsidiarity provides that charity begins at home, that is, those closest to us and whose need is best known to us should be cared for first. Thus it is not unjust that a family seek the best obtainable care for family members or that physicians give special attention to their regular patients with whom a special relationship of trust has been built, as long as no one else is treated unjustly. The same principle, however, requires that those who have responsibility for a larger group (as does any health care facility open to the public, even if privately owned) should attempt to distribute resources to protect the basic rights of all but to give the greatest care to those who have most need and will benefit most.

Special Difficulties in Triage

One of the most difficult problems in applying this kind of justice arises when a choice must be made between supplying a few patients with expensive and lengthy treatment that may only keep them living for awhile in very restricted activity (for example, kidney dialysis or heart transplantation), and supplying a larger number of persons with simple treatments (for example, a vaccine or dietary supplement) that may keep them normally active for many years. On the one hand, in the second case the benefit for the many is great, while in the first case the benefit for the few is small; but on the other hand, for each of the few the need is very great indeed, and the benefit (from their point of view) is very real. Nevertheless, it seems that in the social distribution of health care, priority should be given to that kind of preventive medicine or treatment of acute disease that will raise the general standards of health, especially for the young, over elaborate modes of treatment for the aged or seriously handicapped because it helps more people and enables them to lead a more beneficial life. At present the problem with our national health care program is that there are no priorities for expenditure of funds. Thus the more dramatic and colorful programs, such as transplant and dialysis, receive ample funds, while the more basic preventive programs, such as prenatal care and vaccinations, receive insufficient support. For example, although public health departments offer free vaccinations, because of restricted funds they are often unable to implement programs that effectively contact poor children who consequently go unprotected.

Even more difficult questions arise when the triage principle is extended to problems of health care distribution on a global scale. An adequate discussion of this topic exceeds the scope of this book, but we believe that American health care professionals must think about health in global terms. This problem of social triage was dramatized by Garrett Hardin in his proposal of a "lifeboat ethics."[11] He argued that because of the crisis of the population explosion and world hunger, the developed countries are faced with a hard choice. To continue to send medical aid and food to underdeveloped countries will only increase their overpopulation, with the result that even more people will starve than are starving now. Consequently, Hardin advocates that either food be given only with the condition that these countries institute very stringent (even compulsory) population controls, or all foreign aid be terminated.

Hardin further argues that the developed countries would be foolish to lower their own standards of living and health for the sake of poorer countries, since they need all they have to raise healthy, well-educated children who are the only hope of the human race for the future. No matter how much is given to poorer countries, they can never produce such children.

If Hardin is right in believing that the crisis is so near that only short-range solutions are possible, then it is doubtful that anything at all can be done about the situation, since social policy seldom can move so rapidly. However, most experts believe that, in the long range, various possibilities still exist for bringing world population and food resources into balance. The present situation has come about because the developed countries have introduced modern medical technology into the underdeveloped countries, not merely for humanitarian reasons, but to further their policies of political and economic colonialism. Unwittingly, the advanced countries, by introducing modern medicine, also upset the ecological balance and produced a rapid population growth, without at the same time producing the standard of living which in developed countries motivates and facilitates responsible parenthood. Thus, justice demands that the developed countries help restore the balance which they themselves destroyed.

The United States and other wealthy countries need to undertake such a restoration of justice not only for the sake of poor countries, but also for their own self-preservation. It is quite unrealistic for the wealthy nations to suppose, as Hardin does, that they can sail away in their lifeboat and leave the rest of the world to sink. There is no place to sail to and no oc an to absorb the millions who look enviously to the wealth we hoard. Nor is it true that these countries are without power, since the ultimate weapon may turn out to be not the atom bomb, but sheer numbers.

Thus, in the social triage situation the fundamental principle must be equal justice for all members of the world community, even the least privileged. If resources are scarce, then these resources must first be assigned to those members of the community who can use them best and most justly for the good of all. But whoever makes this selection must avoid the danger of being judges in their own case. Even according to Hardin's argument, would it not be wiser to attempt to select from *all* countries those citizens on whom the future of the race can most securely depend, rather than waste these resources on so many in the United States who consume much and contribute little?

7.4 Conclusion

Research and allocation of scarce medical resources are prominent ethical issues in health care because they affect or influence all aspects of it. The ethical difficulties concerned with research usually result from neglecting subjects' rights to informed consent. For this reason, people who are more easily manipulated, such as children, prisoners, and the elderly, require special protection under the law and in the ethical norms recognized by legitimate researchers.

In regard to allocation of scarce resources the United States has been ambivalent, seeking whenever possible to avoid the ethical challenge of making difficult choices. Thus, when it became obvious that some people might not receive treatment for end-stage renal disease, the federal government decided to fund a transplant and dialysis program for anyone needing treatment. No norms to evaluate the program were ever offered. The same situation seems to be developing in regard to organ transplants; who has a right to receive the scarce organs, since there is public pressure to try to supply organs for all even when the chances of success are slim and the costs exorbitant. Is it time to set some ethical standards for allocating scarce resources?

Footnotes

1. Jay Katz, Alexander Capron, and Eleanor Swift Glass, *Experimentation with Human Beings* (New York: Russell Sage Foundation, 1972).

2. *Ibid.*

3. "Final Regulations for the Protection of Human Research Subjects," *Federal Register* 46(16) (Jan. 16, 1981).

4. For a complete listing of documents concerning research with human subjects consult *Summing Up: Final Report on Studies of the Ethical and Legal Problems in Medicine and Behavioral Research* (Washington, DC: U.S. Government Printing Office, March 1983); and the various studies of the National Commission for the Protection of Human Subjects of Biomedical and Behavioral Research, U.S. Department of Health and Human Services, 1981, esp. *The Belmont Report*, cf. footnote 5.

5. Commission for the Protection of Human Subjects of Research, "The Belmont Report: Ethical Principles and Guidelines for the Protection of Human Subjects of Research" (Washington, DC: U.S. Government Printing Office, 1978).

6. Helsinki (1975) and Nuremberg (1946) Codes for Human Experimentation, *Encyclopedia of Bioethics*, vol. IV, pp. 1764ff.

7. Paul Ramsey, *Fabricated Man: The Ethics of Genetic Control* (New Haven: Yale University Press, 1970).

8. William May, "Proxy Consent to Human Experimentation," *Linacre Quarterly* 43 (1976): 73-84.

9. *Research Involving Children*, National Commission for Protection of Human Subjects of Biomedical and Behavioral Research, U.S. Government Printing Office 0577-0004, March 8, 1983, Fed. Register, DHHS, M 45 CFR, 46.

10. Quoted by Stuart Hinds, "Triage in Medicine," *Triage, Medicine and Society* 3 (1975): 6-22.

11. Garret Hardin, "Living on a Lifeboat," *BioScience* 24 (1974): 561-568.

Study Questions

1. Explain the conditions for informed consent, how it differs from proxy consent, and the practical difficulties that might arise when physicians and researchers seek informed consent.

2. What are placebos? Under what conditions may they be used in experimentation with human subjects? When should researchers interrupt the protocol to discontinue use of placebos?

3. If each human being has an equal right to health care, when a disaster occurs such as a plane crash or train wreck why may greater medical attention be given to some less seriously injured victims than to others who are more seriously injured? Could triage be applied to individual nations in regard to the world food supply?

Cases

1. Baby Fae, a newborn infant with a severe heart defect which would cause her death within a few weeks, received the heart of a baby ape in an organ transplant operation. An editorial in the *Journal of the American Medical Association* (12/13/85) severely criticized this transplant. From an ethical perspective, what conditions need to be verified to ensure that a transplant of this nature would be acceptable?

2. You are a researcher seeking a cure for AIDS (Acquired Immune Deficiency Syndrome). Desiring to test a vaccine you and your colleagues have developed, you seek to infect yourself with the AIDS virus. Discuss this action from an ethical perspective.

3. The neonatal care unit at Children's Memorial Hospital has six respirators available and eight newborn infants in need of pulmonary assistance. What ethical norms would you use to determine which infants will be able to utilize the respirators?

Chapter 8
Sexuality and Reproduction

8.1 Responsible Parenthood

The principle of personalized sexuality discussed in Chapter 6 recognizes that human sexuality has four principal values: pleasure, love, reproduction, and symbolism. In keeping with a Christian view of what it means to be truly human, created by God in the divine image, the principle also maintains that these four values are so interdependent that, although in a given act one or other of the values may predominate, it is harmful to human dignity (and therefore unethical) to use our sexual powers in any way that separates these values from each other. We are the products of biological evolution, but that evolution has been guided by a wise and loving Creator. Human sexual nature is a wonderfully designed and integrated complex which we cannot disrupt without risking serious harm to the fulfillment of the person in community, just as we cannot upset the ecological balance of our environment without grave risks to life.

Humanists, however, because they believe that we are products of blind evolutionary forces acting without purpose, argue that the connection of these four sexual values is merely a matter of chance. They see no reason why, without any major risk, we may not use medical technology to separate these values when such separation seems to free us from inconvenient restrictions on our behavior. Thus they favor contraceptive technologies, which make it possible to separate sexual activity for the sake of pleasure or for the expression of love from reproduction. Nor do they see any ethical problem in artificial reproductive technologies which separate reproduction partially or totally from sexual activity.

Christians faced with the development of such technologies today are often puzzled why the Catholic Church continues to oppose such apparently advantageous and harmless methods of bringing biological reproduction under rational control. To object to such technologies as unnatural seems absurd, since all technology is artificial by definition. Surely the Church cannot suggest that we give up all technology and return to the state of primitives. Moreover, if God has given us creative intelligence, are we not supposed to use it to human advantage? When the health and sanity of women are threatened by pregnancy, why can we not use modern medical knowledge to prevent such risks? Moreover, today the very existence of the human race is threatened by the population explosion, which must soon be brought under rational control. Is it not impossible to do this except by contraception and sterilization (unless we resort to abortion)? Surely it cannot be ethical to doom millions to overcrowding and starvation. Finally, many couples want to have children but are forbidden by the dictates of the Church to achieve normal parenthood by the miracles of artificial insemination or *in vitro* reproduction. If parenthood is so great a value, why make it impossible for those who so earnestly desire it?

To understand the Catholic position, it is important to recall several of the basic principles discussed in Chapter 6. First, the principle of stewardship and creativity indicates that not only is it not forbidden but it is even demanded that we develop technology to achieve rational control over nature. Therefore the Catholic Church does not reject but favors the development of technology to improve the use of human sexuality to maximize all its values, including reproductive control. But the same principle warns us that technology must be ecological; it must respect the built-in wisdom or teleology of nature, lest it prove self-destructive. This applies in a very special way to sexuality, on which depends the very future of the human race. Each generation has an inescapable responsibility for future generations. In considering any method of controlling reproduction, we must ask whether it furthers or destroys this intrinsic teleology of sexuality.

Also involved is the principle of moral discernment, which shows us (contrary to proportionalism and utilitarianism) that some actions are intrinsically wrong because they are contradictory to basic human needs and therefore may not be used to gain some apparent short-range advantage without in the long range doing harm to the individual and the community. Finally, the principle of the common good maintains that it is wrong for individuals simply to seek their own advantage without regard to its social effects, because individuals cannot be happy without the assistance of society. From these last two principles it follows that in considering technologies of reproductive control we must always ask whether the action in question is ultimately self-defeating, not only for the individual but also for society. Since society is based on the family, methods of reproductive control that undermine the family undermine the whole social order and ultimately injure all members of society.

8.2 Natural Family Planning

Christians regard children, because they are unique persons with irreplaceable qualities, as gifts of God. Although the person is produced by God with the cooperation of the parents through the biological processes of reproduction and as a result of their mutual expression of self-giving love, God alone can complete this work through his immediate creation of a unique human soul in a manner transcending the capability of any natural, biological force. Consequently, we can never claim anything more than a relative control over reproduction, which remains under the absolute control of God. When parents begin to think of their children as products and possessions, this sense of the child as a gift of God is lost and the child begins to lose status as a person with human rights. Consequently, it is never ethical to consider a child unwanted, no matter how defective the child may be or how burdensome the responsibility for its care.

When people, married or not, engage in sexual intercourse, they have the responsibility to love and care for the children they beget. Since no method of reproductive control can guarantee that pregnancy will never result from intercourse (even those supposedly sterilized cannot be sure the surgery was performed correctly), intercourse always entails this responsibility. A married couple who are able to beget and educate a family make a generous contribution to society and achieve a remarkable fulfillment in their own personal creative lives, an achievement that fully compensates for the sacrifice of many less important values.

[There can be, however, circumstances both individual and social that make it advisable for a couple to limit their family or even to have no children. These circumstances exist when either partner is incurably sterile, when the woman's physical or mental health is imperiled by pregnancy or the burden of child care, when the parents are incompetent to care for and educate their children properly, when the couple's financial situation makes such care difficult or impossible, and, finally, when overpopulation of a country threatens to reduce resources to a level of universal poverty.]

Overpopulation does not prevail and is not likely to prevail in the foreseeable future in the economically advanced countries, where population growth often approaches zero and natural resources can be much more efficiently employed by the development of new technologies. In underdeveloped countries, however, where the ecological balance has been disrupted by the importation of modern technologies, especially the eradication of contagious diseases and high infant mortality, there can temporarily exist a serious situation of overpopulation. The developed countries who exported these technologies have failed to assist the underdeveloped to raise their standards of living sufficiently to sustain this higher level of population or to bring it under control. People living in poverty are often unable to develop the personal or social discipline needed to motivate or implement reproductive control by any method. The Catholic Church therefore rejects the view that problems of population balance can be justly or even effectively solved by forcing or encouraging people to employ immoral methods of reproductive control, anymore than by resorting to genocide.]

Control of Reproduction

What methods does the Catholic Church propose to achieve a rational control over reproduction? First, it is essential that present social conditions of poverty be overcome to make it possible for couples, without undue pressure, to take full responsibility for their children. This would mean changes in the economy and also in the pattern of life and relationships of adolescents to lessen extra-marital sexual activity, illegitimacy, and premature marriage. Such life patterns favoring sexual responsibility have been achieved before and are still achievable. Second, couples preparing for marriage should be instructed in acceptable technologies of regulating conception through natural family planning (NFP).

Natural family planning is a modern technology of conception control based on the fact that although a woman is physiologically capable of intercourse continuously (with some inconvenience during the brief period of menstruation), she is fertile only for 5 or 6 days out of the menstrual cycle, at the time of ovulation. If the exact time of ovulation can be determined, a couple wishing to have a child greatly increase the probability of conception by having intercourse during that time. Couples who do not wish to conceive greatly lessen the probability of conception by abstaining for the 5 or 6 days of the cycle when pregnancy is possible.

The Natural Cycle

This natural cycle in the human species is a God-given, yet evolutionary, adaptation to human survival of great importance. Normally only one ovum at a time is available for fertilization, thus preventing multiple pregnancies dangerous both to mother and child. It also suitably prepares the woman physiologically for pregnancy when this occurs and returns her body to its resting state if pregnancy does not occur. Finally, it enables the woman to be ready for intercourse whenever her mate is (a feature specific to the human species), while other mammalian females are ready only during a seasonal fertile period (estrus). This promotes the bonding that makes the human male not a mere impregnator, but a constant and loving husband and real father who provides sustenance for his wife and child during pregnancy and nursing. Intercourse during the long sterile phase, as well as during the brief fertile phase of the cycle, therefore is not separated from procreation but is part of a pattern of marital life that promotes the optimum conditions for both pregnancy and child care.

When the deliberate exclusive use of the sterile period of a woman's cycle to prevent conception was first proposed, some Catholic theologians thought it was just another form of contraception. They could not see how a couple could knowingly and deliberately limit intercourse to the sterile period without also intending to separate the unitive value of the sexual act from its procreative value. Since it is in this very separation that the sin of contraception consists, why is the deliberate exclusive use of the sterile period not contraception? The irony is that theologians who today dissent from the Church's teaching on contraception use the same argument but draw the opposite conclusion: if it is permissible to use the sterile period in order not to conceive, then why are not all forms of contraception permissible?

Most theologians, however, quickly saw that the use of the natural sterile period was essentially different from deliberately inducing sterility by contraception according to the following reasoning: (1) No particular couple is absolutely obliged to have children to preserve the species, since others will do so; (2) They may in some cases have good reasons for not wanting another child, whom the woman cannot bear without serious injury to herself or the child or for whom they cannot adequately care; (3) They have no obligation to have intercourse during the fertile period, provided that both have sufficient self-control to abstain; (4) They have a right to have intercourse during the sterile period, just as do permanently sterile couples, because this at least achieves the other values of sexuality; (5) They perform the sexual act in a manner conformed to the design of God and nature, since the cycle of sterility and infertility in the woman is adapted to provide the optimum situation for a pregnancy and to bond the parents into a stable and caring family.

Contraception, on the other hand, although it may be practiced by a couple in a way that meets the first four of these conditions, essentially consists in a violation of the last of them: it deliberately disrupts the natural design of the sexual act and of the natural cycle to exclude their relation to procreation. This objective perversion of the act cannot be remedied simply by the couple's subjectively good intentions any more than genuine love between homosexuals can give to their sexual acts the complementarity and fertility of heterosexual acts.

This is why some theologians who have accepted contraception have been forced by the logic of their position to accept homosexual partnerships as equally normal as heterosexual marriage. Pushed a little farther, they would have to conform to the humanist view that all sexual activity between consenting adults is ethical, thus abandoning the Christian conviction that sexuality is a gift designed by a wise God to be used according to his loving purposes, and rejecting the principle of stewardship and creativity as well as that of personalized sexuality.

Signs of Infertility

The effective use of the sterile period to control conception depends on a method of accurately determining the time of ovulation. The pioneering attempt to do this was developed in 1930 by the discoverers of the fertility cycle, Ogino and Knaus. It was called the rhythm method or, more descriptively, *calendar rhythm*. Although theoretically sound, it proved in many cases to be inaccurate and prejudiced many couples and their physicians against the whole project. As a result of further research, two much safer and well-tested methods have now been developed: the *symptothermal* method and the *ovulation* or Billings method. When the term natural family planning or NFP is used today, although it does not exclude calendar rhythm, it usually refers to the symptothermal and ovulation methods.

The symptothermal method uses a number of mutually confirmatory criteria to determine the time of ovulation: changes in the cervical mucus, changes in the position and softness of the cervix and dilation of its opening, and a shift in basal temperature, all of which result from a rise in estrogen in the blood as a result of the ovulation process.

The ovulation or Billings method, on the other hand, uses only the appearance of mucus at the vulva, determined by the woman herself on the basis of a sensation of wetness, and the color and elasticity of the secretion. This alkaline mucus of an appropriate viscosity provides a kind of natural valve that facilitates the movement of the sperm into the uterus and Fallopian tubes at precisely the time when ovulation has produced a mature ovum ready for fertilization, while at other times its absence leaves the sperm to be destroyed by the normal acidity of the vagina. In the presence of this facilitating mucus the sperm can survive for several days, but probably not for more than 6. The most recent studies seem to show that the Billings method for many couples is as effective as the more complex symptothermal method. Even illiterate women can be taught to recognize the mucus signs easily. Further information on natural family planning is available from the family life office of most Catholic dioceses.

Recent research by the World Health Organization on family planning reports 97 percent *method* effectiveness.[1] The figure takes into account those pregnancies that could be explained by a failure of the couple to abstain at a time when they knew by the method they might be fertile. Thus, the method effectiveness rate is as good or better than any known contraceptive method except sterilization. User failures occur in all forms of contraception except successful sterilization. In fact, pregnancies are not always failures, since interviews often reveal conscious or unconscious motivation on the part of couples to achieve pregnancy.

[In addition to methods using the sterile period, breast-feeding may help women conveniently space pregnancies, since lactation alters a woman's hormonal balance and may help maintain an extended period of infertility after childbirth.]Some physicians, by cooperating with social attitudes that scorn breast-feeding, have contributed to an excessive frequency of pregnancies in some women, which in turn has encouraged the spread of contraception.

Effectiveness

Critics are often misinformed about the results of research on natural family planning and even confuse it with calendar rhythm. The objections of those better informed are not against its method effectiveness but against its user effectiveness. The principal argument here is the assertion that women often experience their greatest sexual desire around ovulation. Under the conditions of modern life the most propitious times for many couples to have intercourse may be when abstinence is required.

The experienced advocates and practioners of natural family planning counter this objection by saying that although it may be true that nature encourages intercourse at the fertile period to promote reproduction for the survival of the species, nevertheless, if the couple has sufficient reason to limit reproduction, this disadvantage can be overcome by sensitive lovemaking.

They further argue that natural family planning has many advantages: (1) it places responsibility not merely on the woman, as do most methods, or on the man, as does vasectomy, but on *both* partners equally; (2) many women who use such methods have reported an enhanced sense of personal dignity resulting from an awareness of their own body and its rhythms; (3) abstinence from intercourse can help a couple learn to have confidence in the strength of their love for each other and to express it in a variety of ways, without that preoccupation with "total orgasm" that is proving to be a source of tension for many men and women today; and (4) periodic abstinence removes something of the sexual routine and enhances the experience when it is actually decided on. Although it is true that spontaneity is an element of lovemaking (counselors report that 50 percent of college girls who are sexually active refuse even to use contraceptives for this reason), a truly mature notion of spontaneity is not just being able to have intercourse at any time, but rather knowing how to give oneself to another at the appropriate time, a time necessarily determined by the rhythm of some life style.

Besides these possible subjective psychological advantages, natural family planning has a number of very definite objective merits: (1) when properly practiced, it can be as effective as any method except sterilization and does not have the obvious disadvantages of a sterilizing operation; (2) unlike other comparably effective methods, that is, progesterones and intrauterine devices, it has no medical risks; (3) it is never abortifacient, as progesterones and intrauterine devices can be; and (4) it is inexpensive and does not require regular medical checkups to avoid side effects, but can be effectively taught by simple practical instruction.

A final objection often raised is that natural family planning is too difficult to teach, especially to the uneducated. Proponents answer that this is simply not the case, since it has even been taught to illiterates. They admit, however, that its effectiveness depends on accurate instruction and on the competence of well-trained teachers. Learning the method from books is discouraged unless competent teachers are unavailable. One of the chief reasons these methods have not yet won general acceptance among physicians is that they have not always been taught in a thoroughly professional manner.

Controversy over Contraception

Certain crude forms of contraception by withdrawal, barrier methods, and drugs (mainly abortifacients) were common in the ancient world in which Christianity was born. Although Church teaching on the subject was not precisely formulated because of the state of medical knowledge, its opposition to human intervention to frustrate the natural sexual process, once initiated, was never in doubt. Only in the nineteenth century, with the development of modern gynecology and more effective methods of contraception, was the Church forced to defend and enforce this constant teaching. The popes, in response to inquiries by bishops about how to counsel women who in good faith were engaging in intercourse with husbands who practiced withdrawal or the use of a condom (penile sheath) tended to advise confessors to tolerate such practices, but as such practices became widespread, the popes began to urge a more active opposition to all forms of contraception. Finally, in 1930 in reply to the action of the Lambeth Conference of the Anglican Church in officially approving the practice of contraception, Pius XI in the encyclical *Casti Conubii* vigorously reaffirmed the traditional position, precisely formulated it, and insisted on its enforcement in the sacramental ministry.

In the same year Ogino and Knaus announced their discovery of the fertility cycle, which gave rise to the controversy on whether the rhythm method was just another form of contraception. This controversy subsided when Pius XII in 1951 declared that the use of the sterile period was not contraception, and could be justified, sometimes even for the entire duration of a marriage, by sufficient reasons of health or inability to care for and educate children.

The development of antiovulant drugs (the pill) in the 1950s raised a new issue. A noted moralist at the University of Louvain, Louis Janssens, proposed arguments for the view that antiovulants were not contraceptive but could be used to induce the natural sterile period in a controlled manner. This view was still under debate by theologians when Pope John XXIII appointed a Study Commission on Family Population and Birth Problems with a wide representation of experts to advise him. Vatican II reaffirmed traditional principles on marriage with a strong emphasis on its procreative aspect, but it also formulated this teaching in a more personalistic manner by avoiding language that would imply that the love of married people is a mere means to procreation rather than in itself a superabundant value of which children are the overflow and completion. Some wanted the Council to define the sin of contraception more precisely to settle whether it included the use of the pill, but Paul VI preferred to delay any judgment until the Study Commission had finished its work.

The Pope added an executive commission of 16 bishops to the Study Commission, which in 1966 submitted three reports: a document favorable to the practice of contraception in some situations (signed by 9 of the bishops), another opposing all forms of contraception as intrinsically evil (signed by 3 of the bishops; the others abstained), and a rebuttal of this latter document by the signers of the former. The majority document itself characterized its work as a study prepared as a result of the Pope's willingness to engage in dialogue with experts and as materials for his consideration. Thus the Pope had before him both sides of the issue on which he had the responsibility to judge. This he did after two additional years of reflection and consultation with other theologians. His encyclical *Humanae Vitae*, published in 1968, gives evidence that he had listened to both sides and had incorporated in his own encyclical a good deal from both documents, but he was unable to accept the proposal of the majority report to abandon the Church's traditional rejection of all contraceptive acts as intrinsically evil. Instead he declared:

> Therefore in conformity to these principles of a human and Christian teaching on marriage, we must again declare that the direct interruption of generation already begun as a legitimate way of regulating the number of children, and especially abortion, even for therapeutic motives, are to be altogether rejected. Equally to be excluded as the teaching authority of the Church has frequently declared, is direct sterilization of a man or a woman, whether this be temporary or permanent. *Likewise is every act to be rejected which, either in anticipation of the conjugal act, or in its accomplishment or in the development of its natural consequences, proposes, whether as an end or a means, to render procreation impossible.*[2]

An analysis of the documents of the Study Commission reveals an underlying difficulty that was never greatly discussed in the press. Not only did the opinion of the majority abandon Janssens' effort to prove that the pill was not contraceptive and approve contraception as such (at least in some cases), but it adopted (not by name, but in fact) the ethical methodology of proportionalism. Nor was this strange, since Joseph Fuchs, a leading proponent of this methodology, was a prominent member of the theological committee that prepared the document that received the votes of the majority of the consultants. Consequently, neither this document nor the rebuttal of the minority objections made any attempt to answer the question of whether contraception is intrinsically unethical, since proportionalists do not admit that any concrete moral norms, if stated in neutral language, are without exception. Thus if Paul VI had accepted the reasoning by which the majority arrived at its conclusion, he would have had to abandon the concept of intrinsic morality and adopt proportionalism. In Chapter 6 we argued that this methodology cannot be made consistent with the Scriptures or Christian tradition.

Dissent

The minority report also attempted to establish that, although its conclusion that contraception is intrinsically wrong has never been infallibly defined by the *extraordinary* teaching authority, it belongs to the body of undefined but definable and therefore also infallible doctrines taught by the Church with its *ordinary* teaching authority (see Chapter 3). In the rebuttal by the majority, however, it was pointed out that ordinary teaching, even when universal and continuous, must also be taught by the Church as at least implicitly revealed by God if it is to be definable and that the minority document had not proved this to be the case. That issue was not settled by Paul VI or any subsequent papal document, so that it may still be freely discussed. Nevertheless, the arguments for its definability are impressive and have been augmented by the endorsement of the papal teaching by the World Synod of Bishops in 1981.[3]

Those who continue to dissent from this papal teaching seem to do so for two reasons.[4] First, they have adopted the proportionalist methodology and hence deny the possibility of any concrete exceptionless norms, including that against contraception. Second, they feel their position is confirmed and the papal position nullified by the *sensus fidelium* (consensus of believing Catholics, laity as well as clergy), since a high percentage of Catholics today practice contraception. Consequently, the dissenters are convinced that eventually the Pope will listen to the Holy Spirit speaking through the consensus of the laity and "catch up with the signs of the times."

As to the first of these grounds for dissent, it may well be asked whether contraception has been so widely accepted by theologians because the proportionalism that justifies it is a sound methodology or rather that proportionalism has been widely accepted by them because it justifies contraception. The minority document clearly pointed out that, if this method were adopted to defend contraception, it would soon logically lead theologians to accept as sometimes permissible masturbation, premarital sex, and homosexual activity. The majority in their rebuttal roundly denied this would happen, but the prediction has proved true.

As to the second, it is essential to be precise about what the *sensus fidelium* is. Just as the Pope and Council teach infallibly only when they witness to a doctrine as revealed by God (or necessarily connected to it) and transmitted as such through the sacred tradition of the Church, and not when they merely express their opinions or act on them, so the consensus of the faithful is not infallible when it is merely an expression of majority opinion or practice, but only when it is a witness to a doctrine as revealed by God and transmitted as such through the Sacred Tradition of the Church. If the Church ever defines that contraception is morally evil or morally good, the Church—faithful people, bishops, and Pope together—must be able to witness that this truth has been at least implicitly revealed by God from the apostolic age and handed down in the tradition of the believing community as revealed. We do not know, however, of any study that has attempted to ascertain the *sensus fidelium* in regard to contraception as distinguished from popular opinion and practice.

It is true that the gap between papal teaching in sexual matters and popular opinion and practice among even Catholics of good will is distressingly wide at present. Has it not often been so throughout history? And is it only in the field of sexuality that this gap exists? Are popular Catholic opinions and practices any more than superficially in conformity with Church teaching in matters of social justice and peace?

Subjective Considerations

Must we conclude that Catholics, perhaps the majority in the United States, who practice contraception are in the state of sin and must be excluded from the sacraments? In pastoral practice today the Church in most countries seems to be using what has been called *gradualism*. Gradualism is recognized in the teaching of the Synod of Bishops in 1981 as recognition that people do not achieve moral maturity all at once, and must strive for it over time.[5] Hence, their subjective guilt may be diminished if they sincerely suppose they are unable to follow the objective norms of morality. Pope John Paul II, in the same document, has distinguished between the law of gradualism, which rightly requires those who minister to others to respect their good will and the developmental stage of their subjective consciences, and a gradualism of the law, which is the false notion that the laws of God do not always and everywhere objectively oblige.[6] Those who speak or act in the name of the Church, not only priests but religious and Catholic lay-persons who serve in Catholic institutions and the institutions themselves, as corporate persons must clearly witness to Catholic ethics as interpreted by the teaching authority of the Church, even when they honestly think that teaching should be revised. At the same time they should not judge others, including their fellow Catholics, to be guilty of sin, especially in matters where there is obviously a great deal of subjective confusion. The media in reporting the Church's teaching on contraception and sterilization have compounded confusion by giving wide publicity to the views of prominent dissenting theologians.

Humanae Vitae itself urges confessors, while never condoning or advising contraceptive practices, to seek to keep married people receiving the sacraments.[7] Consequently, it seems that at present most confessors do not refuse absolution to those whom they can judge to be confused or dissenting in good faith or forbid them to receive communion. Confessors should, however, not neglect to encourage generosity in the transmission of life as well as natural family planning as the right solution for couples who have sufficient reason to limit their families. Moreover, they should take every appropriate opportunity to educate their people in a correct and credible understanding of the Church's teaching. Catholic health care facilities and professionals thus have a special obligation to inform those they care for of the advantages of this method and breast-feeding and the risks of contraceptive methods. The policies of Catholic institutions should, of course, be in line with the *Ethical and Religious Directives*[8] in this as in other matters. The teachings of the Gospel have often appeared utterly unrealistic but in the long run have proved the only true realism.

Although all forms of contraception are unethical, it is important, besides considering the general objections to them, to consider the particular problems raised by different current methods.

8.3 Sterilization

The most radical form of contraception currently in use is permanent sterilization. Male sterilization by vasectomy involves cutting and tying the ducts through which the sperm, produced in the testes, enter the semen. Although the man remains sexually potent, he is incapable of impregnating a woman. Female sterilization usually consists of cutting and tying the Fallopian tubes, in which the ovum is fertilized and through which it passes into the uterus. Both procedures are relatively simple and risk free, although there is some evidence that both may have medical complications. In some cases it is possible to reverse sterilization, but success cannot be ensured.

When sterility results merely as a side effect of a medical treatment directly aimed at specific disease, it is said to be indirect sterilization. It can be justified usually by the principle of totality because there is a proportionate gain for health. Thus diseased sex organs can be removed surgically or can be treated by drugs or radiation therapy even if treatment results in sterility. Direct sterilization has as its purpose contraception. According to *Humanae Vitae* it is intrinsically unethical and contrary to the principle of totality which requires that no basic human function may be sacrificed unless this is necessary to save the person's life. Nor is this principle satisfied to prevent a life-threatening pregnancy, since such a pregnancy can be avoided by natural family planning or in extreme cases by total abstention.

As a form of birth regulation, the chief disadvantage of sterilization is that it is usually permanent. Individuals deprived of their basic human capacity to reproduce may be subjectively quite satisfied with this condition, since at the time they wish to be able to continue sexual activity without risk of pregnancy. Nevertheless, objectively the ability to reproduce, even when not actually used, is a great personal gift that relates the individual to the community and its future. The sense of power, of life, and of belonging this creates is reflected in the religions and philosophies of all cultures. The Old Testament testifies to this by treating sterility in man or woman as a tragedy (1 Sm 1:5-6; Hs 9:14). The considerable number of sterilized persons who request medical help to restore their fertility clarifies how great a risk they took in choosing this method of contraception at a time when it may have seemed to them expedient.

Indira Gandhi's efforts in India to enforce a sterilization program on people of an ancient culture illustrated both how tempting this method is to a government seeking a quick solution to the problem of population control and how deeply it is resented and feared. The meaning of complete sexual power is still alive among otherwise powerless people. Our highly technological American milieu is singularly insensitive to deep human needs, which are unconscious or suppressed by cultural influences. The fact that the majority of the sterilized responded on a questionnaire that they experienced only a feeling of relief and freedom as a result of their operation is not necessarily a reliable indication of its deeper consequences. Social and psychological research on such effects is still superficial, and the present ecological crisis warns of the gradual long-term risks of what at first appeared to be harmless and effective technologies.

Involuntary sterilization is an obvious violation of the principle of free and informed consent. Fortunately, in 1979 the United States Department of Health, Education, and Welfare issued guidelines for federally funded institutions that ensured such consent for sterilization of any persons confined to such institutions. These rules include a moratorium on the sterilization of all mentally incompetent persons under the age of 21 and a 30-day waiting period for all others. Nevertheless, it is clear that there can be considerable pressure for sterilization of even mildly retarded persons and of the poor, especially blacks and Hispanics, allegedly for eugenic reasons, but really to reduce the costs or trouble to parents and the public of "unwanted children."

Sterilization is often recommended for the mentally retarded on the grounds that it protects them from sexual exploitation or irresponsible parenthood. Indeed there may be some cases in which, for instance, the guardians of a severely retarded girl may be justified in having her permanently sterilized or given antiovulant drugs if there is evidence that she will be exploited by others. In such cases the sterilization is indirect, since the girl's engagement in sexual activity is not free but amounts to rape. But in most cases the fact that the retarded have been sterilized makes them more available for such exploitation and relieves their guardians of their responsibility for proper training and protection. The mildly retarded, who are often the chief object of sterilization efforts, can learn self-control. The human dignity of all such persons forbids their guardians from solving the often difficult problems of their care by a quick mechanical solution.

Other Contraceptive Methods

The other methods of contraception, although less drastic than permanent surgical sterilization, also raise special questions. The most effective method, along with natural family planning and sterilization, is the use of various antiovulant drugs (oral contraception).[9] Some of these drugs (notably the "morning after pill") are not antiovulant but prevent the implantation of the already fertilized ovum and hence are abortifacient. The antiovulant drugs are permissible if the purpose is truly to correct some pathological condition or even to prevent conception in cases where rape has occurred or probably will occur (see section 8.5 on rape). With such exceptions the use of antiovulants to prevent conception from voluntary intercourse cannot be justified, as is clear from the principle of personalized sexuality, since it separates the unitive or love value from its procreative value by deliberately destroying the natural relation of the sexual act to reproduction.

In addition to this essential reason for rejecting their use, the antiovulants profoundly disturb the woman's physiological balance and consequently have multiple side effects. Although advocates of contraception and even government health agencies continue to declare certain doses of the antiovulants safe, the evidence also continues to accumulate of the variety (over 60 have been identified) and seriousness of these side effects.[10] Some antiovulants are dangerous or even fatal to those suffering from circulatory disease, especially for women past 35. Moreover, despite apparent ease of use, these contraceptive drugs must be taken under medical supervision, which is not always accessible to the poor. Efforts to produce safe temporarily sterilizing drugs for males have not been successful.

Among the other contemporary methods of contraception are the intrauterine device (IUD), the diaphragm, various spermicidal sprays and gels, and the condom. It is not entirely clear how the IUD works, but it is probable that it is effective not as a contraceptive but as an abortifacient, preventing the implantation of the fertilized ovum. Moreover, its use can result in serious infection and permanent sterility.[11]

The diaphragm, condom, and especially the spermicides are all subject to frequent failure (although the diaphragm, when properly fitted and in place, seems generally effective). Of all the forms of contraception, only vasectomy and the condom place the burden of responsibility on the male, and the latter is unesthetic and liable to fail. Such barrier methods, while they do not affect human physiology as do the antiovulants, obviously alter the symbolism of the sexual act as one of total self-giving, which perhaps is one of the reasons for the reluctance of many young people to use them, even at the risk of pregnancy. They introduce a repulsive mechanical element into lovemaking contrary to its natural pattern. The still more fundamental ethical objection to them is that which holds against all forms of direct contraception, namely, that they separate the essentially interdependent values of sexuality and thus pervert the naturally good, human act of erotic love. *stop*

8.4 Artificial Reproduction

Persons want children not only to continue the human race, but also because human sexuality finds its complete expression of love not simply in orgasm but ultimately in family life. Further evidence of this is found in the demands by infertile parents to adopt children and even to resort to artificial insemination or *in vitro* fertilization.

Artificial insemination is any process by which fecundation of an ovum takes place not as a result of the act of sexual intercourse, but as the result of sperm being deliberately introduced into the vagina in some other way. The sperm used in artificial insemination may be from the husband of the woman who wishes to conceive; if so, the process is referred to as homologous insemination, or artificial insemination by the husband (AIH). If the semen is from another man, it is known as heterologous insemination, or artificial insemination by a donor (AID).

Although the feasibility of artificial human insemination was known in the last century, it was not practiced to any significant extent until the 1930s. Today it is not unusual. People who have children in this way, however, usually do not care to reveal the fact, and hence it is difficult to collect accurate statistics. Judging from the number of scientific and popular articles written on the subject in the last few years in the United States and elsewhere, many thousands of children are conceived and born through artificial insemination.

The process is comparatively simple. Semen is collected, usually by masturbation, into a sterilized container. Sometimes the semen may be frozen and used at a later date, but frequently it is used within a few hours. If the semen of a donor is used, usually some attempt is made to screen him to avoid transmitting a debilitating hereditary or viral disease. Results of screening, however, are at best uncertain. The semen is introduced into the vagina as close as possible to the day of ovulation by a syringe or plastic cap placed at the cervix. Recent studies show that conception results in about 60 percent of the cases; in a higher percentage if insemination is repeated over a number of cycles.

People who request artificial insemination are usually married, childless for a number of years, and unwilling or unable to adopt children. Sometimes not sterility but fear that the husband may transmit hereditary deficiencies leads them to resort to AID. Physicians who perform this procedure often refer to it as therapy, although it can hardly be called a healing process. Some physicians refuse to inseminate single women, nor will they inseminate a married woman if the purpose of having a child is to hold the marriage together. Moreover, some require a series of psychological tests and inquiries to determine whether the couple will be able to handle the strains and tensions in married life that this procedure may cause. Even these minimal standards, however, are not observed by all physicians who practice artificial insemination.

From a legal point of view, artificial insemination is in an ambiguous position. Some countries have laws that treat heterologous insemination (AID) as adultery. In the United States no laws have been enacted regarding it, but several bills, some favorable and some unfavorable, have been introduced in state legislatures. Some of the favorable bills would legitimize children born of AID and bestow the usual rights of inheritance on the child so conceived. These rights are subject to challenge, especially in the case of AID children. Although the courts of the United States have no established jurisprudence in regard to artificial insemination, the courts tend to approve AIH but to consider AID contrary to public policy and good morals.

AID

Following the teaching of Pius XII,[12] most Catholic theologians reject artificial insemination by donor (AID) as a method of solving the very serious problem of a childless couple who intensely desire children. The use of an active element from a third party in the generation of the child involves a violation of the nontransferable and inalienable rights to personalistic procreation that married partners give one another. A woman needs to bear children as a man needs to be a father. It is obviously not an absolute need, however, and it does not justify the risk that her husband will be unable (even if he originally consents) to accept the child whom he knows to be another man's without unconscious hostility, nor the risk that the child will suffer from this disruption of the basic order of the family, which is so deeply ecological and a work of God's providence. Furthermore, she does an injustice to the donor, since although he is willing he is being sexually exploited much as a prostitute is, he is the true father of the child and responsible for it, and yet he is induced (usually by payment) to surrender his responsibility in a dehumanizing way. It is especially deplorable that medical students frequently play this degrading role for a little extra money. In one reported case, a single donor became the biological father of as many as 50 children. Moreover, this gives rise to the possibility of the spread of unknown genetic defects and to the deleterious effects of unrecognized incest.

The fact that some studies of AID parents report a high level of subjective satisfaction on the part of the parents does not tell us much about the ultimate effect of AID on the child or on society. Usually a time comes in a child's life when he or she feels that his or her very existence depends on the secure love of the parents for each other and their identification with the child. The recent decision by a so-called *surrogate mother* to retain her child indicates the strong nature of this bonding. While undoubtedly it is better for a child to be adopted by a loving family than to be raised in an institution, the adopted child may suffer some disadvantage compared to the natural child. This is evidenced by the frequently reported cases where adopted children feel a great need to discover their biological parents. Such needs cannot be reduced to purely conscious factors but arise from unconscious sources not under voluntary control.

AIH

When, however, it is the wife and not the husband who is infertile and it is possible to use the husband's semen (AIH), the case is less clear as far as Catholic theologians are concerned. Some Catholic theologians believe AIH can be permitted either because they dissent from Pius XII's teaching[13] or because they believe his condemnation falls only on the use of masturbation to obtain the semen. They argue that as some justify contraception by saying the act remains remotely ordered to procreation, so in AIH the artificial procreative process remains remotely ordered to the unitive act of love. The partners express their love regularly by intercourse, trying to conceive, but since they cannot, they use an artificial process to achieve pregnancy.

Undoubtedly it is legitimate to use medical art to remedy infertility and probably even to promote fertility if such intervention does not change the essential character of the act so that the child is still generated by the actual expression of unitive love. It is difficult, however, to establish convincingly that this essential significance of parenthood is retained when insemination is physically separated from the act of unitive love. Some argue that it is the couple's love for each other that motivates their use of artificial insemination. That is true, but the artificial procedure is not an equivalent of the marital act of union, which God and nature have given an intrinsic symbolism and meaning that AIH completely lacks. No one would say that the technical procedure of AIH or AID is an act of lovemaking!

Moreover, the acceptance of AID opens the way to a host of other ethical problems, all of which tend to undermine the family as the basic, natural foundation of society. If AID is licit, then would it not also be licit to inseminate women in order to modify or improve the human species, or to supply surrogate mothers? Why could not single women be inseminated if they thought having a child would lead to greater personal fulfillment? Moreover, if conception outside of intercourse is fitting for human beings, why not approve conception in a test tube (*in vitro* fertilization) when both egg and sperm become subject to human manipulation? In the latter case, the fertilized ovum might be placed for gestation in the womb of the woman whose egg is used, in the womb of another woman, or in an artificial placenta.

Judging these matters, as in the discussion of contraception, requires returning to the basic principle of the inseparability of the unitive and generative meaning of sexuality. The objection to contraception is that it deprives the act of sexual love of its relation to procreation, and Catholic theologians defending it must show that this relation is not essentially removed. Similarly, but conversely, the issue regarding artificial insemination is whether the procreative process is in this way separated from its relation to the expression of sexual love.

Fertility Testing

Approximately 15 percent of all married couples in the United States are unable to achieve pregnancy. This number will probably increase in the future because of the increased use of IUDs and contraceptive pills. Research shows that frequent use of such contraceptives often reduces fertility even after their use is discontinued.[14] Women are infertile because of ovulation factors (25 percent) or because of occluded fallopian tubes (25 percent). Endometriosis is another frequent cause of infertility in women, although it can sometimes be successfully treated and fertility restored. If the man is infertile, it is usually because sperm are less numerous or motile than normal. Also, the cervical mucus may be hostile to the sperm, that is, acting as an antibody.

Tests that seek to determine the cause of a woman's infertility offer no ethical difficulty. Moreover, therapy, such as medication to cure endometriosis, does not involve any unethical procedures. The same is not true in testing for fertility and therapy to overcome male infertility. It is not illicit to obtain a sample of semen from intercourse by use of a perforated condom, but it is unethical to obtain it through masturbation, because according to the principle of personalized sexuality, sexual powers can be used morally only in the marital act. This does not rule out the effort to devise means that would facilitate the act of intercourse performed in a natural manner to attain pregnancy. It must be admitted that at present insufficient research has been done to discover morally acceptable ways of overcoming male infertility.

In Vitro Fertilization

The wide acceptance of artificial insemination has led to a further step toward artificial reproduction, namely, *in vitro* fertilization (IVF). (The more accurate term is *in vitro* fertilization and embryo transplant—IVF-ET. However, the shorter term, IVF, is usually used to designate the total process.) One or more eggs are surgically removed from a woman's ovary, fertilized with her husband's sperm in a laboratory dish, and developed in the dish for a few days, after which the tiny embryo (or, more commonly, several embryos, to increase the chances of success) is transferred into the woman's uterus in the hope the pregnancy will proceed normally. Often the procedure must be repeated several times before pregnancy is achieved, if at all. So far, when such pregnancies have been reported in the media, the children born have been reported as normal. But the success rate is not high and the media does not report on the expense and frustration for disappointed couples.

It seems clear enough that in this procedure, even more than in artificial insemination, there is a complete separation of reproduction from lovemaking. Besides this essential defect, the procedure raises other serious problems. What of the many fertilized embryos that may be produced but that do not implant or are not carried to term? It is true that even in natural reproduction many embryos also are lost, but not as the result of technology deliberately designed and used. Again, would it not be better to devote the extensive resources being used to develop and make available this complicated and fallible remedy for sterility to the discovery of solutions to overcome sterility itself? Finally, does not this process promote the false attitude that the child is not a gift but a product and a possession who exists primarily to satisfy a parental need rather than for his or her own sake? The English bishops in a thoughtful study of IVF reached the following conclusion:

> What concerns us about IVF is this: it involves a severing of procreation from sexual intercourse. A proper act of sexual intercourse is an act by which in physical enjoyment of their friendship husband and wife give expression to their commitment to each other and to shared life and common concerns. Even when engaged in, with the specific hope that a child will result,

such sexual intercourse remains essentially an expressive act of love, not an exercise in skillful production. If their hope for a child is fulfilled the child will be a gift embodying the parent's act of personal (i.e., bodily, emotional, intelligent and responsible) involvement with each other. Procreation will thus have been an extension of the parent's whole common life and of the fully personal act which most vividly expresses that common life.[15]

Another point to be considered is what reasonably may be called "the right of a child to its own parents." A child has no rights before it is conceived, but once conceived it has a natural right to that intimate relation to its parents which arises from the fact that they are its biological parents by intercourse within marriage, an intercourse that fully expresses their mutual love. The adopted child, although far better off than an orphan, still lacks the complete implementation of this natural right, as is apparent from the many cases of adopted children who, despite the great love shown them by their adoptive parents, are extremely anxious to locate their biological parents. The child begotten by AID is deprived of this relation with one of its biological parents. Even the child begotten by AIH or *in vitro* fertilization is deprived of the fullness of this relation, since he or she is not the fruit of an act of love but of a technological procedure. This human right obliges parents not to bring children into the world except in a way that endows them with this intimate relation to their parents. Children commonly fear that they are really adopted and thus may be someday rejected by their "parents." When it becomes routine for children to be produced in one of these artificial modes, *all* children may wonder if they really have parents, or were begotten by unknown fathers, or manufactured in a laboratory.

The essential ethical consideration in any intervention in the reproductive process is that the child be brought into existence by the natural love act of the married couple. Consequently, there seems to be room for further discussion on a number of possibilities on which the teaching authority of the Church has not yet passed official judgment. For example, when sterility is the result of an obstruction of the Fallopian tubes, it may become possible to remove a mature ovum from the ovary and return it to the tube beyond the obstruction adjacent to the uterus where it would be accessible to the sperm in normal intercourse. Or, if necessary, a portion of the semen deposited by the husband in normal intercourse might be used to fertilize the ovum *in vitro* before returning it to the uterus, or both sperm and ovum might be placed in the uterus together so that fertilization would take place there. Obviously, it would be better to devote research to preventing and repairing pathology of the Fallopian tubes than to the development of such complicated, even if licit, techniques.

Another possibility might arise when a woman is able to conceive in the natural way but unable to carry the child to viable term. It would seem that the natural process would be assisted rather than subverted if the child were transferred to an artificial womb and its life thus protected.

Would it also be licit to transplant an embryo naturally conceived from the uterus of its mother to a foster mother for the good of the child or because of serious danger to the mother? Would the foster mother be justified in thus lending her womb to carry the fetus of another? Although one study group has rejected this form of artificial gestation, some say that it does not seem beyond the realm of ethical intervention. Certainly, it would not constitute mutilation of the woman's sexual organs, nor would it destroy her personal bodily integrity. It would be similar to the age-old custom of the wet nurse. Such procedures, like child adoption, can be justified only by real necessity, since they deprive the child of some elements of the intimacy of its normal relations to its mother. Unfortunately, the use of "surrogate mothers" is also open to depersonalizing commercialization.

8.5 Rape

Rape is one of the more common social crimes. Because many rape victims hesitate to expose themselves to shame and notoriety, and because false charges of rape are often filed, it is difficult to ascertain with any degree of accuracy the number of rapes committed annually in the United States. When crimes of violence are tabulated, however, the percentage of rapes increases each year. There is evidence that rape is motivated by hostile impulses—a desire to assert the aggressive power of the rapist and to humiliate the victim—more than a desire for sexual pleasure. Strange to say, some people would actually defend rape in some cases and justify it within marriage on the grounds that it meets masculine needs. Without or within marriage, however, it is contrary to the meaning of sexuality as an expression of mutual love for the sexual act to be performed against the woman's will. A woman in *immediate* danger of pregnancy due to rape may protect herself by taking antiovulant drugs, and it has recently been argued that this would also apply to a woman subject to rape in marriage, e.g., where she has sufficient reason to avoid pregnancy but her husband refuses to practice natural family planning.[16] Pope John Paul II recently pointed out the sinfulness of the husband who even in thought considers his wife a mere sexual object, without regard for her free personhood. Such behavior is a part of wife abuse, which is at last being exposed to public concern.

An actual victim of rape should be given the most sensitive and charitable care possible. Such victims often complain justifiably that they are treated by the police and medical personnel alike as though they were responsible for provoking the attack, thus compounding the grave injustice the woman has suffered. Many cities now have formed rape treatment task forces, not only to help educate police and medical personnel concerning humane treatment for rape victims, but also to prevent the crime by alerting the public to the signs of impending attack and to the measures that might ward it off. Hospital procedures developed by such task forces are designed to accomplish four things:

1. To offer the psychological support and counseling that the woman needs to work through the trauma of the attack and its aftermath. Often this will require follow-up treatment with a counselor or psychologist.

2. To provide medical care for injuries or abrasions that might have occurred.

3. To gather evidence to be used if the rapist is apprehended and prosecuted. This usually consists of a careful examination of the vagina, pelvic area, and clothing.

4. To provide treatment to prevent possible venereal disease and pregnancy.

This last point, preventing pregnancy, raises special ethical problems. Since it is more probable that the woman is in the sterile portion of her cycle and because the trauma of rape has an antiovulatory effect, it seems the chances of conception after rape are very low statistically.[17] But becoming pregnant is a very serious concern to the victim, and she deserves every help that medical professionals can give her, provided that help is ethical. Of course, in many cases, it will be possible to ascertain that conception is not likely. If conception is a possibility, since the victim is in no way responsible for it, she has the right to use any ethical means to avoid it. A woman who has consented to intercourse takes responsibility as a free person to use the sexual act in keeping with its intrinsic significance of love and procreation. The rape victim, however, has no such responsibility because she has not consented to the sexual act. Hence she has assumed no responsibility to give proper meaning to the sexual act that has been unjustly forced on her. Thus she or the people caring for her may use any available medical procedure to prevent conception before it has occurred. However, if the woman has already conceived she cannot take any action to abort or destroy the fertilized ovum directly or request others to do so, nor may they cooperate with her in doing so. While she has the right to protect herself from the effects of the aggression, she does not have the right to do so at the expense of the life of an innocent child. Nor is there any proportion between the child's right to life itself, and her right to be free of the injury done her, grave as this is. Finally, a woman does not restore her personal dignity and integrity by destroying the life of another person who is her own child, but rather by caring for that child and thus demonstrating to herself and to others her great dignity as a person, a woman, and a caring mother. This teaching of the Church is based on the sacred value of both the mother and her child equally.

Ethical problems arise in the treatment of rape victims when methods are proposed that do not only prevent conception but that may be or are abortifacient. As already noted, such methods are illicit because the woman is protecting her rights at the expense of the rights of a child already in existence. On the other hand, when there is *doubt* whether conception has in fact taken place, the probability should benefit the woman's rights. This means, therefore, that as long as it is truly doubtful that the woman has conceived, she can take means to prevent conception, even if these means might in some cases indirectly be abortifacient if conception has taken place without her knowing it. But once it becomes certain or highly probable that conception has occurred, she must then give the benefit of the doubt to the rights of the fetus to life and avoid any serious risk of abortion.

Formerly, when discussing licit methods of attacking the sperm before conception, Catholic moralists recommended (with some limitations as to time) dilation and curettage (D and C), vaginal douche, or intrauterine douche. Today, from both the medical and moral points of view, none of these methods seems to be acceptable.

The vaginal douche may be used for cleansing and sanitizing purposes to prevent venereal disease but is unlikely to prevent conception. Conception takes place ordinarily in the Fallopian tubes, not in the vagina or uterus, and recent studies show the sperm usually enters the tubes between 5 to 30 minutes after intercourse. Hence, the vaginal spermicidal douche might attack some of the sperm remaining in the vagina but would be ineffective for most of them. The intrauterine douche is considered too dangerous because the fluid it introduces could flow through the Fallopian tubes into the peritoneal cavity and perhaps cause serious infection. Competent gynecologists do not employ this procedure today.

The theologians who formerly allowed dilation and curettage realized that the scraping of the womb made it impossible for an already implanted zygote to survive or for a fertilized ovum to be implanted. But they argued that the principal purpose of this action was to eliminate the sperm, and if this were done soon enough after the attack, the principle of double effect could be used. Given the new evidence of sperm motility, it no longer seems reasonable to say that curettage is a specific remedy to remove the sperm when the significant sperm is probably already out of the uterus.

Most rape protocols used in hospitals or trauma centers today recommend the use of progesterone/estrogen pills in high doses, for example, OVRAL, seven times a day for three days. Although some of these pills are marketed primarily as anovulant pills, they render the endometrium hostile to implantation of the fertilized ovum. A recent statement of the hierarchy in England allowed such treatment (the "morning after pill") *provided the woman had not ovulated recently!* One might question, however, the need to use such strong pharmaceuticals if it is clear that the woman has not ovulated and thus would not become pregnant as a result of the rape. If the woman had become pregnant the direct effect of such high doses would be abortifacient, and thus the principle of double effect could not be invoked as it could be if the anovulant pill were given in normal doses. A true anovulant pill, used in lower doses, could be used with a view to preventing ovulation, but not in such high doses that it would become an abortifacient if conception had already occurred.[18]

Since Catholic health care facilities may be faced with legal difficulties or lawsuits because of their "negligence" in failing to use procedures or prescribe drugs that are abortifacient, they may ethically, in keeping with the principle of informed consent, include in their protocols for the care of rape victims a requirement that victims be informed that such procedures and drugs can be obtained through their private physician or non-Catholic facilities, but that Catholic facilities do not use them because they risk causing abortion. The decision to be satisfied with the Catholic facility's mode of care or to go elsewhere thus remains with the victim.

The fact that once a woman has suffered rape little can be ethically done at present to prevent the relatively few pregnancies that result does not mean that Catholic facilities cannot give such women the best of care, not only immediately following the violence, but in the period of psychological recovery and, if it occurs, pregnancy. Catholic professionals also should be actively involved in research on this question and in social movements to combat the frequency of rape in our violent society.

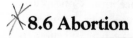 8.6 Abortion

A thorough analysis of the ethics of abortion must consider the question, "When does human life begin?" After considering this question, we shall study the pertinent theological and social factors.

The biography of any human person also includes remarkable morphological and functional changes. The difference in morphology and behavior of the newborn, the preadolescent, the mature adult, and the senile are not as startling as the differences between a caterpillar and a butterfly, but they are remarkable indeed. Yet the practicing physician does not doubt that he is the same person as the medical student whose trials and learning experiences he so well remembers, and as the young boy who first dreamed of being a doctor, and as the infant whom he cannot recollect but whose scars and immunities he still bears in his adult body and understands as part of his own medical history. Nor does he doubt that the child whose prenatal existence he first confirmed, whom he helped deliver, and whose health he has assisted to adulthood and beyond is the same identical person.

Thus a definition of human personhood begins with the notion of the person as a conscious, intelligent, free adult, but it must include the entire biography of the unique organism whose personhood is fully self-conscious and fully evident in morphology and behavior only at certain periods of that biography. This means that even if personhood is defined behavioristically, not only *actual*, here-and-now performance must be taken into account but also the capacity or *potentiality* for behavior.

The term *potentiality* has many senses in current usage. It is necessary to distinguish some of them, since confused uses of the term are at the bottom of many current arguments about the origin of the human person. First, any kind of stuff or material has the potentiality for being made or formed into an unlimited number of very different kinds of things. In this sense, the subatomic particles are potentially all the things that make up the universe, and the gaseous nebula from which the earth's galaxy originally came was potentially the human race. Potentiality in this sense of mere "stuff" is something *passive*, as clay in the hand of the sculptor.

But there are other senses in which potentiality is conceived *actively* as the power to mold and develop passively potential material. Thus the sculptor has the active potentiality (i.e., capability) to form clay into a variety of figures. It is this active sense of potentiality which is especially useful in understanding living organisms. At any given moment of its biography an organism has both a structure and a variety of functions. These functions are active potentialities that depend on the existence of the structure as an actuality; for example, a bird has the power to fly only when its wing structures have been actually developed. But what is more important is that basic to all the functions of an organism is the potentiality for *self-development*, that is, to elaborate its own structures and thus to acquire more diversified functions. This capacity for self-development is the function that gives unity to all the others and guarantees the biographical identity of the organism.

Obviously this potentiality for self-development, like any function, presupposes some kind of organic structure, but it is necessarily a minimal structure, since on its relatively simple foundation the organism is able to elaborate itself into its adult complexity. Modern embryology has shown clearly that this minimal or initial structure must be understood in an epigenetic, and not in a preformist, way. This means that the original, simplest structure is not a miniature model of the completed, elaborated structure, but does contain the information necessary to develop it. It is entirely inadequate to think of the genetic endowment of an organism as a small mock-up of the adult. Even to call it a blueprint is misleading because no blueprint can ever copy itself, let alone produce a building. Rather, a developing organism contains the potentiality for active self-development, a potentiality based on a minimal actual structure, yet containing all the information necessary to produce a maximum actual structure.

Thus the zygote or fertilized ovum of a sexually reproducing species is not a "blob of protoplasm"; it is a complete, unified structure, although that structure is very simple compared to that of the adult into which it will develop itself. This simple structure somehow contains all the information and all the active potentiality of self-development necessary to live its whole biography of interaction with its environment. It is this minimal structure which makes it actually a member of a definite species. The zygote of a cat, biologically speaking, is not potentially a cat; it is actually a member of the cat species with the potentiality of becoming a perfectly self-developed cat. Of course, only the adult cat can carry out all the various functions of cat life because only at maturity is the cat structure elaborated and diversified to the point that it has all the active potentialities of cat life. From the beginning, however, the cat zygote had the basic active potentiality to develop all these structures and the functions following on them.

When these distinctions are applied to the origin of the human person, it is obvious at once that it is a mistake to argue that if the fetus is a human being "potentially" then so are the ovum and sperm. Biologically, the ovum and sperm are not complete organisms, nor does either possess the genetic information necessary for self-development into a human being because they are haploid (i.e., they have only half the requisite set of chromosomes and genes). Thus it seems difficult indeed for a scientifically educated person to doubt that he or she has been the same person with a continuous biography, since that unique zygote began to develop itself into this adult who can look back over this personal history and acknowledge it as his or her own.

Delayed Hominization

An argument that some offer against this conclusion is that of the Aristotelian theory of delayed hominization, which has greatly influenced Catholic thought because of its adoption by the medieval theologians Albert the Great and Thomas Aquinas. Aristotle argued that until an organism has developed to the point that is has a central organ with the minimal structure required for psychological functions it should be considered a vegetative, rather than an animal, being. For Aristotle, this "primary organ" was the heart. According to modern biology it is the central nervous system and especially the cerebrum. Since the cerebrum is observable in the fetus only toward the end of the third month, this would mean that prior to this stage the embryo or fetus is not even an animal organism and *a fortiori* not human.

The weakness of this argument is that it defines incorrectly the minimal structure necessary for the organism to be a human person in the sense already explained, that is, an organism that actually has the active potentiality to develop itself into a human adult capable of intelligent and free activity. We now know, as Aristotle and Aquinas did not, that before the appearance of the brain as the primary organ of the fetus a sequence of primordial centers of development in the embryo goes back continuously to the nucleus of the zygote, which has contained from the beginning all the information and active potentiality necessary to eventually develop the brain and bring it to the stage of adult functioning. Thus, while it is true that the developing fetus first exhibits vegetative (physiological) and animal (psychological and motor) functions and finally (long after birth) specifically human functions, it possesses from conception the active potentiality to develop all these functional abilities. The minimal structure necessary for this active potentiality of self-development (even on the basis of Aristotle's and Aquinas' philosophical principles) is all that is required for an organism to be actually a human person, not the brain structures necessary for adult psychological activities.

Theological Considerations

Abortion is the termination of a pregnancy with resulting death of the human fetus. Abortion may occur spontaneously, in which case it is usually called a miscarriage, or it may be caused deliberately and then it is called an induced or procured abortion. Catholic theologians also distinguish between those procured abortions which are *direct* and those which are *indirect*. A direct abortion is one in which the direct, immediate purpose of the procedure is to destroy the human fetus at any stage after conception or to expel it when it is not viable. Most procured abortions are direct. An indirect abortion is one in which the direct, immediate purpose of the procedure is to treat the mother, but in which the death of the fetus is an incidental and secondary result that would have been avoided if possible. Two examples of indirect abortion are surgery for ectopic pregnancy and surgery for a cancerous uterus when the woman is pregnant.[19]

Today it is generally conceded by Catholic theologians that such indirect abortion may be justified by the principle of double effect: (1) because the act itself is directly for the purpose of treating the mother and hence ethical; (2) because the mother and physician do not have any unethical circumstantial intention, that is, they would save the child if they could; (3) because the death of the child is not the *means* by which the mother is treated, but only a result of the treatment (i.e., it is not a cause but a side effect of the treatment); and (4) because there is a proportionate reason if the treatment is necessary to save the life of the mother, especially since the child is doomed anyway.

The real area of difficulty, therefore, concerns *direct* abortion, of which many millions are now performed each year in the world. On this subject there is an age-old controversy. Although in all human cultures people have valued, loved, and protected their children and this care has been recognized as one of the most basic of ethical responsibilities, direct abortion has also been widely practiced. A study of primitive cultures shows that motivation for abortion in these cultures is highly varied, including not only pragmatic reasons but also religious and symbolic reasons arising from unconscious urges, such as hostility to male domination. This was also true of the ancient civilizations, although here economic and demographic factors came more and more to prevail, so that in the Greco-Roman world in which Christianity arose, abortion and infanticide in some places produced rates of reproduction below the zero-growth level. For these cultures, it can be generally said that abortion and infanticide were not strictly distinguished. In Roman culture, for example, an infant did not have legal status until accepted by the *pater familias*; hence the tradition that the illegitimate are in effect nonpersons.

Jewish Teachings

In contrast to these views is the attitude in the Jewish Scriptures. For the Jews all human life has as its author the One God whose creative power produces the child in the mother's womb and brings it step-by-step to full life. The parents play only an instrumental role in this creative process, so that from the beginning a direct, personal I-Thou relation exists between the Creator and the human being whom he is creating just as truly as he created Adam. Several of the prophets of Israel express the profound religious conviction that it was God who formed them in their mother's womb for a special purpose. These texts led to later theological speculations among the more mystical or philosophical Jewish thinkers on the time of the "infusion of the human soul," speculations which agreed with Greek philosophical tendencies that enhanced the respect for the dignity of the unborn. In any case, Orthodox Jews are convinced that when the child of a Jewish mother becomes a "living soul" it is destined for the Kingdom of God, although this membership in the Chosen People requires that it be sealed after birth by circumcision for the male. Thus, death in the womb does not exclude salvation.

Jewish thought in practical ethics, however, has been dominated by the legislation of the Torah, which in time was elaborated by the system of rabbinical interpretation, which became normative for post-Biblical Judaism. The Torah inculcates a high respect for human life, and the rabbis insisted that since the principle of justice is "an eye for an eye, a tooth for a tooth, a life for a life" (Ex 21:23-25), one cannot sacrifice one human life for another unless that other is an aggressor or criminal in some way. Consequently, Judaism has resolutely opposed any form of infanticide and has required Jews to accept martyrdom rather than to kill the innocent.

In conflicts where the mother's life is endangered, however, the rabbis taught that the child could be considered an "unjust aggressor" or "pursuer" against whom the woman could defend herself. Hence, in such cases, induced abortion was permitted, and the child was not considered to have a full right to life until birth, or "when the head or half the body emerges." This reasoning was confirmed by the fact that the Law in Exodus 21:22 does not set capital punishment but only a monetary fine for one who causes an abortion by striking a pregnant woman. Rabbinical casuistry led some to stricter views, which drew the line at the stage when the fetus was of human form (as evidenced by the Hellenistic Septuagint translation of Exodus 21:22), while others wished to draw the line 30 days *after* birth if the delivery was premature. There were also wide differences on what degree of danger to the mother justified induced abortion, some even accepting psychological reasons as sufficient justification when they threatened the couple's married life. Underlying all these debates, however, is the basic Jewish conviction of the high value of marriage and of children in view of the preservation of the Chosen People.

Jesus did not repudiate the Jewish Scriptures, nor even their rabbinical application, but he gave them his own characteristic interpretation by stressing that God's care extends to every human being no matter how sinful, ignorant, or ritually unclean. Jesus preached the good news of God's love for the "little ones," the outcasts rejected by secular and religious authorities, including powerless little children whom he declared should be given special respect as privileged members in his Father's Kingdom (Mk 9:33-37). Far from being un-Jewish, Jesus' attitude represents the deepest prophetic spirituality of Israel.

Christian Teachings

The Christian Church, confronted with the widespread Greek and Roman practice of infanticide and abortion, evaluated such customs in the light of this teaching of Jesus on the dignity of children. Luke, in his infancy narratives based on Judeo-Christian sources, takes up the Old Testament theme of the prophetic vocation and pictures John the Baptist as called to his mission by the Holy Spirit in Elizabeth's womb. In striking parallel to this, Jesus as the new Adam is created by the overshadowing Spirit in the virgin earth of Mary's womb, where he is already Lord, the Holy One, the Son of God. Thus, the Old Testament conviction that God is the creator of human life from the moment it begins, so that the human person is defined primarily by this unique I-Thou relation to its creator rather than by the legal provisions of Exodus, came to be the guiding theme of Christian thinking about the unborn child.

In the practical moral exhortations of the New Testament Epistles, abortion is never explicitly mentioned, but in the *Didache*, a manual of Church discipline written in the same period, probably in Jewish-Christian circles, it is explicitly forbidden. This opposition to direct abortion has remained, despite some controversy over subordinate issues, what John Noonan, Jr., calls "an almost absolute value" throughout the history of the Christian Church.[20] One difficulty in regard to this position arose from contact with Greek thought and took the form of the question, When is the human soul infused into the body? Platonists believed that this human animation was at conception, but the Aristotelians, more concerned with biological processes, believed (as has already been explained) that it could not be at conception when the embryo is (as they thought) simply unformed menstrual blood, but must be at about 40 to 60 days of pregnancy when the fetus has definite organic form. Those influenced by Stoic philosophy even believed it was only at birth that the child breathed in the "vital spirit."

Christian thinkers respected all these views of ancient biology, but the great authority of St. Thomas Aquinas led to the general acceptance of the Aristotelian theory that ensoulment takes place when the fetus has a definitely human form, between one and two months of gestation, which still has its defenders. Nevertheless, for Aquinas, abortion was a grave crime because it interrupted the creative work of God in nature, although it was not murder in the technical sense if it took place before ensoulment. Hence Catholic teaching traditionally regarded early abortion as a crime equivalent to murder, but not identical with it.

A second difficulty arose from the question of whether the gravity of the crime of abortion was aggravated because it prevents the child from receiving the baptism that Christ required for salvation. Today the Catholic Church still insists on the importance of infant baptism even in emergencies such as spontaneous abortion, but theologians generally no longer conclude that this practice implies that unbaptized children cannot be saved.

Other controversies have arisen over the correct way to deal with conflict situations where the mother's life seems threatened. As already noted, rabbis permitted therapeutic abortion, and some Catholic theologians in the past also favored this view, as do some Protestant churches even at present. Recently, some Catholic theologians are also attempting to revive this opinion. Since as far back as 1679, however, popes have repeatedly repudiated the notion that the killing of one person could ever be a means of therapy for another because such a practice seems utterly inconsistent with the equal dignity of human persons. Nevertheless, this disagreement on how to deal with conflict cases does not negate the basic agreement among all the Christian Churches (1) that abortion is contrary to the will of God who creates each human person and (2) that if abortion is ever permissible in a conflict situation (and this is denied by some), it can be justified only by the most serious reasons.

Authoritative Teaching

As to why the Roman Catholic Church has taken a strict view on the subject, the most authoritative recent statement on this subject is the *Declaration on Procured Abortion* issued by the Congregation for the Doctrine of the Faith (1974), as well as the important statements by the bishops of the United States (National Conference of Catholic Bishops, 1974). These documents are elaborations of the condemnation of abortion by the Second Vatican Council, which linked it with infanticide (*Church in the Modern World*). The *Declaration* argues as follows:

> The first right of the human person is his or her life. A person has other goods and some are more precious, but this one is fundamental—the condition of all the others. Hence it must be protected above all others. A society or public authority may not in any form recognize this right for some and not for others: all discrimination is evil whether it be founded on race, sex, color, or religion. It is not recognition by another that constitutes this right. This right is antecedent to its recognition; it demands recognition and it is strictly unjust to refuse it. Any discrimination based on the various states of life is no more justified than any other discrimination. The right to life remains complete in an old person, even one greatly weakened. It is not lost by one who is incurably sick. The right to life is not less to be respected in the small infant just born than in the mature person. In reality, respect for human life is called for from the time the process of generation begins. From the time that the ovum is fertilized, a life is begun which is neither that of the father nor the mother. It is rather the life of a new human being with his or her own growth. It would never be made human if it were not human already (nn. 11-12).

Note that this authoritative Catholic position does *not* depend on the arguments already given that human personhood begins at conception, but rather on the following proposition:

> From a moral point of view it is certain that even if a doubt existed whether the fruit of conception is already a human person it is an objectively grave

sin to dare to risk murder. "The one who will be a human being is already one" (Tertullian; n. 12).

The reason for this is further given in note 19 of the *Declaration*:

This declaration expressly leaves aside the question of the moment when the spiritual soul is infused. There is not a unanimous tradition on this point and authors are as yet in disagreement. For some it dates from the first instance, for others it could at least precede implantation. It is not within the competence of science to decide between these views. It is a philosophical problem from which our moral affirmation remains independent for two reasons: (1) supposing a belated animation, there is still nothing less than a *human* life preparing for and calling for a soul in which the nature received from the parents is completed; (2) on the other hand it suffices that this presence of the soul be probable in order that the taking of life involve accepting the risk of killing a human being, who is not only waiting for, but already in possession of his or her soul.

It would be exaggerated to say that these various documents, even those of the Second Vatican Council, are definitive and infallible judgments of the pastors of the Church on revealed truth, but the strength and unanimity of the teachings are very great. Furthermore, Connery's study shows that the issues involved have been well debated over a long period and that the advance of medical knowledge, far from weakening the Church's position, has tended to reinforce and sharpen it.[21]

Social Considerations

A Woman's Right to Decide. Of course, frequently a pregnant woman may in good faith believe that not to have an abortion will do more harm (not only to herself but to others) than to have one. Magda Denes has documented this in a very sensitive way from interviews with women in an abortion clinic.[22] Some of the considerations frequently cited in favor of a woman's right to make this decision for herself are as follows:

1. A woman has to bear the risk and burden of pregnancy, delivery, and child care, which she will hardly be able to sustain unless to do so is her own choice.

2. Sometimes in the case of very young, inexperienced, or retarded women and in the case of incest or rape, a woman has little or no responsibility for the pregnancy, yet she must bear the consequences.

3. Even when she has shared in the responsibility for the pregnancy, she nevertheless has the right to a normal sex life on which her marriage and care of other children also depends, yet contraception does not give her complete control over pregnancy. Therefore, she has the right to use abortion as a last resort.

4. For a woman to bear an unwanted child is a disaster for the child as well as for herself, because no matter how she may try, she may not be able to provide the child with the psychological atmosphere it needs, and as a result of her own psychological tensions may be led to child neglect or abuse.

5. A woman who discovers she has a defective child, and especially a genetically defective child who may perpetuate the defect, has an obligation

not to bring a child into the world whose life will be one of suffering and a burden to society.

6. Nor can a woman depend on help from society to care for her unwanted child, nor to provide for its adoption. Such help is often insufficient and given on degrading conditions.

7. Nor should women be forced to obtain an abortion from an illegal and probably dangerous abortionist, perhaps at the risk of death and perhaps of future sterility.

8. Modern women should be free to fulfill their duty of contributing to the solution of the very serious modern problem of population control by using abortion as a backup when contraception fails or is unavailable.

9. Women should not be inhibited in their use of this right of choice by suffering interference from others who attempt to impose their own religious value systems on others or to arouse neurotic guilt feelings in those who choose abortion.

The advantages for the woman and for society are very tangible, and in a concrete situation many may concur, and the opposite disadvantages of pregnancy seem so overwhelming, especially if the woman is poor, already heavily burdened with children, and physically or psychologically ill, that she may very well believe that there is no other way out. As Rachel Conrad Wahlberg puts it, "Those who are involved personally with an unwanted pregnancy tend to discuss the philosophical, medical, or moral questions. Those who face nine months of pregnancy and 15 to 20 years of child raising are more concerned with the immediate crisis."[23] Instead of judging them, Christians must seek ways to assist women to escape such anguishing dilemmas, while at the same time showing an equal compassion for the helpless child.

Rights of Child. The right of the mother to compassion, however, is based on the same grounds as the child's right to life, so that human sympathy and justice must be given to both. Hence, some of the effects of permitting abortion must also be considered.

1. By choosing to abort the child, the mother seeks to defend her own rights by destroying another human being, an action that is radically unjust to another and that is contrary to her own moral dignity as a person. It is true that the continued existence of the child places a woman in a unique relation to another person existing within her own body, yet the harm she suffers from this is (except in the most extreme case) only a relative harm for which other remedies may be sought, while the fetus suffers the absolute loss of the right to live, for which no remedy is possible.

2. The legalization of abortion in difficult cases has in fact encouraged the widespread practice of abortion in much less justifiable cases, because it becomes the easy way out. Hence, the preponderance of evidence is that the social approval of abortion will imperil many more lives of children than social disapproval, even taking into account the prevalence of illegal abortions. Furthermore, children raised in a society where it is known that abortion is permitted, or that their mothers have had an abortion, lack the important psychological assurance of unqualified parental acceptance if the child once born is found defective.

3. Women are encouraged and even forced by society to act in a way contradictory to their love and care for their own and others' children. It is risky to suppose that apparent social approval of abortion will do more than cover up the deep conflicts that this introduces in a woman's self-regard or in society's appreciation of the dignity of women as persons. Furthermore, the physical risks of abortion (including sterility) are not negligible, nor is the argument that they are less than the risks of childbirth significant, because this abstracts from the fact that legalized abortion has resulted in the death of many more fetuses than women who would have died in childbirth or from legal abortions.

4. Abortion policies tend to exclude the father from his proper responsibility for pregnancy and for the child and from his role of supporting his wife and sharing her burdens. Hence, he, too, is degraded as a person and burdened with deep conflicts.

5. Some unmarried women, mentally retarded women, and victims of rape and incest need the protection and care of society, which is too likely to dispense itself from this obligation simply by providing abortion as a solution. The same is true of poor women whose rights to raise a family are ignored by the encouragement of abortion to keep down welfare expenses.

6. The family institution, which is basic to society, is further weakened when the value of parenthood and of the child as a gift of God is undermined by the spreading practice of abortion, today over 1 million a year in the United States. There is little evidence that such practices encourage an attitude of responsible parenthood but rather that they promote irresponsibility by providing an easy way to escape its consequences. Hence, although very effective in population control, abortion is not a sound long-term solution for a long-term global problem.

7. Easy abortion encourages in society and in individuals an attitude of low regard for the human person as such in favor of a merely functional evaluation of persons in terms of their actual, present contribution to economic productivity and subjective well-being. This goes contrary to the advance of the concept of the dignity of the person and of inalienable rights on which modern democracy is based.

Thus, authoritative Catholic documents consistently support the moral norm that direct killing of innocent human beings can never be ethically justifiable. This does not necessarily exclude capital punishment, since a criminal is by definition not an innocent, although Catholic theologians today generally oppose capital punishment. Nor does it exclude killing an aggressor in self-defense or in war, provided that the moral object intended is to stop the aggressive act, rather than the direct killing of the aggressor. One obvious exception to the norm, however, has been proposed by some critics of the authoritative Catholic teaching against direct abortion, which they believe reduces the position to absurdity, that is, the case where a physician can only save the mother by killing the child, but seems required by this rule to let both die.

This criticism can be answered in several ways. Thomas J. O'Donnell provides a detailed analysis of the so-called medical indications for therapeutic abortion and shows that today the medical profession has solved this dilemma by providing the physician with the means to save both mother and child or at least to deal with the problems of both when both are at risk without attempting to choose the life of the mother against that of the child.[24] Germain Grisez answers it by a more careful formulation of the principle of double effect, which he believes permits the doctor in extreme situations to kill the child *indirectly* in saving the mother.[25] All these authors agree that the rule against direct killing of the innocent child is without exception and that in practice physicians may not sacrifice the life of the child to that of its mother but must do whatever they can for both.

8.7 Sex Therapy and Sexual Research

One authority estimates that in 75 percent of marital discord, the inability to engage in satisfactory sexual expression is a contributing factor, although perhaps it is as often an effect as a cause. What should be not only an expression but also a source of deepening love and commitment, rich in tenderness and joy, can be a source of profound depression and alienation. According to Masters and Johnson, famous sexual therapists, the most common forms of sexual dysfunction for men are premature ejaculation, impotency, and secondary potency difficulties; for women, the most common forms are vaginismus or orgastic dysfunction.[26] Contrary to the beliefs of some psychoanalysts, sexual dysfunction need not be a sign of a deep or severe psychic pathology, but can be the result of various relatively superficial maladjustments that impede spontaneity. Thus, sex therapy has a more limited objective than psychoanalysis or marital therapy. These latter two forms of assistance seek to help people with sexual dysfunction, but they concentrate more on the underlying conflicts and destructive interpersonal behavior that may give rise to such dysfunction. In sex therapy, however, the dysfunction is treated directly, and the therapy is complete when the couple is able to achieve a satisfactory sexual response.

At the larger centers, the common sexual dysfunctions of married people are treated through an integrated combination of instruction and actual sexual experiences in which the couple explore a more relaxed, personalized approach to sexual relations freed from anxieties about "performance." The instructions are usually given by a man-woman team, while the actual experiences are engaged in privately by the couple in their home or a hotel near the therapy center. At the beginning of therapy a thorough history is taken and a complete physical examination given. After therapy, which commonly consists of about 10 days of instruction, a follow-up is made to see if the couple has successfully integrated the new approach to sexual relations into their ordinary living. Over 80 percent success is commonly reported by such centers, which is remarkable considering the relatively short period of therapy compared to that required to meet other types of marital problems in marriage counseling.

As a general rule, most centers and private therapists accept only married couples for treatment. Some sex therapists, however, Masters and Johnson included, will accept single persons. At one time Masters and Johnson made use of paid surrogate partners for single persons and in special cases for married persons, but they have discontinued this much-criticized practice.

The principle of personalized sexuality indicates the importance for married couples to be able to express and deepen their love by satisfying sexual relations. The clinical experience of sex therapists today seems to show that when couples have good interpersonal relations, effective communication of attitudes and feelings, and a positive and anxiety-free attitude toward bodily intimacy and sensual enjoyment, sexual dysfunction is rare and special training unnecessary. In present-day culture, however, many men and women find interpersonal communication, even at nonsexual levels, difficult and are inhibited in the spontaneous expression of their feelings both by inhibiting fears and by exaggerated competitive attitudes. Hence, much of the need for sex therapy could be obviated by adequate preparation for marriage.

From a Christian point of view this education ought to stress the intimate relation between the various meanings of sexuality as sensual satisfaction, as love and completion between man and woman, and as the source of the continuing life of the family and society. Above all it should show how permanent self-giving is the heart of the matter. When couples learn to communicate with each other honestly and lovingly, sexual adjustment is usually easy, since intercourse is itself a form of intimate communication.

There is no doubt, therefore, that sex therapy may be necessary and ethically acceptable for married couples who need to overcome difficulties of miseducation or personal sexual development, provided that the prescribed sexual actions are performed with the married partner and in view of the expression of marital love through complete sexual union and not as a substitute for it.

Ethical Norms

Given the importance of the human activity involved, the need for definite ethical standards for sexual therapists is obvious. First, the same confidentiality required for anyone offering therapeutic treatment must be observed. Second, the persons involved should not be asked to perform actions that are immoral or that are contrary to their conscience. Hence, use of surrogate partners as well as activities that are intentionally and directly masturbatory must be rejected. Third, therapists must not engage in sexual activity with patients. Unfortunately, studies show that these moral standards are sometimes violated. Disregard of these principles will not only harm the patients, but will also destroy respect for sexual therapy and those who pursue it as a profession.

It is unfortunate also that sex therapists often seem to approach their task from a purely scientific-technological point of view. One noted psychiatrist completes her study of some of the literature with the lament, "There is a conspicuous absence of the word love." We cannot help but wonder, therefore, whether this approach may still further the depersonalization of human sexuality from which our culture suffers.

Sexual Research

What has just been said of sex therapy also applies to sexual research, including diagnostic procedures that may be used to determine the normality of sexual response. Such research is legitimate and necessary in order to understand better the nature of human sexuality and the physiological or psychological pathological conditions to which it is subject. However, such research must be in accord with the principles for psychological research with human subjects, which means that the experiences must be designed to be therapeutic or truly educational and not depersonalizing or reinforcing patterns inconsistent with the total health—moral and spiritual as well as biological and psychological—of the human person.

8.8 Conclusion

Sexuality influences every phase of human function: the biological, the psychological, the social, and the spiritual. For this reason, sexuality has an intense effect on human health. Balanced sexuality disposes for human health. Many people have criticized the Catholic Church for being overly concerned about human sexuality, but the Church, through its teaching on sexuality, is trying to help people develop healthy personalities and lead them closer to God. Others challenge the Church's teaching on sexuality as being outmoded. Truly, Church teaching is not in keeping with those who envision sexuality solely as a source of pleasure. Nor is it in keeping with a dualistic view of the human person. Church teaching, following Christ's teaching, leads to an integrated and balanced experience of sexuality, compatible with human health in the full sense of the term.

Footnotes

1. Evelyn Billings, MD, *The Billings Method* (Melbourne, Australia: Gordon and Gotch, 1985), p. 219.

2. Pope Paul VI, Encyclical Letter on the Regulation of Births (*Humanae Vitae*), June 30, 1968, p. 1.

3. Pope John Paul II, "The Christian Family in the Modern World," Nov. 22, 1981, in A. Flannery (ed), *Post Conciliar Documents* (North Port, NY: Costello Publishing, 1982).

4. Francis Murphy, *Catholic Perspectives on Population Issues II* (Washington, DC: Population Reference Bureau, 1981), p. 24.

5. Pope John Paul II, "The Christian Family in the Modern World," Nov. 22, 1981, in A. Flannery (ed), *Post Conciliar Documents* (North Port, NY: Costello Publishing, 1982), n. 34.

6. loc. Cit., n. 25.

7. op. Cit., n. 25.

8. United States Catholic Conference, *Ethical and Religious Directives for Catholic Health Facilities* (Washington, DC: United States Catholic Conference, 1978).

9. Christopher Tietze, "Ranking of Contraceptive Methods by Levels of Effectiveness," *Advances in Planned Parenthood* 6 (1970): 117-126.

10. See *Index Medicus*, "Contraception Adverse Effects," for a list of contemporary articles reporting side effects.

11. Janet Daling, "Primary Tubal Infertility in Relation to the Use of an Intrauterine Device," *New England Journal of Medicine* 312 (1985): 937-941.

12. Pope Pius XII, "Allocution to the Delegates at the Fourth International Congress of Catholic Doctors, Sept. 29, 1949, in *The Human Body* (Boston: St. Paul Editions, 1960), p. 118.

13. Pope Pius XII, "Allocution to the Second World Congress on Fertility and Sterility," May 19, 1956, in *The Human Body* (Boston: St. Paul Editions, 1960), p. 389.

14. See *Index Medicus* and Janet Daling, pp. 937-941.

15. *In Vitro Fertilization Morality and Public Policy* (Catholic Information Services, Abbots Langley, May, 1983), p. 24.

16. E. Bayer, *Rape Within Marriage* (Lanham, MD: University Press of America, 1985).

17. American Academy of Pediatrics Committee on Adolescence, "Rape and the Adolescent," *Pediatrics* 72 (1980): 738-740.

18. Lloyd Hess, "Treatment for Rape Victims in Catholic Health Facilities," *Ethics & Medics*, Vol. 10, n. 11-12; "Report of British Bishops," *Origins*, 3/13/86; Vol. 15: n. 39, p. 634-638.

19. United States Catholic Conference, *Ethical and Religious Directives for Catholic Health Facilities* (Washington, DC: United States Catholic Conference, 1971).

20. John Noonan, Jr., *The Morality of Abortion*, "An Almost Absolute Value in History," (Cambridge: Harvard University Press, 1970), pp. 1-59.

21. John Connery, *Abortion: The Development of the Roman Catholic Perspective* (Chicago: Loyola University Press, 1977).

22. Magda Denes, *Necessity and Sorrow: Life and Death in an Abortion Hospital* (New York: Basic Books, 1976).

23. Wahlberg, Rachel Conrad, "The Woman and the Fetus, One Flesh?" *Christian Century* 88 (1971), pp. 1045-1048.

24. Thomas J. O'Donnell, *Morals in Medicine* (New York: Alban House, 1979).

25. Germain Grisez, *Abortion: The Myths, the Realities, the Arguments* (Washington, DC: Corpus Books, 1970).

26. William H. Masters and Virginia Johnson, *Human Sexual Inadequacy* (Boston: Little, Brown, 1970).

Study Questions

1. What are the four values of sexual activity and in what sense is it unethical to seek these values separately?

2. What is the Church's teaching in regard to generation and limitation of children?

3. What is the most basic reason underlying the Church's teaching in regard to contraception?

4. Debate the issue: Tubal ligation to prevent serious physiological difficulties resulting from pregnancy, such as renal disorder or heart trouble, should be considered direct sterilization.

5. Evaluate the various natural and manipulated forms of human generation from the viewpoint of a child and from the viewpoint of the qualities which make up a balanced adult personality.

6. Write a rape protocol for a Catholic hospital.

7. Media persons often say, "Abortion is an emotional issue." In what sense is this true and how would you convince another that it is more than an emotional issue?

8. Write a mission statement for a sexual dysfunction clinic in a Catholic medical center.

Cases

1. Joe hesitates to marry Sarah because of his understanding of Church teachings to which he wants to be faithful. He tells Sarah that the Church teaches that married people should be ready to accept as many children as God sends, hence, they should wait 8 years before getting married until both are 33 and unlikely to have many children. Can you help them through a more accurate explanation of the Church teaching in regard to marriage and children?

2. Frank and Esther, wishing to limit the size of their family, consult their family physician concerning effective methods. Not knowing anything about natural family planning he suggests contraceptive methods. Wishing to follow the teaching of the Church they come to you, a sexual counselor, for help. What sources of information would you suggest to them?

3. Father Dave, a kindly priest who wishes to simplify life's problems, says "Follow your own conscience," when asked about the use of contraceptives. Is this advice adequate or could you suggest a more complete pastoral answer which Father Dave might use?

4. A Catholic hospital follows the *Ethical and Religious Directives* and does not allow direct sterilizations. A group of obstetricians threatens to boycott the hospital unless it at least will allow sterilizations after Caesarean sections. Could the Catholic hospital allow sterilization in those circumstances on the grounds that they would be justified because of the principle of material cooperation?

5. In the United States there are regulations which prohibit generating fetuses for the sake of research. But in some countries, physicians at IVF clinics do research upon fetuses which they have no intention of placing in a womb. After the research is completed the fetuses are destroyed. What is your ethical evaluation of this practice?

6. Cora is pregnant as the result of rape. She decides to have an abortion, but insists it not be done by the injection of a saline solution or any other method that would attack the child itself. She argues that if the child is expelled simply by inducing premature labor it will be ethical, since she never consented to "lending" her womb to the child, and she is simply insisting that it leave like a tenant who has not paid the rent. Is her argument sound?

7. Anne went into septic shock in the seventh month of her pregnancy. It is virtually certain that she will die from this condition if the source of infection is not removed. In removing the source of infection, her unborn child would also be removed and may die. Is this a direct or indirect abortion?

8. A young man seeks to persuade a young woman that the only way they can be sure that they will be compatible as marriage partners is to have sexual intercourse frequently before marriage. Do the findings of sexual research and sexual therapy offer any information which would support or disprove the arguments of the young man?

Chapter 9

Reconstructing Human Beings

In recent years, medical technology has moved from the mere capability of repairing the human body to new capabilities of remodeling the body by surgical reconstruction (sexual reassignment) and even by genetic reconstruction, which alters not only an individual but also all his or her descendants. Some of these new capabilities are already practical; others, still futuristic. We shall discuss many of them in this section, applying the principles of stewardship, human dignity, and totality to the issues of genetic reconstruction and screening; the principles of totality and human dignity to organ transplants; and the principles of personalized sexuality and totality to sexual reassignment.

9.1 Human Dominion Over Nature — *Ethical justification*

Concern in the area of genetic manipulation prompted the President's Commission on Ethics in Medicine and Biomedical Behavioral Research to publish two studies, *Splicing Life* and *Screening and Counseling for Genetic Conditions*. In general we agree with these studies, but we shall add the Christian perspective to this new technology.

A basic axiom of medicine has always been the Greek dictum, *Art perfects nature*, which implies that a human person can be healed (or patched up) and developed to maturity but cannot be essentially remade. Today, however, we must face the questions: Is it right for persons to become their own creators? Can and should human nature be remade? Can genetic engineering hasten the processes of evolution by eliminating troublesome wisdom teeth or appendixes or at least by some type of surgery at a very early age, before trouble arises? Might the technology of the future greatly reduce the complexities of the digestive system, which so often becomes diseased, and can human beings be fed in some simpler way, perhaps by a more effective intravenous method? Might all human beings be sterilized and reproduce artificially?

These issues are largely futuristic but can by no means be ignored, since the first steps are already being taken into this forbidding if not forbidden territory. Three levels of physical remaking are possible. (1) Surgical procedures might replace existing organs with transplants, biological constructs, or artificial organs that are not mere substitutes for natural organs but that expand old or introduce new functions into the body. To reiterate, the digestive system might be replaced with a new way of nourishing the body, and much of the reproductive system might be eliminated and children could be produced in a test tube and incubated in an artificial womb. There are possibilities of expanding the human senses to make seeing or hearing possible beyond the present range of sight and vision. (2) Embryological development might be influenced by drugs or surgery to mold the development of the phenotype (the actual body) while not changing the genotype (inherited characteristics). Thus, conceivably, the phenotypic sex of a child could be determined at will despite the genotype by altering the course of development very early in embryonic life. (3) Ultimately genetic engineering might be employed to actually produce any gene combination in the fertilized ovum, thus creating human beings by "recipe."

The basic ethical issue here is seen by some theologians as the question of the extent of man's dominion over nature. This is a classical way of posing the issue, but it is perhaps too much influenced by the Greek image of God as a jealous monarch who becomes angry when Prometheus infringes on his prerogatives. Others see such attempts to improve on man as an insult to the work of the Creator whose masterpiece is the human person or at least as a fatal temptation to pride.

Today, however, in considering radical human development, two theological points must be stressed. (1) God is a generous Creator, who in creating human beings also called them by the gift of intelligence to share in his creative power. Consequently, God does not want humans to leave fallow the talents he has given them, but encourages them to improve on the universe he has made. (2) Such improvement is possible because theology can accept the idea that God has made an evolutionary universe in which man has been created through an evolutionary process that is not yet complete. Thus, God has called humankind to join with him in bringing the universe to its completion, and in doing this he has not made humans merely workers to execute his orders, or to add trifling original touches on their own, but has made them genuine co-workers and encourages them to exercise real originality.

It is important to remember, however, that human creativity depends on a human brain. Any alteration that would injure the brain and hence a person's very creativity would indeed be disastrous mutilation, especially if this were to be transmitted genetically, thus further polluting the gene pool with defects which might be hidden and incalculable.

It is generally admitted that knowledge of this wonderful brain is still in its beginnings. The complexity of the brain is beyond any other system imaginable, and this complexity is reduced to a relatively small organ capable of self-development from the embryo and of self-maintenance, but not of self-restoration. The human brain may be near the limit of complexity and integration possible in organic, living systems.

This is certainly not so true of other organ systems, and it is possible to imagine that someday in other environments it might become necessary, for example, to replace the human lungs with other ways of obtaining oxygen or adapt our digestive systems to new forms of nutrition. In principle it would seem that such changes would be ethical (1) if they gave support to human intelligence by helping the life of the brain and (2) if they did not suppress any of the fundamental human functions that integrate the human personality. Thus, alterations that would make it impossible for human beings to directly sense the external world at least as effectively as we now do with "five senses" would be contrary to the principle of totality. So would alterations that would make it impossible for human beings to experience the basic emotions, since emotional life is closely related to human intelligence and creativity. Again, alterations that would make human beings sexless and incapable of parenthood would also be antihuman.

Thus we propose the following norms for genetic manipulation of human beings:

1. Genetic engineering and less radical transformations of the present normal human body would be permissible if they improve rather than mutilate the basic human functions, especially as they relate to supporting human intelligence and creativity. Transformation is forbidden, however, if human intelligence and creativity are endangered and if the fundamental functions that constitute human integrity are suppressed.

2. Experimental efforts of this radical type must be undertaken with great caution and only on the basis of existing knowledge, not with high risks to the subjects or to the gene pool.

9.2 Organ Transplants

Two types of organ transplants are possible, one involving an organ or tissue taken from a dead person and given to a living person, and the other involving an organ taken from one living person and given to another living person. Transplanting an organ or tissue from a dead person to a living person presents no ethical problem. With few exceptions, religious groups as well as humanistic ethicists have recognized the worth and ethical validity of such transplants. If some serious question arises concerning this type of transplant, it stems from factors other than the transplant itself. For example, concern has been expressed about the worth of heart transplants, most of it arising either from the great expense of money and personnel involved in a medical procedure that brings very little substantive value to society or from fear that in some cases the organ donor had not actually died (see p. 196 on brain death). But these concerns are not focused on the transplant as such. Pope Pius XII summed up Catholic teaching on transplants involving an organ from a dead person thus:

> A person may will to dispose of his body and to destine it to ends that are useful, morally irreproachable and even noble, among them the desire to aid the sick and suffering. One may make a decision of this nature with respect to his own body with full realization of the reverence which is due it...this decision should not be condemned but positively justified.[1]

There are far more difficulties, however, and less consensus concerning an organ transplant between living persons. The main question, whether a person can endanger his life to save the life of another by means of an organ transplant, involves the principle of totality.

Gerald Kelly, SJ, a leader in the development of medical ethics in the United States, wrote, "It may come as a surprise to physicians that theologians should have any difficulty about mutilations and other procedures which are performed with the consent of the subject but which have as their purpose the helping of others. By a sort of instinctive judgment we consider that the giving of a part of one's body to help a sick man is not only morally justifiable, but, in some instances, actually heroic."[2] In developing the rationale for an opinion favorable to transplantation, Kelly maintained, "It is clear from reason and papal teaching that the principle of totality cannot be used to justify the donating of a part of one's body to another person. Moreover, since man is only the administrator of his life and bodily members and functions, his power to dispose of these things is limited." But Kelly sought to delineate as clearly as possible the limits of this dominion, especially insofar as organ transplants are concerned.

Functional Integrity Required

Hence, Kelly asked, is there any other way in which this seemingly worthwhile and Christian action could be justified? He suggested that the principle of fraternal love, or charity (our principle of common good), would justify the transplant provided that there was only limited harm to the donor. Although it was not unanimously accepted, some theologians agreed with this opinion and developed it more clearly. Distinguishing between anatomical integrity and functional integrity, they stated that the latter, not the former, was necessary in order to ensure human or bodily integrity. Anatomical integrity refers to the material or physical integrity of the human body. Functional integrity refers to the systematic efficiency of the human body. For example, if one kidney were missing from a person's body, there would be a lack of anatomical integrity, but if one healthy kidney were present and working, there would be functional integrity because one healthy kidney is more than able to provide systemic efficiency. If a cornea were to be taken from the eye of one living person and given to another, however, the case would be different. Not only would anatomical integrity be destroyed, but functional integrity would be destroyed as well. The loss of sight in one eye severely damages vision, especially insofar as depth perception is concerned. Hence, in this case more than anatomical integrity is involved.

This distinction between anatomical and functional integrity, which we have incorporated in our formulation of the principle of totality, explains why the Church has approved blood transfusions and skin grafts and why theologians have approved elective appendectomy if the abdominal cavity is open for another legitimate reason. In these situations, loss of anatomical integrity may occur through loss of blood, skin tissue, or an internal organ, but no loss of functional integrity occurs.

Clearly, organ donation is not an obligation; rather it is something chosen in the freedom of charity. Motivated by the same charity, one could decide not to offer an organ. Such a decision would not be unethical. For this reason, it is imperative that a donor's free and informed consent be obtained. Given the fact that the more successful transplants are between members of the same family, familial or social pressure to offer oneself as a donor may at times be severe but the courts (rightly, we believe) refuse to compel such donations.

Hence, organ transplants between two living persons are licit if the donor's functional integrity is maintained, but we would caution that great care be taken in weighing the merely potential benefit against the actual risks. Consent should not be given unless the prognosis is good, because some recipients of kidney transplants die within a short time because of "rejection," even if the transplant is "successful." Therefore, it is necessary to weigh the value of such a brief prolongation of life against the lifelong risk to the donor.

In addition to the rationale put forward by Kelly and others to justify transplants between living persons, some Catholic theologians go a step farther and seek to justify these procedures either by expanding the principle of totality or by treating the whole process as a curative action, even though two people are involved and one will be injured. In so doing, they destroy the limits so carefully delineated by Kelly and others to protect human integrity. The human unity of body and soul is ignored by these theories, and the body is treated as merely something used by the person, the parts of which are at the disposal or "over against" the person and thus may be sacrificed by the person for any higher good. Falling heir to Cartesian dualism that renders appreciation of the body-soul unity of human nature impossible, one author even concludes that both eyes may be donated "for the good of another person."

Finally, arguments for the gift of human body parts lose their force when it is a question of sale, even the sale of blood. Such a sale is ethically objectionable for two reasons: (1) it is contrary to the dignity of the human body and depersonalizing, and (2) all those who need such a gift should receive it, rather than only those who can pay. Recently the U.S. Congress passed laws against selling organs when it passed a bill to establish better methods of harvesting and distributing human organs.

Although often discussed, there has been no method determined for just and ethical distribution of available organs. Most medical centers where organ transplants are performed seek to follow ethical policies by determining the seriousness of the recipient's malady and likelihood of survival and proceed on a first-come, first-served basis (see p. 111). There have been notable exceptions to fair distribution. Occasionally, a parent or a loved one has publicized the case of a child or spouse and, through media attention, has been able to receive a transplant before others who have been waiting longer. Clearly, procurement and distribution of organs is an ethical issue for which some national policy is needed and seems gradually to be developing through particular legislation.

to a living person does not offer any intrinsic ethical problem. Transplanting organs from one living person to another is also ethically acceptable provided that the following criteria are met:

1. There is a serious need on the part of the recipient that cannot be fulfilled in any other way.

2. The functional integrity of the donor as a human person will not be impaired, even though anatomical integrity may suffer.

3. The risk taken by the donor as an act of charity is proportionate to the good resulting for the recipient.

4. The donor's consent is free and informed.

5. The recipients for the scarce organs are selected justly.

9.3 Sexual Reassignment

A special type of reconstructive surgery recently introduced is transsexual surgery, a procedure by which the sexual phenotype of a male is altered to resemble that of a female, or vice versa. Such surgery, along with hormonal treatment and psychotherapy, is called *sexual reassignment*. Some physicians believe it to be helpful in dealing with the puzzling and painful condition called *transsexualism* or, more accurately, *gender dysphoria syndrome*, which is characterized by great anxiety over one's phenotypic sex and socially imposed gender role. Such procedures, involving as they do a radical mutilation, namely, castration and construction of a pseudovagina for a male, mastectomy and hysterectomy (sometimes also the construction of a nonfunctional pseudo-penis and testes) for the female, along with hormonal treatments with possible serious side effects, obviously raise the ethical question of whether the attempt to change a person's biological sex is ever a legitimate aim of medical care.

Catholic moralists have always admitted that in cases where a child is born with ambiguous genitalia, the parents should raise the child as belonging to that sex in which it is most likely to be able to function best. Nor does there seem to be any objection to the use of surgery or hormones to improve the normal appearance or function of such a person in accordance with the sex in which he or she is to be or has been raised. The reasoning behind this position is that a person must "live according to nature" insofar as this is humanly knowable.

Sexual Development

Recently, however, knowledge of sexual development has vastly increased, and sexual ambiguity is seen as far more complex and common than formerly thought. The *biological* determination of sex depends on the presence or absence of the Y chromosome in the one-cell zygote which in the beginning constitutes the human person. When present, it produces the H-Y antigen as early as the eight-cell stage of development, and the person begins to move toward maleness; otherwise, all zygotes develop into females. All embryos originally have undifferentiated gonads and two sets of sexual ducts, the Wolffian and the Mullerian, but at seven weeks the male gonads differentiate and begin to produce hormones that destroy the Mullerian ducts and cause the development of the male genitalia; otherwise the Wolffian ducts are absorbed and the gonads and the Mullerian ducts develop into the female sexual system. At the same time the differing hormonal balance in the two sexes causes certain differences in the male and female brain, in particular preparing the female brain to regulate the menstrual cycle. It has been established for some animals, but not certainly for humans, that these neurological differences also result in behavioral differences in the two sexes.

All these biological determinations are at work before birth. After birth it is probable, but not yet proved, that *biophysical* events at the unconscious level, similar to the imprinting demonstrated in animals, also promote sexual differentiation, such as the way the mother cares differently for a female than a male child. Finally, at the conscious *environmental* level, the person learns his or her own *gender identity* and assumes a *gender role* in society. In this long and complicated process many things can go wrong at each stage, with the result that in the human population a whole spectrum of conditions exists between the normal masculine and feminine conditions, meaning by "normal" a condition determined by the intrinsic teleology of sex optimal for species survival.

Transsexualism

Among these possible abnormalities, *homosexuality* is a highly varied condition, probably having many etiological factors, in which a person who is phenotypically unambiguously male or female and in no doubt about his or her gender is conscious of greater sexual attraction to those of his or her own sex than to others and who, consequently, is unable to enter into a satisfactory marriage. *Transvestism* is a condition in which a person, usually heterosexual in orientation, is more comfortable sexually while wearing clothing symbolic of the opposite sex; it is probably a form of fetishism. *Transsexualism* differs markedly from the foregoing by gender dysphoria syndrome, i.e., an anxiety, sometimes reaching suicidal depression, as the result of the obsessive feeling that one's "real" sex is the opposite of one's phenotypic sex.

Sexual reassignment would be acceptable ethically if it were possible to demonstrate that transsexualism is similar to the situation of a person born with ambiguous genitalia. At present we do not believe that this can be shown to be the case for several reasons. First, it has not yet been established that the cause of gender dysphoria syndrome is biological. No such cause is obvious at the level of either the genotype or phenotype, and as yet the evidence is tenuous that the reason transsexuals feel from early in their lives that they have "a soul different from my body" is due to some developmental accident in the central nervous or hormonal systems. At present, it remains more probable that the determining causes are at the psychological level of development, although some biological predispositions may exist. J. K. Meyer, an expert in this field, went so far as to state, "I have seen any number of men who would like to live as females and vice versa; I have not seen one with a reversal of core gender identity."[3] Other candidates for surgery can only be diagnosed as suffering from *secondary* gender dysphoria, which is stress related and results from "failures of other gender identity adaptations, such as transvestism, effeminate homosexuality, gender ambiguity." Consequently, the gender ambiguity in question appears to be primarily psychological and should thus be treated psychotherapeutically, rather than surgically.

Second, contrary to what is often stated, when candidates for transsexual surgery are required to undergo preparatory psychotherapy, many are found to be ambiguous about really wanting it and in the end decide against it. Moreover, most transsexuals who have been carefully diagnosed appear to be suffering from serious psychological problems, sometimes subtle and not immediately recognized, other than their gender dysphoria. Even after surgery they continue to need at least some psychotherapeutic support, although their frequent difficulty in forming stable personal relations makes this follow-up difficult.

Third, although when this type of surgery was first introduced there were enthusiastic reports of its success, as experience accumulates there is now no solid agreement as to whether it does much good. Recently, Johns Hopkins University, noted for its leadership in research in this field, announced the suspension of its program for further reassessment as a result of a report by Meyer and Reter that concluded that this type of surgery offers no advantage over psychotherapy.[4]

Fourth, from a theological point of view it is clear that surgery does not really solve these persons' existential problem, since it does not enable them to achieve sexual normality and be able to enter into a valid Christian marriage or have children. Since many of these individuals are somewhat asexual, their problem is not primarily sexual satisfaction but the relief of the burden of anxiety, which can usually be at least considerably lightened by psychotherapy. Hence studies so far reported by no means give assurance that sexual reassignment solves the more general character problems from which most of these persons suffer.

We conclude that, based on the present state of knowledge, this type of surgery is unethical. Certainly compassion should be extended to this small but greatly suffering group of human beings, but it should take the practical form of psychotherapy and pastoral guidance. It is unfortunate that the widespread publicity given to sex-change surgery and the exaggerated reports of its success have created an increasing demand among troubled people, most of whom would not be accepted for such surgery by any reputable clinic.

9.4 Genetic Screening and Counseling

The right of married couples to beget children is conditioned by their capability to provide for them. Prospective parents therefore must consider these factors: (1) their own need to have children as the completion of their mutual love, (2) their own capacity to care for these children, and (3) the risks that each particular child may suffer from grave handicaps that require special care, including the possibility that this child will be faced in its turn with the question of whether he or she should pass on defective genes to the next generation. Some significant risks of defect exist for *every* child and could not be eliminated no matter what means would be utilized. Thus, in all cases parents must decide whether they have the capacity to care for a potentially defective child. Furthermore, it is the duty of the genetics counselor and of society to assist the parents in accepting and meeting reasonable risks. For genetics counselors or society at large to encourage in parents the attitude that they should not have children unless the children are perfect and require the least care possible is as reprehensible as to encourage parents to reproduce fatalistically with no account of their genetic compatibility. Genetic screening and genetic counseling may occur before conception of a child, or when the child is still in the womb. Because many ethical issues are common to pre-conception and post-conception screening and counseling, we will consider both forms simultaneously.

Screening

The medical specialty of diagnosing inherited or genetic defects and their treatment, as well as the task of screening populations for these defects, and of counseling couples who are or may become parents of defective children is developing rapidly, and special institutes dedicated to it are being founded throughout the United States. Techniques of diagnosing genetic defects post-conception at early stages of human development are being perfected, such as amniocentesis, by which some genetic defects can be determined by examining the amniotic fluid in which the fetus floats in the womb. Sonography and chorionic sampling are also used in genetic screening. Sonography uses sound waves to "picture" the infant and is noninvasive. Today, sonography is often combined with amniocentesis to ensure that the needle introduced through the abdomen of the pregnant woman to gather amniotic fluid does not injure the infant. The chorion is the outer envelope of the fetus. Chorionic villi are the waste matter of the chorion. Chorionic sampling uses chorionic villi gathered from the mouth of the vagina to determine the infant's genetic pattern. This procedure is less invasive than amniocentesis, enables diagnosis of genetic abnormalities earlier in pregnancy, and thus is less dangerous for the infant and will probably replace amniocentesis as the process is perfected. It should be emphasized that although amniocentesis when properly performed is now a relatively safe procedure, nonetheless, its risk of producing a miscarriage or injuring the fetus is not negligible when we consider that it is the life or health of a human person who cannot give consent which is being risked (see page 88).

Amniocentesis is often a first step toward abortion.

Why such advances in genetic screening are medically important is evident from the following statistical considerations:

> There are more than 3,000 single-gene defects identified at present.[5] Moreover each of us carries between five and eight mutant lethal equivalents (genes), which we are all able to transmit to subsequent generations. Thus, we are all mutants, in the strictest sense, although only about 5 percent to 8 percent of us actually manifest some form of genetic mutation. An estimated 0.5 percent of all live births are attended by chromosomal imbalances such as trisomies and chromosome maldistributions....Three-quarters of these, or 0.29 percent, are deleterious defects. (Also, an estimated 9 percent of all early embryos are chromosomally abnormal, most of them lethally so.) Major single-gene mutations—homozygous and heterozygous—such as the autosomal dominants and recessives and the x-linked disorders occur in 1.8 percent of the general population. The polygenic conditions such as diabetes mellitus, gout, and some allergies occur in 1.7 percent to 2.6 percent of all live births. (These figures appear to remain fairly constant throughout the globe.) Add the figures, and we have the 4.8 percent to 5 percent incidence of genetic disease in all live births.[6]

In view of these facts, some scientists in the name of preventive medicine advocate *genetic screening* of the whole population for four purposes: (1) for scientific research, since such research is necessary to achieve full understanding and control over human inheritance; (2) to assist responsible parenthood so that carriers of genetic defects may not pass them on; (3) to make possible early therapy before the malfunctioning of defective genes has caused extensive damage; and (4) to give the parents the option of aborting the child when the defect is serious and no therapy is yet known.

The first three reasons are certainly legitimate, but persons who perform antenatal screening must be careful not to promote abortion or to cooperate in other ways through direct counseling of abortion. The possibility of cooperation in abortion, however, should not prevent a Catholic health care facility from instituting a pre-conception or post-conception screening program. Such programs must be conducted prudently, however, since serious questions may be raised. First, the research purposes of genetic screening must be regulated in the same way as any other kind of research on human subjects. Thus, it seems that since amniocentesis involves significant risk (at least in 1 percent of cases), it cannot be used for research purposes unless proportionate benefits exist for the fetus.

Therapy for infants still in the womb is a possibility; for example, hydrocephalus may be treated before birth. Therapy of this type justifies amniocentesis, and the potential for treating genetic anomalies before birth is increasing. Some ethicists maintain that the benefit that comes to the parents from amniocentesis—either knowing that the child is normal or being able to prepare themselves for the birth of a debilitated child—would justify the amniocentesis. We would maintain that benefit to the parents *per se* does not justify amniocentesis, but insofar as the parents may better care for the newborn child, we would admit an argument allowing amniocentesis.

Most screening techniques used *postnatally*, that is, after the birth of a defective child, involve the withdrawal of an insignificant amount of body fluid or tissue and are harmless. Nevertheless, informed consent is required in all such cases. Even when consent is given, care must be taken about how the information is used. If the results are made known to subjects, there is danger that they may misunderstand or exaggerate the seriousness and possible consequences of their condition or the condition of their children. If the results are known to others, there is danger of stigmatization, that is, that victims will be regarded by others as humanly inferior or dangerous. For example, it is unfair to label those blacks who are carriers of the sickle-cell trait, or those Jews who are carriers of the Tay-Sachs syndrome, diseased or defective.

Hence, the use of screening to promote responsible parenthood is in general a laudable purpose, since there can be no doubt that couples should not bring into the world children for whom (with the reasonable assistance of society) they cannot adequately care and that the care of defective children presents special burdens. Consequently, prospective parents have the duty to seek the scientific information useful to such decisions, and society has the duty to assist them in obtaining such information.

But extreme caution is necessary if the program involves *negative eugenics*. Proponents of this type of screening argue that modern medicine has upset the ecological balance by saving the lives of more and more defective persons who would have died before they could reproduce. Thus negative eugenicists maintain that the load of defective genes in the gene pool is increasing and a much higher level of genetic disease may soon occur in the population. But as Marc Lappe has written:

> The consensus of the best medical and genetic opinion is that whatever genetic deterioration is occurring as a result of decreased natural selection is so slow as to be insignificant when contrasted to "environmental" changes, including those produced by medical innovation.[7]

Hence, if only those persons who themselves suffer from a particular disease are prevented from reproducing, this would not eliminate heterozygous carriers who would continue to transmit defects dependent on recessive genes. Moreover as defective genes are eliminated from the gene pool, they are constantly replaced by mutations caused by environmental factors. Thus preconception genetic screening programs must be carefully designed. A task force of the Institute of Society, Ethics and Life Sciences[8] has suggested guidelines for these programs, which can be summarized as follows:

1. The attainability of program aims should be pretested by pilot proj-

ects and other studies, and the program should be constantly evaluated and updated.

2. Community participation in planning and executing the program should be secured to educate the public on the true significance and legitimate use of the information obtained.

3. The information obtained should be made available according to clearly stated policies known to those participating before they consent, and their privacy should be carefully protected.

4. Screening programs should be voluntary. The rights of parents to make their own decisions about the use of the information in family planning should be protected and care taken to avoid stigmatizing them or their offspring.

5. Information about screening should be open and available to all, with priorities given to well-defined populations suffering from frequent defects.

6. Programs should not be instituted unless the tests used are able to give relatively unambiguous information, and this should be precisely recorded.

7. The general principles with regard to experimentation with human subjects, such as informed consent, protection from risks, and so forth, should be observed.

8. Persons to be screened or have their children screened should be informed before they consent of the nature and cost of therapy and its risks or that no therapy is available.

9. Counseling to help the subjects understand and deal with the information should be provided.

We would also add that it is important to consider whether the cost in money and personnel in administering such programs give them high priority in view of the rarity of most of these conditions. It must be recognized, however, that in some cases (phenylketonuria, for example) the testing per subject is quite inexpensive, while the cost of caring institutionally for even a few mentally retarded children who might have been successfully treated and enabled to develop normally, may be very high.

Counseling

If genetic screening programs are to be voluntary, then the question becomes chiefly that of counseling parents as they attempt to decide how to use this information in planning their families. Like screening, genetic counseling may occur before or after a child is conceived.

Genetic counseling may be characterized as a process of communication that attempts to deal with the human problems associated with the occurrence, or risk of occurrence, of a genetic disorder in an individual or family. This process involves an attempt by one or more appropriately trained persons to help an individual, couple, or family:

1. To comprehend the medical facts, such as the risk of occurrence or reoccurrence of a disorder, the possibilities for diagnosis, the probable course of the disorder, and the available therapies;

2. To appreciate the ways in which hereditary and environmental factors contribute to the disorder and the extent to which specified relatives are at risk for being affected or for producing an affected child;

3. To understand the medically and ethically acceptable options for dealing with a positive diagnosis, as well as the reasons why other options are medically and/or ethically unacceptable;

4. To choose the course of action that seems appropriate to the clients in view of their own values and goals and to act in accordance with that decision; and

5. To make the best possible adjustment to the disorder in an affected member of the family or to the risk of a recurrence of the disorder.

A family comes to a genetic counselor because of fears about possible defects in children or about their responsibilities for future pregnancies. Usually these fears have arisen because of positive test results in mass screening or because of a record of genetic disease in parents, previous children, or near relatives.

Some argue that if serious reasons exist to believe a fetus is gravely defective, the parents should be persuaded to agree to abort the child if this suspicion is confirmed by amniocentesis. We believe that counselors should not recommend abortion as a solution. If the parents declare a definite and firm intention to abort, the counselor should present other options and avoid formal cooperation in an abortion, since the counselor should protect the fetus' right to life exactly as they would protect the rights of a child already born against the infringement of these rights by the parents, however well-intentioned they may be. A counselor, however, in doing whatever possible to avoid abortion should exercise great prudence, avoiding threats, pressures, and recriminations, because they will only aggravate the situation. Indeed, undue persuasion may lead to a malpractice claim. In sum, if abortion is in question, the counselor should respect the conscience of the parents while doing everything possible to protect the child.

It remains true, however, that couples have the duty of responsible parenthood, and society has a legitimate concern to support and encourage this responsibility. The genetic counselor therefore has the function of helping prospective parents prepare themselves for the possibility that a fetus will be defective and to plan ways to provide for this eventuality. The counselor also has the task of helping them decide whether they will or will not have children.

Problems also arise with regard to counseling adults who have a genetic defect that will eventually become a serious handicap or lead to early death; for example, Huntington's chorea, which in middle life results in progressive neurological degeneration. The counselor realizes the need to inform the victim of the danger of transmitting the defect to the next generation, yet hates to burden the victim with knowledge of his or her own doom. Undoubtedly as people become more aware of the existence of genetic defects, it will become impossible to keep such knowledge from them. It would seem that all individuals should have the freedom to decide whether they wish a diagnosis. Nevertheless, we would argue that individuals who seriously suspect they have such serious defects would be wise to have the matter settled by a reliable test and to adjust their life plans accordingly.

9.5 Genetic Reconstruction

This issue of parents' need and right to have children or even to *order* the sort of child they want is also at the base of the host of new problems that loom on the horizon concerning genetic engineering or, to use an expression that has less pejorative connotations, *genetic reconstruction*. This is the effort to repair genetic defects at their genotypic source in the genes and chromosomes rather than in their phenotypic effects and, further, to control and produce at will new combinations of genetic traits in offspring.

One of the simplest forms of such engineering would be to determine at will the sex of the fetus by selecting sperm that do or do not have the Y chromosome that determines maleness and then using selected sperm for artificial insemination or *in vitro* fertilization and implantation. Even if a technique could be invented to promote or suppress the production of one or the other type of sperm in the father without interfering with the normal process of sexual intercourse, the social and ecological consequences of such intervention could be counterproductive.

Sexual Selection

Biologists are convinced that evolutionary selection has developed the process of sexual differentiation by a genetic mechanism of the sort we find in the human species because this ensures an approximate 50-50 distribution of the sexes. Some additional mechanism not fully understood even produces a slightly higher number of male zygotes to offset the higher mortality of males. Studies made in the United States show that most young couples now want two children, preferring a boy first but, once the boy is assured, then a girl. While this preference is probably cultural and subject to cultural modification, it is possible it also has a sociobiological foundation in the greater mortality of males. These studies predict that if sex selection was widely adopted there would first be a marked rise in male births that would then level to a 50-50 distribution. It seems, therefore, that the promotion of sexual selection might not be seriously deleterious to society, although it certainly would have risks and would have few, if any, social advantages over leaving it to nature. Its only advantage would be that parents would have freedom of choice, provided that overall they use this choice to have equal numbers of boys and girls.

Ethically speaking, is this free choice of a boy or a girl an advantage to the child? After all, parents should not let their subjective preferences operate at the expense of their children in this matter, just as it is unethical for them to insist that the child be a physician or a lawyer if this is not truly in the child's interests. Christian teaching shows that it is important to children to be accepted by their parents as a divine gift to be loved for what they uniquely are and not merely because they conform to the parents' hopes or expectations. At present, society is becoming more aware of the immense injustice and harm done to women by culture patterns and structures that constantly say to a girl, "You should have been a boy." Sex selection by the parents will either reinforce this male preference pattern or, if parents can be reeducated to equal preference, it will still say to the individual child, "You are loved because you conform to your parents' preferences." This seems an injustice to the child and further reinforces the cultural message that children exist primarily to fulfill their parents' needs rather than for their own sake. This implication is already built into many cultural structures, and people have an ethical responsibility to fight against it.

The same consideration applies to more complex forms of genetic reconstruction. If the purpose of such techniques is therapy for an individual fetus, the only ethical issue is the proportion of probable benefit to risk. The issues already discussed, however, concerning *in vitro* fertilization and artificial insemination and implantation arise if these techniques can be used to produce a healthy embryo only at the expense of creating a number of embryos from which one will be selected and the others allowed to perish.

Research directed to performing genetic therapy, that is, seeking to cure genetic anomalies in the early stages of prenatal life, are underway at several research centers throughout the world. Although methods for using this knowledge on humans have not yet been developed, considerable progress has been made in splicing genes and influencing the genotype of lower forms of life. Because these efforts are therapeutic, when they are ready for human research, they will be welcome and subject to the same ethical norms as other research protocols (see p. 106).

Superior Human Beings

What if the purpose is not therapy for an existing fetus, but the future production of superior human beings? A suggested method is to recombine genes in the nucleus of a zygote, probably by using viruses that can incorporate a section of a chromosome derived from one nucleus and fixing it in a chromosome of another (transduction). Thus, it might be possible to produce a human being according to recipe, with the height, complexion, physiological traits, and mental abilities desired. While this is still very remote, we would not rule it out ethically merely on the grounds that it would be usurpation of God's creative power, since we believe that God wishes to share this creative power with human persons insofar as they are capable of using it well (principle of stewardship).

Grave ethical difficulties, however, do arise over whether society has either the knowledge or the virtue to take the responsibility for creating these superior members of the race. Attempts to define *superior* eugenically are so ambiguous as to be arbitrary. Because humans are evolutionary and historical beings, *superior* does not mean a being superior in one age and culture, but rather a being with capabilities of meeting the challenges of new and unpredicted situations. Genetic variation assists this flexibility, while the production of many identical human beings or the favoring of certain supposedly superior types amounts to a restriction on this genetic variability. Furthermore, all the difficulties already raised about the way in which such techniques tend to separate the child from its relations to parents and family arise once more.

Hence, the following conclusions can be drawn:

1. It is more feasible, technically and ethically, to improve the human condition by improving the environment and development of the individual, that is, the *phenotype*, than by modifying genetic endowment, that is, the *genotype*, and priority in research and investment of medical resources should be given to the former effort. Genetic research is extremely important, however, to understand the interactions of genotype and phenotype.

2. Presently proposed methods of genetic reconstruction of human beings involve *in vitro* fertilization and other procedures that are ethically objec-

tionable because they separate reproduction from its parental context and involve the production of human beings, of whom some will be defective because of experimental failure and who will probably be destroyed. This contravenes the basic principles of ethical experimentation with human subjects.

3. Proposals to improve the human race by sex selection, cloning, or genetic reconstruction are ethically unacceptable in the present state of knowledge. Unless limited to very modest interventions, they would restrict the genetic variability important to human survival, and they would separate reproduction from its parental context.

4. If the foregoing problems can be overcome, it will be ethically desirable to develop and use genetic methods for therapy of genetic defects in existing embryos, keeping in view the risk-benefit proportion.

The principle of stewardship throws light on many of the problems of human reconstruction. Natural law should not be conceived of as a fixed pattern of human life to which human beings are forever confined. Rather, the Creator has made human beings free and intelligent, and it is precisely this intelligent freedom that *is* human nature and the foundation of natural moral law. Human intelligence, however, is not disembodied but depends on a brain and a body that have a specific structure. In caring for their total health, persons not only have the right but the obligation to understand their psychological and biological structure and to improve themselves even in ways that may seem novel to past generations. Such improvement is good stewardship of the share in divine creativity with which God has endowed mankind.

At the same time, persons must use this creativity with profound respect for God's existing creation and especially for their own psychological and biological mode of existence, lest by tampering with their brains or the rest of their personalities they should undermine the freedom and intelligence on which this creativity depends (principle of totality). Consequently, the use of surgery and genetic manipulation to improve their bodies is ethically good, provided that they take full account of such risks and are not carried away by a false ambition to work technical miracles without regard to their real meaning for human living. In particular, Christians should be concerned that such innovations do not weaken the fundamental relations within the family or the sense of the child as a unique gift of God.

9.6 Conclusion

As human power over our genetic constituents increases, the ability to change human design and function will also increase. Hence it is extremely important that we start to ask the important questions about human reconstruction now. Are there limits to the power we have over human engineering? Do we have the right to do something simply because we have the power to do something? Science can destroy the world and all its people as well as improve life for every person. The choice is an ethical one. We believe that an ethical choice for the future of human development should follow the Christian principles applied in this chapter.

Footnotes

1. Pope Pius XII, "Allocation to Eye Specialists," May 14, 1957; *The Human Body* (Boston: St. Paul Press, 1960), p. 637.

2. Gerald Kelly, "The Morality of Mutilation: Toward a Revision of the Treatise," *Theological Studies* 17 (1956): 322-344.

3. J. Meyer, "Psychiatric Considerations in Sexual Reassignment of Non-Intersex Individuals," *Clinics in Plastic Surgery* (1974): 275-283.

4. *Science* 1979, 9/21/79, p. 10.

5. V.A. McKusick, *Mendelian Inheritance in Man* (Baltimore: Johns Hopkins University Press, 1982).

6. John A. Osmundsen, "We Are All Mutants—Preventive Genetic Medicine: A Growing Clinical Field Troubled by a Confusion of Ethicists," *Medical Dimension* 2 (1973): pp. 5-7.

7. Marc Lappe, MD, "Moral Obligations and the Fallacies of Genetic Control," *Theological Studies* 33 (1972): 411-427.

8. "Ethical and Social Issues in Screening for Genetic Diseases," *New England Journal of Medicine* 286 (1972): 1129-1132.

Study Questions

1. Explain the statement: "An artificial means of improving human function is an acceptable method of cooperating with God the Creator."

2. If one person may freely give a kidney for transplant to another person, would it violate the principle of totality to give an eye to another person?

3. Explain the various stages of sexual development and indicate factors at each stage which might inhibit a person's normal development.

4. Write a protocol for a genetic screening program in a Catholic hospital.

5. "As human power over our genetic constituents increases, the ability to change human design and function will also increase," (p. 169). Design "a new human being" incorporating the changes in design and function which you think would improve human life.

Cases

1. As a research scientist working with DNA splicing you are requested to participate in research that will improve human hearing by changing the genotype of the human person. What conditions would you stipulate concerning the research project before joining the team that will carry on the research?

2. Don and Dan are identical twins. After Don suffers kidney failure, Dan is requested by his brother's wife to donate one of his healthy kidneys to Don. Does Dan have any obligation to surrender one of his healthy kidneys to his brother? Under what condition would you defend Dan's decision not to surrender his kidney?

   [handwritten margin note: Preserve functional integrity you can donate the organ]

3. Dr. C, a surgeon, is a member of a medical-psychiatric team accepting patients for sexual reassignment. The team carefully screens each patient and performs surgery in only 20 percent of the cases. The others are treated through psychotherapy. Dr. C maintains that sexual reassignment is ethically acceptable for some people because it relieves the psychological pain and makes life somewhat more manageable for the patient. Dr. C and his team ask you, CEO of a Catholic hospital, to grant privileges to perform their specialty in your health care facility. Please respond.

   [handwritten margin note: Tremendous violation of phys. integrity for a mental condition.]

4. You and your spouse each have a nephew who has Down's syndrome. What criteria will you use to determine whether you will have children? Would you take part in a genetic screening program before conception occurs?

5. A research scientist from the U.S. seeks to cure a genetic defect in a native of Africa by means of recombinant DNA (gene splicing) that supplements a defective gene in the genotype of the patient. A federal agency declares his efforts unethical and cancels his research funds. When and under what conditions will such research be ethically acceptable?

Chapter 10

Psychotherapy and Behavior Modification

Human beings suffer from psychological as well as physiological impairment. When the psychological function of the human personality is not working properly, the person needs therapeutic help to overcome or tolerate the illness or malady in question. In order to present the ethical issues associated with mental therapy, we shall first discuss how psychological illness, often called mental illness, differs from physiological illness. Then we shall discuss the main methods of therapeutic assistance for psychological dysfunction, namely, psychotherapy and behavior control. Finally, we shall consider chemical addiction, a very common form of psychological illness in our society. While the ethical principles used in this section in regard to ethical therapy stress the need for the therapist to recognize the subject's freedom (principles of faith), the principles of hope are also important for recovery. For example, a person with chemical addiction must be aware that recovery is impossible unless the principle of growth through suffering is internalized.

10.1 Mental Sickness

In dealing with ethical problems in psychiatric medicine a very special problem arises: What is the difference between mental illness and ordinary physical illness? In our model of human personality the *psychological* dimension is closely interrelated with the *physical* dimension but also clearly distinct from it as well as from the ethical and spiritual dimension. The failure in the history of medicine to make these distinctions has been a source of vast confusion, and this remains a source of current controversy.

Thus, a group of antipsychiatry psychiatrists has made a strong, if exaggerated, case against the whole concept of mental illness and the medical model of psychiatry. These psychiatrists argue that the concept of mental illness is completely invalid and that the greater number of psychiatric illnesses are really social maladjustments between the behavior of a nonconformist individual and the demands of a social system. The cause of these maladjustments is to be located in the modern social system, which is unable to deal with individual differences.

The novel of Ken Kesey (and even more the movie based on it), *One Flew Over the Cuckoo's Nest*,[1] dramatized the way in which patients, even those self-committed to a mental institution, can be reduced to robotlike conformity by the "system." The tragedy of this story was that the "monster" Nurse Ratchett was in fact a dedicated, well-meaning, and highly professional person who quite unconsciously had become a manipulator of people. Clearly in such cases it is not the individuals who are sick, but a system that fits both patients and health care professionals into a mutually destructive gestalt.

Thus, Richard M. Restak has argued in *Pre-Meditated Man* that most of the problems of bioethics are not really ethical in the ordinary sense, but *political*, that is, questions of power or whose will concerning human behavior is to prevail.[2] The line between normal behavior and abnormal behavior thus turns out to be only a question of who is deciding what *they* want *us* to do. This warning should be heeded, but the outcries against the system should not be allowed to confuse the problem of medical care. Thus, it is necessary to hold firmly to the fact that there is such a thing as human behavior that is dysfunctional and that is caused by organic and physiological defects. There can be no doubt that not only lesions of the central nervous system, but also a wide variety of physiological disorders, can make it difficult or impossible for human beings to sense and perceive the world correctly, to live in a state of emotional balance and sensitivity, to think clearly, and to make decisions free from uncontrollable impulses. Moreover, there is increasing evidence that there may be a genetic basis for mental illnesses, particularly for schizophrenia and manic-depressive psychosis.

Medical Model

Many people require psychiatric care that is impossible without hospitalization. This need gives some credibility to the medical model of care for individuals who are mentally ill. However, extreme caution must be taken within practical limits to protect the patient's human rights, especially as regards both voluntary and involuntary commitments and retention, the right of treatment during the patient's stay, and even the right to refuse some forms of treatment. Thus, psychiatric care must include an effort to help patients develop skills to cope with the social situation in which they must live after leaving the hospital and which they ordinarily cannot much alter. It is essential that Christians recognize and respond to the need for a profound social transformation of culture so that it will be able to meet the needs of so-called deviants who are precisely the "little ones" to whom Jesus went out. But it does seem misleading to continue to use a medical model for all mental illness if this means the same model as is used for organic disease. Psychotherapy as such is a different kind of therapy than that used for physical disease. To treat patients by talking with them or guiding them in recalling and reenacting past experiences is very different from treating them with drugs.

Mental illness, therefore, in the strict and proper sense results from faulty development and use of human cognitive and affective capacities. Physical and physiological impairments may contribute to this faulty development and function because they inhibit the adaptive capacity of the person.

Thus, psychotherapy is sometimes more like education or reeducation than it is like the medical model of treatment, if by "education" is meant not the mere acquisition of information but rather the learner's own growth toward self-understanding and control that the therapist facilitates but does not originate. Psychotherapy is based on the assumption that the mentally disturbed person has at least some capacities for normal mental life but that these capacities have not been properly developed, are malfunctioning, or are being poorly used because of abnormal fears and faulty perceptions of reality.

10.2 Psychotherapeutic Methods and Goals

There is, however, a very important difference between psychotherapeutic or mental health education and other types of education. *Education* in the ordinary sense of the word as a function of an academic institution is the development of human capacities at the rational or conscious level, what we have called in Chapter 1, the ethical or social level of human function. Psychotherapy deals with psychic processes less conscious and free than rational thought, just as education at the spiritual level deals with psychic processes that transcend the level of discursive rational thought. Physical education as such deals with the training of processes that are physiological rather than psychic.

Psychotherapeutic Methods

At present there is a plethora of psychotherapeutic methods, but two very different conceptions of human psychological development are reflected in the two main current schools of psychotherapy. These are "insight therapy" and "action therapy." In practice these therapies overlap, but they have different theoretical and clinical sources. The insight therapies derive largely from Freud and the psychoanalytical school, although they have now moved on to include a great variety of therapeutic methods other than psychoanalysis, and especially to take into consideration the social group aspect of behavioral disorders. What characterizes these therapies is that they aim at helping individuals *understand* ("have insight into," "get in touch with") their own behavior and its affective sources and thus learn how to deal with life situations in an effective way. Thus, psychotherapy of this type deals with lack of coordination between the rational level (and in the case of the therapy of Jung, perhaps also with the spiritual level) and the psychological level of the personality. Normal persons have this coordination between rational and subrational processes, while neurotic or psychotic persons do not.

On the other hand, action therapy is the outcome of the behaviorist school of psychology, which rejects or bypasses the whole notion of the subconscious because it does not consider the notion of consciousness to be of any great help in psychological theory. Human beings behave as they do because they live in a physical and social environment that has educated them to behave in a certain way by a kind of education that consists in an ordered series of rewards and punishments (positive and negative reinforcements) that favor some forms of behavior and eliminate others. Action therapy, therefore, is a process of reconditioning the person to a more self-consistent and socially acceptable type of behavior. Its methods do not depend on growth in insight in the subjects, need not explore how their malconditioning has arisen or even how the therapy works, but are aimed simply at removing undesirable behavior patterns and developing new ones.

These two points of view, often obscured by bitter polemics, are not necessarily contradictory. Action therapy reflects the fact that human behavior, which at first may be conscious and deliberate, quickly takes on a patterning and becomes automatic and subconscious. Thus, when a person is learning to drive a car or play the piano, each motion is conscious and deliberate, but once the habit is acquired these actions can be performed without conscious attention. This applies also to motivation, because in general it is easier and more pleasant to perform in a habitual manner and more difficult and even painful to go against a habit or routine response.

Furthermore, in psychosocial development the formation of such habits in the child precedes the time when the person is mature enough to have full self-consciousness and control. The action therapies, based on a highly developed theory of learning through conditioning, seek to reeducate the patient by extinguishing undesirable patterns of behavior and establishing or strengthening desirable ones.

The insight therapists agree with the action therapists that the human being has many automatisms and that aberrant adult behavior is basically due to faulty conditioning in early childhood when the organism is highly impressionable and the power of the ego to resist environmental influences is low. The emphasis of insight theories, however, is on the emergence of the ego or self as controlling behavior in an adaptive manner in the face of the natural and social environments. Consequently, for the therapist simply to correct faulty habits in the client only treats symptoms. The real problem is to help patients develop a strong ego and to understand how they came to have faulty habits so they will be able under their own choice to form better ones. Hence, it requires at least some measure of exploration of the past and a growing insight into one's own personality structure.

It seems, therefore, that the two therapies can complement each other. Clients who have acquired insight into their own behavior and unconscious motivation may still need to be taught how to recondition themselves and to be aided by others in so doing. Thus, insofar as it is distinct from medical therapy, psychotherapy is not so much a process of healing a defective organic structure as of reeducation, not at the level of fully rational behavior, but rather at the level of automatic, conditioned, or subconscious behavior. Its purpose is to free the individual from undesirable patterns of behavior, especially those inconsistent with normal behavior, so that rational free decisions become easier.

Goals of Therapy

This raises the very serious question of what is *normal*. The action therapists say that the criteria of successful psychotherapy of any type can be summarized as follows:

1. Relief of undesirable symptoms (e.g., excessive anxiety);
2. Increased productivity in the person's work;
3. Adjustment and satisfaction in sexual relations;
4. Better interpersonal relations; and
5. Increased ability to endure the stresses of life.

Robert Harper, after surveying the bewildering array of insight therapies current when he wrote (the situation has not much altered since), concludes that most therapies must settle for the following results to consider themselves successful:[3]

1. The patient's weak ego is supported by the therapist's stronger ego.

2. The patient's lack of realism is corrected by the therapist's more realistic attitude.

3. The patient comes to see that many things he or she fears are not so terrible.

4. The patient learns to be more patient in solving problems, and less impulsive and panicky.

5. The patient acquires a greater or new faith or "life-myth" from the example of the therapist, who represents a hope for health.

6. The patient gets a more objective perspective on his or her problems from discussing them with the therapist or with a therapy group.

7. The patient focuses his or her floating anxieties on the outcome of the therapy process, so as to feel less isolated and helpless.

At present, psychotherapeutic methods do not have a clear record of efficiency. Psychoanalytical methods are extremely time-consuming and expensive. The action therapists have argued that the insight therapists have very little objective proof that their methods succeed better than natural processes; furthermore, the success they have seems largely independent of the mode of therapy and mainly dependent upon the personal relation with a therapist who is a sensitive, realistic, and caring person.

The action therapists claim to have a better and more demonstrable record of success, but on examination this success mainly appears in the rather restricted areas of phobias, and its permanence is often questioned. Furthermore, it fails to achieve the ultimate aim of developing a strong autonomy in the patient. At present it must be concluded that mental illness is very complex and knowledge about it and ability to cure it still very limited. Nevertheless, there is no doubt that therapy is sometimes successful. Perhaps this is not so different from any other areas of medical care, let alone of ethical and spiritual guidance. It can never be stressed too much that all modes of therapy are only of service to facilitate the inherent power of the human beings as organisms and persons to heal themselves.

Therefore, using the aforementioned goals, we can describe mental health as psychological freedom based on a realistic perception and understanding of the world, and it involves self-understanding, self-consistency, and self-control. By *self-control*, however, we mean a realistic self-control, that is, one based on a realistic recognition and practical provision for one's intrinsic needs as a human being. *Mental health is a prior condition requisite for dealing with ethical problems of moral right and wrong, since only to the degree that a person is free can there be the possibility of moral choice and moral responsibility.*

Human Freedom

It is important, however, in view of the multidimensional and integral character of human personality to emphasize that no human being is *totally* free. Human freedom is limited (1) by innate biological structure, determined genetically and by various accidents of development, with its innate needs or drives, (2) by unconscious conditioning of the sort already described with which therapy deals, and (3) by one's knowledge of the world and self, set largely by the culture in which one lives and the scope of one's experiences and education. Psychotherapy deals principally, but not exclusively, with limitations on human freedom that arise from the level of unconscious conditioning.

At the psychological level, the area of freedom is very limited in the psychotic, who is out of touch with reality. But most psychotics probably have some areas of freedom, at least sometimes; this is why they can be reached by psychotherapy or chemotherapy, as the case may be, which aims to extend this area gradually. Neurotics are decidedly more free but have some areas of unfreedom that do not occur in normal persons. The normal person also has a limited area of freedom, but its limits lie near the level of the necessary determinisms of automatic and routine behavior compatible with normal freedom.

Freedom demands not only trust between persons but within social groups. Recently, methods of *group* therapy are becoming more common, not only because of the expense of individual therapy but because mental illness is in part a disturbance of social relations and can be adequately treated only through learning social communication skills. In particular, family therapy in which a family is treated as a dynamic system whose malfunction is reflected in the psychological problems of individual members gives promise of a radically effective approach to many mental problems that originated in the family.

Such methods raise some special ethical issues, chiefly those of confidentiality and of adequate professional control. The frank communication required within the group can easily lead to an abuse of the privacy of individual members, and if the therapist does not remain fully in charge and sufficiently sensitive to the needs of every member, some especially fragile participants may be more hurt than healed by the experience.

Modern therapy has tended to move from the treatment of sexual neuroses, common as a result of the Victorian refusal to recognize basic biological needs, to the treatment of anxiety, common in this century as a result of excessive demands of a work-oriented society that fails to recognize human needs for leisure and intimacy. Hence, therapy deals more with neuroses of emptiness or lack of meaning as a result of society's failure to recognize the creative and spiritual sides of personhood. In all these cases, psychological therapy can only go so far to awaken the person's full capacity for freedom.

10.3 Ethical Issues in Psychotherapy

Punishment

On the basis of the distinctions just made, the first point about the ethics of psychotherapy is to reject any use of psychotherapy as *punishment* (although it must be admitted that the neurotic patient may at first perceive it as punishment no matter what the therapist intends). Punishment and reward (in the proper sense of the terms) belong only to *ethical* acts, that is, free, responsible acts. This, of course, requires penological reforms by which the courts decide first on the facts of a criminal action and then separately on the *moral* responsibility of the person who has committed the act. In this second decision, expert testimony from psychiatrists should be admitted, but it should be directed toward determining whether the defendant's freedom was so limited by psychological factors as to remove his or her freedom with regard to this particular class of acts.

It must be remembered that the essential question in judging moral responsibility is not rationality in the sense of knowledge, nor in the sense of capacity to reason logically, nor is it voluntariness (i.e., whether one wills an action), but *moral freedom*, (i.e., the capacity to consider alternatives with their consequences and to choose one or the other without external or internal compulsion). This moral freedom can be destroyed either by such mental confusion as makes it impossible to consider alternatives or by an emotional compulsion (overwhelming fear, pain, or passion) that compels the choice of one alternative, or perhaps by a pathological incapacity to foresee the consequences of one's actions or to appreciate them emotionally (sociopathy).

Therefore, psychiatrists called on in court for expert testimony, insofar as the present confusion of the law permits them, should be primarily concerned to make clear to the jury why in their expert opinion the accused's chronic or temporary psychological condition did or did not render him so unfree that he cannot be held responsible for the act of which he is accused, or if he is partially or remotely responsible for it, then in what degree or in what respect.

It is also important that when a defendant is acquitted on the basis of lack of responsibility, then the court in an entirely different process should decide the question of involuntary commitment for treatment or of confinement to prevent the person from harming others or themselves. Such confinement, however, should not be dealt with as if it were punishment, since it would be unjust to punish someone for acts for which he or she was not morally responsible.

The question then arises whether psychiatrists should play any role in the process of punishment itself. It seems that their role should be limited to two functions: (1) psychiatrists could diagnose prison inmates who develop mental illnesses and require occasional treatment exactly on the same basis as for medical ills; and (2) psychiatrists could act as consultants to penologists in setting up prison routines that make for good mental health and discipline, but they should not be engaged in staffing these services.

One authority states that the difficulty is that psychiatric professionals (1) do not like to take the time to gather the necessary data to apply their own scientific criteria for mental illness criterion and (2) confine themselves in court to stating their *conclusions*. What is necessary is (1) that they gather the data on which a judgment can be made by the lay jury, and (2) that they present this data to the jury in such a way that the jury can make its own judgment of the validity of the expert conclusion. Only in this way can the adversary process be applied so that juries can decide between conflicting expert opinions.

Informed Consent

Granted that therapy has been carefully distinguished from punishment, which has no part in the therapeutic profession, what of the problem of the patient's informed consent? Clearly, here as in other medical questions the patient's free and informed consent is required if he or she is competent. The special problem, of course, is that mentally disturbed patients (1) may be unable to understand the purposes or risks of the treatment and (2) may not be truly free to make a decision even if they understand, either because personal freedom is removed by irrational fear of the treatment or of the consequences of refusal, or because of masochistic tendencies that lead a patient to submit to treatment out of a desire to suffer or be humiliated, or simply because of a narcissistic desire to be the center of attention.

Patients once self-committed to a hospital may then find themselves in a situation where in fact freedom to withdraw from highly traumatizing treatment is no longer practically possible. Yet every psychiatric institution must be dedicated to the proposition that it is therapeutic only to the degree that it really respects and seeks to enlarge the patient's capacity for freedom. If it lessens this capacity, it is countertherapeutic; it is making people ill rather than well.

On the other hand, where it is rightly judged that free consent, at least in the area of treatment, is impossible, then commitment must be made by the patient's guardian, and with scrupulous observance of due legal process. It is obvious that the guardian (usually a member of the family) may be biased, either because of selfishness, ignorance, and more often through unconscious factors that may very well be part of the client's own breakdown.

If the treatment is carried out without the patient's consent, then a primary objective of this treatment must be to bring the patient as soon as possible to the level of mental integration where at least some self-determination becomes feasible. This means, of course, that the use of drugs or psychosurgery simply as a method of controlling patients or tranquilizing them cannot of themselves be legitimate therapeutic objectives. Undoubtedly, those who have to care for patients who are out of control are strongly tempted to pacify them so that they "don't make trouble." This, of course, is permissible in order to prevent the patient from harming him or herself or harming the therapist or others, but such self-defense is not *therapy*. It is only preliminary to therapy.

Transference

The use of insight therapies raises a whole series of ethical problems. The first of these is the process of *transference*. Psychodynamic therapy depends in some measure on patients' becoming dependent for the time of treatment upon the therapist. Without this profound dependency, patients are not freed from their anxieties and inhibitions sufficiently to let themselves become conscious of their true motivations. The termination of therapy is marked by the fact that patients have become sufficiently autonomous and under self-control that they no longer need the therapist.

This vulnerability of patients obviously invests the therapist with special ethical responsibilities. The first of these is that therapists must not violate the trust placed in them. This requires that a therapist carefully maintain professional secrecy, be truly concerned for the patient, prompt in appointments, and reasonably available for consultation. It means also that therapists are honest with patients and do not lie to them or break promises. Furthermore, the therapist must avoid manipulating the patient in the sense of seeking personal gratification from the treatment rather than the patient's benefit. This does not demand, of course, that the therapist have a superhuman objectivity; rather, it simply means that the therapist is worthy of trust.

Abreaction

A second issue sometimes raised by Catholics is whether the process of *abreaction* is not dangerous, since the patient in free fantasy revives the memory of former temptations or sins, of illicit sexual activity, or of hostility and destruction. Is it legitimate thus to again put oneself in the "occasion of sin" where sinful consent is possible? It is true that such dangers may occur in therapy (just as they can in examining one's conscience in preparation for confession), but if they do, they are usually the result of poor therapy. The purpose of psychoanalytic abreaction is precisely to return to some error of the past where the patient failed to resolve a problem correctly and to help the patient now face it in a clearer light.

Value Systems

Perhaps the biggest issue of psychotherapy is whether the therapist is permitted to change the client's value system. The common answer is that a therapist should not change this system but should try to adjust the patient to the system. This answer, however, is somewhat disingenuous. As the existentialist psychoanalysts have pointed out, distortions in the patient's value system often underlie the disorder. Furthermore, the source of many problems is the patient's superego, which is, in part, the value system of the parents or society that has been incorporated into the unconsciousness of the child. On the other hand, it is clear that if the psychological and ethical dimensions of human personality are distinct, as we have argued, then it cannot be the therapist's role to indoctrinate the patient in a value system.

In answer to this difficulty we must say that there are certain values on which the very relation of patient to the therapist depend, and they must be reinforced by therapy. Thus, the therapist must help the client to become more trustful, more honest, more hopeful, more courageous, more patient, and more realistic.

The effort of the therapist then is to extend the area of freedom for patients. As patients become freer they must make some free ethical decisions and will do so according to their own *conscious*, rational system of values. At this point the therapist is nondirective in the sense that it is not the therapist's task to give the patient ethical advice, but only to help the patient be free of illusion and neurosis in making decisions.

It may mean the therapist sometimes thinks that the client's decisions are not ethically good, objectively speaking. In such a case, the therapist may point out that the client's decisions are questionable, or refer the client to an ethical counselor (a clergyman or lawyer or a friend), but the therapist should be careful not to take any responsibility for the person's decision. Thus, the therapist should refer the client to ethical or spiritual advisers if it becomes apparent that the client's value system is inconsistent or inadequate.

Thus, persons undergoing therapy should not change their system of values, divorce their partners, give up their religious vocation, or change their religion or their professional vocation merely under the influence of the psychotherapeutic process. Such changes should be made only when a real degree of psychological freedom has been reached and then under guidance that acts as a countervailing force to the possible ideology of the psychotherapeutic tradition. Thus, the tendency to erect one of the many forms of therapy (including the various mystical cults now so popular) into a religion is a violation of the lines between the psychological level of personality and the ethical and spiritual levels and is doomed to end in disillusionment.

Psychoanalysis and Hedonism

A deeper problem, however, is raised by Philip Rieff in his book, *The Triumph of the Therapeutic*, and by others.[4] Is it possible that the whole system of insight therapy as it originated with Freud has a built-in system of values or ideology which it inculcates? Thus, many have accused psychoanalysis of being essentially a product of the middle class in opulent capitalist countries. Freud himself saw all of civilization as the imposition of social controls on man's infinite and even contradictory drives. Consequently, every social system is a delicate balance between the repressive controls necessary for social life and work and the explosive drives of the id. If Rieff is correct, the inherent ethic of psychoanalytical theory is to produce autonomous, hedonistic, goalless, conscienceless persons—the very sort which ethicists have always condemned as selfish, loveless, and empty. Obviously, such persons are individualistic in the extreme, uncommitted to any social goals except the achievement of freedom to do what they please. Rieff's interpretation of psychoanalysis emphasizes Freud's belief that civilization, that is, social life, is always repression, not fulfillment, of fundamental human needs—a necessary evil.

These accusations are very serious ones. They demand (1) on the part of the community of therapists a serious examination of social conscience and a purification of the theory, training, and practice of therapists who must become conscious that the goals of therapy must be related to higher social and spiritual goals and (2) on the part of clients that they trust their therapists not as omnipotent parents, but only for their limited skill, and that they also receive guidance at the ethical (political and social) and spiritual levels from others as soon as they become sufficiently free emotionally to do so.

It would be very unfair to blame either Freud or his disciples for these unfortunate consequences of an excessive faith in the power of psychotherapy in its present state of development. Freud's great contribution to understanding human behavior is established; and a fruitful historical development of psychoanalysis has already taken place, building on his work and giving it greater balance. Current psychoanalytical theory is concerned with the social as well as the individualistic aspects of human personality and is contributing to other models of human maturity. Consequently, there is no reason to doubt that in the future psychoanalysis could help Christians to be more truly Christians, or Humanists to be more truly Humanists, by becoming freer to commit themselves to their own systems of values and to interpret them in a way consistent with the facts of human experience.

10.4 Behavior Control

In addition to the use of insight and action therapies, it is possible to alter and control human thought, feeling, and behavior by drugs, surgery, and psychological conditioning. Behavior control might be described as "getting people to do someone else's bidding." In this sense, behavior control has existed since the beginning of time. In the more restricted sense, however, the sense in which we shall use the term in this section, *behavior control* is any medically indicated treatment, procedure, or process intended to cause a person, with or without his or her consent, to discontinue an activity that is personally or socially undesirable or to conform to a desirable pattern of behavior. As this description indicates, behavior control is not necessarily contrary to a person's intention or desires, but it signifies that some force over and above internal human motivation has been used in the interest of changing an activity pattern. The purpose of this control may be therapeutic (e.g., the use of drugs can sometimes actually correct a physiological malfunction that is producing abnormal behavior) or it may simply be aimed at controlling antisocial actions. For example, a person trying to overcome the habit of alcoholism may use Antabuse (disulfiram) to help conquer the habit. Although the use of this drug is voluntary, it is still a form of behavior control.

From an ethical point of view, behavior control has become a serious problem because of the increased efficacy of surgical procedures in controlling behavior, the vastly increased panoply of psychoactive drugs that modify emotional responses, and the increased tendency to impose conformity to societal norms. These procedures are not only comparatively new, they are swift and efficient, and their effect on a person can be deep and lasting. Hence, they have greater potential for good or evil than many of the techniques of scientists and physicians in the past centuries, and there is a temptation to attempt the solution of problems by altering the person rather than attempt to transform the social environment.

Principally three forms of behavior control are prevalent today and are associated, either closely or remotely, with medical care. They are shock therapy and psychosurgery, psychoactive drugs, and psychological conditioning. After describing the first three forms of behavior control associated with medical care, we shall present some ethical principles that may be used to evaluate their use.

1. *Shock Therapy and Psychosurgery.* Since the 1930s, there have been experiments with many types of treatment of psychological dysfunctions by means of profound stressing of the central nervous system through chemicals or electricity. Many therapists and therapeutic institutions reject electroshock, but it is still considered by others as worthwhile therapy, especially for involutional depression, where it often has dramatic results in patients who otherwise require protracted hospitalization.

Psychosurgery is surgical destruction of certain parts of the brain for the purpose of treating psychiatric conditions. Arguments on the ethics and merits of psychosurgery vary from severe condemnation to considerable enthusiasm. One of the results of this surgical procedure is a blunting of human emotional responses. Because of the dramatic effects of this form of behavior control, psychosurgery fell into disuse when psychoactive drugs became more effective for the treatment of severe psychosis. In recent years, psychosurgery has become once again more common throughout the world. Modern procedures using, for example, ultrasound, electrical coagulation, or implanted radium seeds are more localized and less destructive. These procedures are being facilitated by new techniques for imaging brain structure and activity. A more sophisticated form of controlling human activity, but one which can be classified as psychosurgery, is electrical stimulation of the brain (ESB) and involves implanting electrodes in the human brain and controlling actions and responses by means of electrical stimuli.

Despite some indications that present-day psychosurgery is helpful for severely depressed patients, and despite the potential use of ESB in helping people with organic brain disease, some scientists and physicians denounce all forms of psychosurgery. On the other hand, those who argue for the use of this form of therapy do so for the following reasons: (1) it has sometimes proved very successful in the treatment of patients with epilepsy or Parkinson's disease, for whom drugs do not satisfactorily control the disorders, (2) it sometimes is the only remedy for intractable pain, and (3) it may be necessary in treatment of certain violent, uncontrollable seizures (some of which are epileptic) since otherwise the patients injure themselves or have to be confined in isolation.

2. *Psychoactive Drugs.* A drug is psychoactive when it has some psychological effect: alters perception, imagination, or emotions; causes alertness, drowsiness, feelings of anger; and so forth. Such drugs are also called psychotropic. Some psychotropic drugs have proved highly effective in psychotherapy: (1) in tranquilizing patients in manic states or in uncontrollable anxiety, (2) in reducing the condition of mental confusion and dissociation, especially in schizophrenia, and (3) in lifting certain types of depression. These effects may be symptomatic, rather than truly curative, but at least they may hasten the natural recovery from an episode. Moreover, they may help return a person more quickly to a more normal way of life and thus prevent the regression that often results from prolonged institutionalization. Also, they make it possible for other types of therapy to be used. The fact that such remarkable results have been obtained by drugs strongly suggests that the physiological factors are of great importance in the etiology of many forms of mental illness. But it is also clear that drugs can never be the total answer to the problems of mental health, which also involves factors of social environment and psychological development.

Some forms of psychoactive agents have been used since the beginning of civilization. Alcoholic beverages were invented at the same time as the invention of cereal agriculture. Extreme ethical concerns over the use of psychoactive drugs, however, did not develop until recent years. In the last 30 years, several pharmacological compounds have been developed or synthesized that alter mental and emotional functioning and are readily available to the public at large. Some of these drugs have demonstrated value to treat specific mental illness, but some others like lysergic acid diethylamide (LSD) have not proved as useful in therapy as was first hoped.

The extent to which psychoactive drugs are used in this society is itself an ethical concern. Antipsychotic, antidepressant, and antianxiety drugs are used not only by people who are severely ill and unable to manage their emotions without medication but also by relatively normal people attempting to control anxiety, tension, depression, insomnia, and other states arising from the stress of life in modern society. Although the psychotropic drugs available for behavior control at present comprise an impressive array, the potential for the future is even more awesome. Gerald Klerman says, "As knowledge of the relationship between brain and behavior increases, it is likely we will develop knowledge of the neurochemical and neuropharmocological bases of memory, learning, mood, aggression, appetite and sexual lust."[5] Hence, not only must psychoactive drugs be evaluated as therapeutic agents, but also future ethical evaluation must consider their potential to improve capabilities and enhance personal pleasure and enjoyment of life.

3. *Operant Conditioning.* Operant conditioning is a form of behavior control that can be used even for normal persons. In fact, B. F. Skinner argues that in the future it will replace all other forms of ethical education and social control. Here we need only point out two aspects of his proposal that have important ethical implications.

First, Skinner denies that human beings possess the power to choose freely between alternate modes of activity, since he is convinced that his experiments have demonstrated that all human behavior is deterministically shaped from birth by environmental forces. According to Skinner, "Freedom and dignity are myths that are preventing us from seeing how continually and subtly we are being shaped by our environment."[6]

Second, in the process of operant conditioning there is no need to let people know their behavior is being changed. Moreover, changes in behavior can be determined for the masses by an elite group of managers. It is evident that Skinner assumes without question that his own humanist values will be inculcated. In other hands, of course, antihumanistic values might be enforced just as effectively. For Skinner, all education is operant conditioning.

Ethical Guidelines

Given these examples of behavior control and modification methods that are prevalent and are becoming more common every day, we suggest several ethical principles that should govern their use, all of which are applications of the more general principle of human dignity in community, which requires that social control enhance the dignity of the members of the community, not reduce them to mere means of political manipulation.

1. No form of treatment may be used that will destroy human freedom. Pius XII stated this well when he wrote:

> In exercising one's right to dispose of oneself or one's faculties and organs, the individual must observe the hierarchy of individual goods to the extent demanded by the laws of morality, so, for example, a person cannot perform upon him or herself or allow medical operations, either physical or somatic, which beyond doubt do remove serious defects or physical or psychic weaknesses, but which entail at the same time permanent destruction of or a considerable lasting lessening of freedom, that is to say, of the human personality in its particular and characteristic functions.[7]

Thus, any form of psychosurgery, personality manipulation, and use of psychoactive drugs that would remove or severely limit human freedom or destroy human personality could not be permitted and may need legal control.

2. If the purpose of the behavior control is therapeutic, then the benefit to the patient must be proportionate to the damage or risk to be endured. A frontal lobotomy, for example, should be performed only as a last resort and with some indication that the patient will benefit. As a general rule, signs of organic brain pathology should be present before psychosurgery is approved.

3. If the purpose of the treatment is therapeutic, the long-range effect of the treatment must be considered as well as the short-range alleviation of some particular difficulty. Simply because a particular therapy alleviates or eliminates

a symptom does not mean that it is ethically acceptable. Most of the drugs currently available for the relief of anxiety and tension carry some danger of dependency, habituation, and addiction. Such dependency diminishes human freedom and dignity and hence is to be avoided. Thus, the practice of using psychoactive drugs to treat psychological difficulties when the disorder lacks a physiological or organic basis must be questioned. Would it not be better to treat the causes of anxiety or depression through counseling or increased self-awareness rather than to depend on pills that merely treat the symptom? Questions such as this are fundamental in developing a philosophy of health care, and they are too often neglected in search of easier, but less beneficial, solutions.

4. If behavior controls are used, the rules of free and informed consent apply, including the right to refuse treatment. Thus, operant conditioning, psychoactive drugs, and psychotherapy should not be imposed on persons unwillingly. Moreover, children, prisoners, and people with a limited sense of awareness should not be subjected to experimental behavioral control, nor should proxy consent be given unless the treatment is truly therapeutic for them.

5. The principle of professional communication as regards confidentiality must be applied with special care in psychotherapy, since the patient's trust in the therapist is of fundamental importance.

6. Experimental research on behavioral control should conform to the norms explained previously in the section on human experimentation.

7. Use of behavioral control procedures to improve human capabilities such as memory, intelligence, and sexual abilities would seem to be licit if free consent is given, if there is no other way to achieve the same goal, and if the action is in accord with the integrity of the human person. In itself, human betterment, or human improvement, is ethically acceptable and beneficial. Care must be exercised, however, to make sure that the basic integrity of the person is not violated and that addiction does not result in the course of seeking self-improvement.

10.5 Addiction

Generally speaking, addiction is habituation to some harmful practice. Although the term *addiction* usually refers to habituation to drugs, one can also be addicted to other detrimental substances or activities: for example, one can be addicted to alcohol or excessive food and also to too much sleep, too much work, and pursuit of sexual pleasure. Although many people use all these things in ways that do not destroy human equilibrium, some persons, for a variety of reasons not fully understood, become addicted to them so that their whole life is more and more absorbed by a single activity that distorts the personality, consumes physical and psychic energy and often results in an intense self-centeredness, personality deterioration, and inability to communicate with others.

One component of chemical dependency, and the most obvious, is its hedonistic character, although persons who are in other respects very ascetic may fall victims to it, precisely because they lack healthy pleasures in their lives. In the face of every difficulty of life, every tension or frustration, the chemically dependent person runs away from the loss of normal satisfaction and achievement by indulging in the physical pleasure, relaxation, and euphoria of the addicting experience. The search for pleasure alone does not constitute addiction, but rather the increasing sense of guilt and helplessness that begin to accompany each overindulgence—with the result that the incipient addict begins to indulge not for the sake of pleasure itself but to blot out the guilt and remorse for the consequences of previous indulgences. Furthermore, this vicious circle is reinforced by the use of psychological coping mechanisms of rationalization and denial that victims need to suppress guilt and pain, so that they become increasingly unable to perceive the real consequences of their behavior. Persons of very different personality types can become addicted, but a common feature is excessive *dependency* needs, not infrequently masked by outward aggressiveness and competitiveness. Moreover, recent research demonstrates that chemical dependency can affect people of all backgrounds. Often the gifted, talented, wealthy, and successful succumb to this severe personality problem.

Chemical dependency or addiction may be broadly classified as physiological or psychological. *Physiological addiction*, which causes a modification or need in the addict's physiological system, usually requires increasing doses of the addicting substance to obtain the same physiological effect. *Psychological dependency* itself results from a learned conditioned behavior pattern that leads the victim to anticipate the pleasure and release of tension, even when the substance does not notably modify the physiological system.

Solutions

Would chemical addiction be less of a problem in this country if it were considered a medical or social problem rather than a moral and legal one? Removing the moral stigma from addiction to alcohol has been helpful in assisting many people to overcome this addiction. Would a similar response to the use of drugs, plus legalization of narcotics for sustaining treatment of addicts, be beneficial over a long time? On the one hand, therapists speak of addiction as a "disease" to reduce its moral opprobrium and to achieve a more sympathetic attitude on the part of nonaddicts; and on the other, an important part of therapy is to get addicts to accept moral responsibility for the harm they have done themselves and others through addiction. This ambiguity can be cleared up if two points are kept in mind. First, chemical dependency is always a psychological disease, since it involves an abnormal behavior pattern accompanied by the neurotic coping mechanisms already described. It can also be a physiological disease because it sometimes produces physiological dependency and usually produces widespread organic changes that greatly aggravate the condition. Second, *voluntary* acts must be distinguished from *free* acts. Addictive behavior is voluntary in the sense that it proceeds from an inner compulsion, but it always involves a restriction of freedom, since the addict becomes less and less able to perceive alternatives of action or to choose among them. In times of addictive need the practical conscience of the addict is concerned totally with the need for a drink or a fix. He or she acts voluntarily, compulsively, but without fully free choice.

Hence, actual consumption of addictive substances by addicts is not always in itself a morally culpable act, and the guilt felt afterward may be unrealistic and neurotic. Even the acquisition of the addiction often proceeds so gradually and subtly that it is difficult to judge that the addict knowingly and deliberately chose addiction. Nevertheless, it would be a mistake to think that the *whole* guilt felt by addicts is illusory. If it were, it would be hard to explain why admission of responsibility has proved so important a part of therapy. The truth seems to be that the real moral responsibility of the addicted person lies in the obligation to ask and receive help from others when this is offered, since therapy cannot be effective until the addict accepts help. Hence, it is a mistake to reduce this complex situation either to a purely moral question or to a purely sociological or medical one. To deny all moral responsibility or capacity to change is to degrade addicts as persons, yet to pass judgment on their degree of responsibility is to misjudge the many ways in which they are victims of forces beyond individual control.

Students of addiction emphasize that the earlier the addiction therapy takes place the better, but they also point out that family and employers commonly contribute to the problem by covering up, excusing, or attempting to endure addictive behavior, hoping that the addict will finally come to his or her senses. In fact this spontaneous self-insight on the part of addicts is very rare, and family, friends, and employers have a serious ethical responsibility to face the facts realistically and intervene decisively and persistently until the addict accepts treatment. Intervention is best done by those who can be supportive rather than judgmental but who can also face the addict with detailed evidence of the seriousness of his or her condition. Human beings grow as persons by facing the difficulties and struggles of life realistically, "bearing one another's burdens" (Ga 6:2) as free people, not as slaves to a pleasure ethic. In saying this, we are not proposing an exaggerated stoicism as the Christian ideal, but a realistic effort to overcome the real causes of suffering, rather than an escape into unconsciousness. Alcoholics Anonymous, which has led the way in the most successful methods of therapy for chemical dependency, has always emphasized that the addict cannot recover without a reaching out for a Higher Power and willingness to repair damage done to others and to be of service to them, especially to fellow victims of addiction.

10.6 Conclusion

Simply because one has ethical goals does not mean that one will always use ethical means to reach those goals. Psychotherapy and behavior modification have the ethical goals of helping people overcome mental illness or harmful behavior. However, both forms of therapy must be analyzed carefully lest individuals' rights be violated or the freedom of the person be weakened or destroyed. Care must be exercised, then, when helping the mentally ill regain their health, so that the person's higher needs and functions are considered.

Footnotes

1. Ken Kesey, *One Flew Over the Cuckoo's Nest* (New York: Viking Press, 1962).

2. Richard Restak, *Pre-Meditated Man: Bioethics and the Control of Future Human Life* (New York: Viking Press, 1973).

3. Robert Harper, *Psychoanalysis and Psychotherapy: 36 Systems* (Englewood, NJ: Prentice-Hall, 1959), pp. 152-155.

4. Phillip Rieff, *The Triumph of the Therapeutic: Uses of Faith After Freud* (New York: Harper & Row, 1968).

5. Gerald Klerman, "Drugs and Social Values," *International Journal of Addiction* V (1970): 2-19.

6. B. F. Skinner, *Beyond Freedom and Dignity* (New York: Knopf, 1971), p. 30.

7. Pope Pius XII, "Allocution to Congress of Histopathology," Sept. 14, 1953; *The Human Body* (Boston: St. Paul Editions), p. 361.

Study Questions

1. Discuss the relationships between mental illness, human freedom, and personal sin.

2. Discuss the meaning of the term, "a normal person," and suggest criteria to determine whether or not a person is normal.

3. Describe the proper attitude of a counselor or psychotherapist to the value system of a neurotic or psychotic patient.

4. Debate the issue: Insight therapy is a more ethical form of healing persons than behavioral control.

5. Describe the process of acquiring addictive behavior and indicate the moral responsibilities of the subject at various stages of the process.

6. What reasons would you give for the increase in use of addictive substances by teenagers and young adults?

Cases

1. A "halfway house" for recovering psychiatric patients is proposed for your neighborhood. Fearing for their safety and property values, your neighbors protest the location of the facility in your area. What arguments would you use to help them reconsider their decision?

2. Dr. Philip is a Catholic psychiatrist who regularly provides counseling for homosexual men. He believes that his responsibility is to assist them in adjusting to their life styles. He does not think that it is his responsibility to try to bring them to conform to Catholic teachings on homosexuality. Are his beliefs morally acceptable from the Catholic perspective? What are the moral responsibilities of a Catholic health care professional in these situations?

3. At a state psychiatric hospital, the standard policy is to send as many people back into society as possible and to sedate those who are confined to the hospital in order to make them more manageable. What ethical norms would you develop for the release of patients and for the therapy of permanent patients if you were the CEO of this hospital?

4. Father Jerry is 40 years old and has been a priest for 15 years. Experiencing severe anxiety about the effectiveness of his priestly ministry and dissatisfaction with his present parochial assignment, he approaches his bishop with his problems. The bishop responds that Fr. Jerry is not praying enough, otherwise he would be a happy priest. Fr. Jerry comes to you as a friend; how would you seek to help him?

5. Mary, a mother and housewife, enjoys several martinis before preparing dinner for her husband and four children. After she burns the main course three nights in a row, Harry, her husband, suggests that she might have a problem with alcohol. Mary violently rejects the idea, but later asks your opinion. What information and help would you offer her?

Chapter 11
Suffering and Death

11.1 The Mystery of Suffering and Death

Health care professionals who assume a position of unlimited power in the process of healing have an unrealistic outlook. They think of themselves as the persons who cure, rather than realizing that it is God who cures and health care professionals who cooperate in this work by using the forces of nature.

"Death was not God's doing; he takes no pleasure in the extinction of the living. To be—for this he created all" (Ws 1:13-14). God had not wished to include suffering and death in man's destiny. Whence, then, came suffering and death? St. Paul says, "Through one man sin entered the world and with sin death, death thus coming to all men inasmuch as all sinned" (Rm 5:12). This original sin was essentially a sin of pride, the will to be like God not by using God's gifts to come closer to God in community, but to use these gifts to set up the human individual in self-centered domination of the world apart from God. It is this misuse of God's gifts from the beginning of the human race to this day that has prevented humankind from overcoming the natural causes of death and transformed what might have been a joyful completion of this life and a serene passage into a greater life, into a blind, terrifying mystery.

Although people have turned their backs on God, he has not turned from them but has offered them forgiveness and restoration. Yet in his mercy, he cannot deny their human freedom but has called them to return to him, not simply by restoring them to their innocent beginnings, but by a long history of struggle and learning from experience, an experience in which suffering is inevitable. For the Christian and for all who travel the same road in less clear ways, God has revealed in Christ the direction of their journey and the power of grace by which it can be traveled. In baptism, according to St. Paul (Rm 6:1-11), through the Cross of Christ man has died and been reborn in a new creation that will be completed in the resurrection of the body in eternal life. Men live now in such unity with Christ that all the events of their lives take on meaning from his life and death. Consequently, both the joy and the suffering of this life have a Christian meaning: its joys are signs of the hope for everlasting life in his kingdom, which is already present here on earth in promise, and its sorrows are a sharing in his Cross through which a victorious resurrection is to be achieved.

Jesus came to conquer suffering and death. In what sense has he succeeded? People still get sick and continue to suffer, and death is inevitable. He conquered sickness, suffering, and death in the sense that he gave them a new meaning, a new power. By believing in Jesus as Savior, by joining suffering and death to his, mankind overcomes the evil aspect of suffering and death. Through his sacrifice, man is able to conquer the evil that is associated with suffering and death. Although the results of original and actual sin are still present in life, they no longer dominate it and they no longer serve as punishment. Rather, suffering and death are transformed into the very actions that help mankind fulfill its destiny.

At one time death was defined as separation of body and soul. Although this definition is correct, it is no longer adequate. In their attempts to specify more clearly what it means to die, modern theologians have concentrated on death as a personal act of a human being—an act that terminates earthly existence but that also fulfills it. Hence, the person is not merely passive in the face of death, and death is different for the just and the sinner. In the view of Karl Rahner, a view accepted and developed by many theologians, death is an active consummation, a maturing self-realization that embodies what each person has made of himself or herself during life.[2] Death becomes a ratification of life, not merely an inevitable process. It is an event, an action in which the freedom of the person is intimately involved. Dying with Christ is an adventure, a consequence of, but not a penalty for, sin. This is a new approach to death, yet it is thoroughly in keeping with the Christian tradition. Indeed, this view of death seems to describe more clearly the experience of Christ, who offered his life, rather than have it taken from him, who completed his love and generosity in the final act of obedience to the Father.

11.2 Determining Death

When biologists speak of the death of any living organism, they refer to that inevitable and critical moment when an organism ceases to function as a specific, unified, homeostatic system and becomes disorganized into a mere collection of heterogeneous chemical substances. From a biological point of view, the death of a human organism is like any death and is determined in much the same way, by various signs that the unifying life functions have ceased. But people believe that human death is something more. Human death has a mystery about it, because at death we lose touch irrevocably with a person who previously was able to communicate and to share our human community of thought, of love, of freedom, and of creativity. Human death is not merely a decay of an organism, it is the departure of a member of the human community.

The world over, people have interpreted this departure of someone known and loved as the separation of a spiritual soul from its body. Certainly, science is unable to close the door on such an explanation. Christians are convinced that the departed will return in their full bodily personhood in a transformed existence, as Jesus did. In any case, people often have the painful responsibility of determining when the death of another has occurred, because the time of death influences many other human decisions such as inheritance, legal and moral rights possessed by the dying person, spiritual care for the dying person, and the possibility of organ transplantation.

Dying is a process, but death is an event. We can be certain this event has not yet occurred as long as a person can communicate through speech or gesture. When such communication ceases, we can only judge by signs that are no longer distinctly and specifically human. Yet we do not dare to conclude that death has occurred merely because such specifically human signs are no longer evident, as becomes very clear when we observe someone wake from sleep or coma.

Consequently, we are morally obliged to treat anybody who is apparently human (even in the fetal state) as a human person with human rights until we are sure that this body has become so disorganized that it no longer retains its human unity. To know this we must be reasonably sure of three things: (1) that the body does not now exhibit specific human behavior, (2) that it will not be able to function humanly in the future, and (3) that it no longer has even a radical capacity for human functions because it has lost the basic structures required for human unity. This third condition is required because medical experience has shown that persons who have been in prolonged, apparently irreversible coma nevertheless have sometimes recovered full human consciousness. Such resuscitation is possible as long as the radical structures of the human organism remain and the causes that inhibit their normal function can be removed. This is why some speculate that in the future the human body may be able to be frozen and revived centuries later.

[margin note: Three signs of death*]*

After true human death some cells or even organs of the human body may for a time (perhaps indefinitely if artificially supported) continue to exhibit some life functions that are not those of the human organism as a unified entity but merely a residual life at a level of organization comparable to that of plants and lower animals. Hence, the essential point about determining human death is not to decide whether *any* life is present, but whether human life in the most radical sense of a unified human person is still present.

Signs of Death

Certainly, some signs of human death were always easy to identify. If rigor mortis or putrefaction occurred, then even nonprofessionals were able to recognize that the human organism was irreversibly destroyed. Other less conclusive signs of human death were the absence of breathing and heartbeat, although it was known that these functions might sometimes be revived by such methods of resuscitation as were then available. When such efforts failed, death was judged certain. Physicians were required to pronounce the patient dead on the basis of such evidence and certify the time of death for legal purposes such as inheritance. Thus, cessation of spontaneous heart and lung function became known as the *clinical* signs of death.

In recent times, two developments have led to the proposal of a new set of clinical signs for determining the fact of human death. First of all, machines have been perfected to aid heart and lung function artificially, or to enable a person to be resuscitated after the heart and lungs have ceased to function for a short time. Often people recover full and spontaneous heart and lung function after being temporarily assisted by such machines, proving that the radical structures of the unified human organism had not been destroyed. On the other hand, it seems certain that such machines are able to maintain heart and lung action, at least temporarily, even after this unity of the organism has ceased to exist, since the heart completely separated from the body can continue to beat, and tissues in a test tube can continue to exhibit some residual life if nourished by an appropriate solution.

Thus, such artificially sustained heart and lung action are not proof that human life still remains, yet as long as they are sustained it is impossible to verify the traditional signs of human death. Therefore, the question arises: Are there other clinical signs that can be used, not necessarily to constitute a new definition of death, but rather as alternative complementary means to establish the same essential fact, namely, the irreversible cessation of spontaneous heart and lung function.

The second, and perhaps more important, reason for seeking new clinical signs of death has been the recent advancement of techniques of organ transplantation, especially of the kidney and heart. Such transplantations are more likely to be successful if the organs are freshly harvested from a body through which blood is circulating, although this is not absolutely necessary. Hence, surgeons prefer to keep the body of a "dead" donor "alive" on a respirator. How, then, is it possible to be sure that the donor is in fact dead?

Is the Person Dead?

First, the traditional cardiovascular clinical signs are basic and sufficient and should be retained; the new brain death criteria should be employed only when such signs cannot be used because the dying person depends on a respirator or other form of artificial maintenance. If brain death is permitted to become the exclusive definition (as is the increasing tendency in some states), no one can be judged dead without elaborate tests in a hospital. Present moral dilemmas about how to determine death are due in large part to excessive reliance on technology, and the excess should be moderated rather than encouraged.

Second, the new brain death criteria must be ascertained by well-trained professionals. Human error and even carelessness must be anticipated and avoided. How can errors be prevented when human life is at stake? The *Harvard Criteria for Brain Death*, a widely accepted document, envisions a process of observation for no less than 24 hours.[3] Moreover, the persons using the electroencephalogram (EEG) must be trained to recognize such conditions as hypothermia and drug-induced coma, which may produce a flat EEG in a patient who can recover, since the flat EEG alone is not an infallible sign of death. Today, shorter intervals of observation are sometimes allowed in protocols approved by various medical groups, for example, 6 hours. The EEG is replaced in some protocols by an angiogram to test blood flow in the cerebellum.

Third, and most serious, is the question about the nature of brain death itself. It is critical that the criteria used to certify brain death establish that the person is dead, not merely dying or in a deep coma. While the medical profession has accepted the general idea of using the brain as the main criteria in some cases to establish human death, just which specific signs should be used to determine that human death has occurred have not been agreed upon by all. Thus, one group of physicians maintains that irreversible cessation of brain functions is not sufficient to signify human death because that does not indicate that the brain has been destroyed.[4] Most neurosurgeons would respond that if the brain has ceased to function irreversibly, then it is destroyed because blood is not circulating effectively, even though the brain may not have lost all signs of cellular activity. Although it is not our purpose to settle any of the differences of opinion in regard to medical matters, it is our theological conclusion that when total and irreversible function of brain activity is clinically proved, then the person in question is dead because the form (soul) is no longer able to inform the matter (body). To date, many states have approved this method of discerning human death in so-called definition of death legislation, and the need for national legislation in this regard has been recommended. The legislation of the various states requires that the signs indicate that total, not merely partial, death of the brain has occurred.

Partial Brain Death

Would it be possible to declare a person dead if only some part of the brain, that is, the higher or neocortical centers on which it appears specifically human thought processes depend, ceased to function? Some are willing to defend this latter view. Thus, the philosophers Robert Rizzo and Paul Yonder state:

> We must ask whether the death of the cerebral cortex or neocortex signals human death, even though other parts may be still functioning for a time....We offer the hypothesis that human death should be related to the cessation of functions distinctly human since breathing, heartbeat and circulation are vegetative processes shared by other animals.
>
> From all clinical evidence the death of the neocortex marks the end of the physiological basis for human consciousness, that is, a consciousness unique in its powers of reflection. It signals the end of the brain as a dynamic integrated whole and presages in most cases the imminent death of other cerebral systems.[5]

Despite some support for the position that cortical death constitutes human death, this position presents several difficulties. First, if people who have spontaneously functioning hearts and lungs, but no other vital signs, are declared dead, what about people who have weak signs of "human life"? If those in a deep and irreversible coma are declared dead insofar as human life is concerned, then what about people who are mentally retarded or senile? Do they show sufficient signs of human life to be kept alive? Or should even minimal care be given only to those who no longer have the functioning signs of human life that are associated with activity of the cortical center of the brain? Persons who argue for the elimination of the retarded, senile, infirm, and debilitated in certain circumstances believe partial brain death should be accepted as a proper clinical sign for human death. But society must go very slowly in accepting such a definition unless it is willing to bury people when they are still breathing and their hearts are pulsating spontaneously.

If the criteria of *partial* brain death were to be used as a sufficient evidence of death, ethical responsibility would require certitude about three matters of fact. First, the radical structures necessary and sufficient to constitute the unified organism of the human person would have to be found in the human brain separated from the rest of the body. This certainly is plausible from what is now known. Second, most of the brain would have to be considered unnecessary for the specifically human functions of thinking and willing but existing only to maintain and move the body and supply the higher brain centers with nourishing materials. This also is plausible, but in the present state of knowledge, far from certain. It is generally recognized today that the brain is a system of subsystems that are intimately interdependent. Although it is possible to localize such functions as speech and sight in particular parts of the brain, this is not proof that only one such part is involved in the function or even that it is its primary center, since inhibition of a merely secondary or auxiliary part of a system may impede its function. Third, if it were certain that these higher centers are sufficient for the radical unity of the human organism, it would be very difficult to determine their exact condition without an autopsy. The mere absence of function would not establish their condition. Perhaps some day it may be possible to determine when in special cases such centers are totally destroyed, but at present this is not the case. ✗

Hence, while we accept total brain death as a sufficient criterion for human death, we do not believe that partial brain death is a sufficient criterion. Thus, we do not believe that death should be certified as long as patients are able to maintain spontaneous breathing and heartbeat, since this constitutes strong evidence that the brain as the seat of the radical unity of the human body is still living, even if it is not evidencing its higher functions. Although even then there may be reasonable doubts, the benefit of the doubt should be given to the survival of the comatose person.

11.3 Truth Telling to the Dying

"What to tell the patient" has been considered one of the more difficult and delicate ethical questions for health care professionals. The principle of professional communication is relevant here. In the not too distant past, some physicians and other health care professionals thought that the less the patients knew about their condition, the better would be the chances of recovery. Moreover, some health care professionals would even withhold information of impending death, fearing that such knowledge might lead a person to despair. Because of an awakened moral sense on the part of health care professionals and a sharper realization that patients have legal and moral rights that must be respected, today there is a much greater tendency to be open and honest with patients concerning their condition. In general, patients have the right to the truth concerning their condition, the purpose of the treatment to be given, and the prognosis of the treatment. The *Ethical and Religious Directives for Catholic Health Facilities* (United States Catholic Conference, 1975) declare:

> Everyone has the right and duty to prepare for the solemn moment of death. Unless it is clear, therefore, that a dying patient is already well-prepared for death as regards both temporal and spiritual affairs, it is the physician's duty to inform him of his critical condition or to have some other responsible person impart this information (n. 8).

Clearly, information concerning serious sickness or impending death is to be furnished even if the individual does not ask for it. Legal precedent as well as moral concern prompts this realization. Hence, physicians and other health care professionals may not defend their lack of communication on the grounds that the patient did not wish to know and did not ask questions. Although health care professionals usually respect patients' rights insofar as providing the proper information is concerned, difficult situations often arise and health care professionals hesitate to tell patients their true condition.

Even though the medical personnel might fear untoward results if patients are informed of their true condition, this does not mean that patients should not be told the true facts. Indeed, health care professionals should remember in these cases the words of Eric Cassell, "The depression in patients that commonly occurs after the diagnosis of a fatal disease seems to stem in part from the conspiracy of silence. The physician can be a great help by simply making it clear to the patient that he is available for open and direct communication."[6] Hence, the medical team, along with a friend of the patient or a member of the family, should work together and dispose the patient so that he or she will be able to accept the truth. Interviews with people who are seriously ill or with dying patients reveal that they do not wish to be kept continually in doubt about their condition; on the other hand, they do not want it revealed to them abruptly or brutally.

Howard Brody assesses the practical situation aptly when he states:

> Telling a patient something takes place over a span of time and is not a one-shot affair. Thus, the shading or phrases used, whether the truth is delivered all at once or in small doses, and the kind of follow-up are all important parts of the ethical decision, as well as "tell" or "don't tell." A decision to reveal a grave prognosis, which may be "ethical" in itself, may become "unethical" if the physician tells the patient bluntly and then withdraws, without offering any emotional support to help the patient resolve his feelings. In fact, the assurance that the physician plans to see it through along with the patient, and that he will always make himself available to offer any comfort possible, may be more important than the bad news itself. In many of the "sour cases" that are offered as justification for withholding the truth, it may well be the absence of this transmission of compassion, rather than the telling of the truth, that produced the unfortunate result.[7]

In summary, increased knowledge of psychology and greater regard for the subjective process that accompanies sickness and dying has changed the ethical question in regard to truth telling. As Elisabeth Kübler-Ross declares: "The question should not be 'should we tell?' but rather, 'How do we share this with the patient?'"[8]

11.4 Euthanasia and Suicide

The word *euthanasia* is derived from two Greek words that mean "good death" or "happy death." For centuries, the term referred to an action by which a person was put to death painlessly, usually to avoid further suffering from an incurable disease or to end an irreversible coma. *Webster's New International Dictionary* (3rd ed.), for example, defines *euthanasia* as "a mode or act of inducing death painlessly as a relief from pain." Euthanasia in this sense is often called "mercy killing" or even "death with dignity." In the more traditional meaning of the term, it could be performed with or without the consent of the person to be put to death. In the Judeo-Christian tradition, euthanasia without the consent of the patient would be murder, and with consent of the patient would be both suicide and murder. Today, the proponents of euthanasia generally defend it in this latter form where the patient's consent is given or at least presumed. Thus, our ethical analysis needs to begin with the question of whether suicide is ever permissible or whether it exceeds the limits of rightful control over one's own life.

It is important to be clear that the issue here is not whether persons who commit suicide are to be morally condemned. No doubt the great majority of persons who take their own lives do so because they are so emotionally disturbed that they act compulsively, or at least their perception of objective reality is so distorted by their anguish and depression that their freedom of choice is greatly restricted. Consequently, either their act is not to be evaluated ethically at all, or at least it may be assumed that they act in good faith and are subjectively guiltless. Indeed many experts in suicidology today seem to take it for granted that all suicides are compulsive and irrational. Can this assumption really be made, or is there the possibility that the decision about whether to live or to take one's life may be a genuine ethical issue for some people who have the capacity to make a free and sane choice? Only in such cases does it make any sense to talk about the *morality* of suicide.

Stewardship of Life

The monotheistic religions of Judaism, Christianity, and Islam have always opposed suicide because they regard life as God's gift that his children are to use as faithful stewards. Moreover, these monotheistic religions, unlike others, hold that eternal life is not the survival of a disembodied soul, nor endless reincarnation, but resurrected life with God. Consequently, Christians cannot escape accounting to God for stewardship of the bodies given them on earth, nor can they reject the body, which will always be part of them. This view was already anticipated by the great Greek philosopher Plato who argued that suicide is a rejection of duty to one's body, to the community of which the person is a part, and to God who gave the person life. In a very different way, another great philosopher, Kant, argued that suicide is the greatest of crimes because it is man's rejection of morality itself, since man must be his own moral lawgiver. To kill oneself is to treat oneself as a thing (a means) rather than as a person.

It is probable that the personal reasons for suicide often underlie the social arguments. Basically persons kill themselves because "there is no other way out." The question, therefore, is whether this can ever be reasonably said to be true. There is no doubt that one can feel this way easily enough, but can one conscientiously judge that it is really the case? Essentially, humans are historical beings oriented to the future. As long as there is hope for a future, suicide is clearly unreasonable. When hope in the future is closed off, suicide may look like a rational thing to do. In a Christian scheme of values, however, hope in God grounds the future. By God's providence even the most painful situations not only can be endured but also may be extremely important events in the completion of earthly life. Christians should wait on the God who gave them life, because he knows best how to prepare them for the mystery of eternal life with him. Even Humanists and Marxists who deny any future life ought logically to reject suicide. No matter how painful their life may be, it is the only value left to them. As long as they live they have some possibility of human experience and action, but if they kill themselves they have chosen nothingness, not rest, nor sleep, just nothing.

Granted that suicide is intrinsically wrong, it also becomes clear that active euthanasia is also wrong, although this is today a widely debated question. When sufferers freely choose to die and ask to be killed, they are not only committing the crime of suicide but are also compounding it by making another a partner in the crime. To yield to such a request is false compassion. To have true compassion for the person who has made such a decision is to realize that the person is hopeless, alienated from community, and doubtful of God's love. The mercy killer in such a case is really adding a final rejection to the many rejections that have already driven the person to that point of despair.

On the other hand, if the sufferer is no longer really free to make a truly human decision, but is pleading to be put out of the pain or depression that has taken away the sufferer's capacity to think straight, then the mercy killer is simply a murderer putting to death someone no longer able to protect himself or herself.

If the motives of mercy killers are examined, their claim that they did it for the victim's sake cannot be easily accepted. The real motive may well be that the relative did not want to accept the responsibility of helping the dying person to the end. Often the killer says, "I loved my mother, I couldn't bear to see her suffer!" It is true in such a case that the killer could not bear to see her suffer, but the quality of that love is not so certain. No doubt, however, sometimes mercy killers are themselves not free enough from tortured feelings to make a sane decision.

11.5 Allowing to Die

For the Christian, human life is a gift from the Creator, control of which implies stewardship, not absolute autonomy. It is like the talents given by the master to his servants, which he expects them to invest to gain him a proper return (Mt 25:14-30). Hence, this gift of human life in this existence must be used to a good purpose. Life in this existence then is not the ultimate value for the Christian. Rather the Christian directs human life to the service of God and neighbor, and ultimately to sharing life with the Trinity in eternity. The time may come, therefore, when someone is reasonably convinced that life is coming to an end, and a prolongation of dying by additional medical treatment would make it more difficult to serve God and neighbor. Put another way, prolonging life may not contribute to the spiritual purpose of life (love of God and neighbor) or would make the achievement of that purpose very difficult. Hence, if further therapy is *useless* or a *severe burden* insofar as attaining the spiritual purpose of life is concerned, the therapy may be refused. It would be better, one might judge, to use the remaining time to compose oneself for death than to extend life in a burdensome manner that would only add to suffering and confusion of spirit for oneself and for relatives and friends. To reject such additional medical efforts is not to reject life itself, or the God who gave it, but simply to reject the means to prolong life which in other circumstances might be judged morally necessary. A decision to allow oneself to die in such circumstances "is not the equivalent of suicide. On the contrary it should be considered as an acceptance of the human condition, or a wish to avoid the application of a medical procedure disproportionate to the results that can be expected, or a desire not to impose excessive expense on the family or the community."[9]

Notice then that the determination of what is *useless* or *burdensome* is not to be made solely by assessing the physiological function, the physical pain, or the monetary expenditure associated with the therapy. Prolonged physiological function, physical pain, and the money involved are to be considered insofar as they affect the individual's ability to serve God and neighbor (strive for the spiritual purpose of life). Unless one keeps the spiritual purpose of life in mind when evaluating life-prolonging measures, ultimately one uses physiological function or economic criteria (cost/benefit ratio) as the sole standard for making difficult ethical decisions.

In the same way, the relatives and the medical professionals who care for the dying person unable to make competent decisions may judge that any further efforts to preserve life will be *useless* or of *no significant benefit* and may even make it more difficult for the person to finish the course of life in peace, composure, and union with God. Hence they can make the decision to terminate the supports that prolong the dying process and allow the person to die more quickly.

Finding the right words to express the judgment that efforts to prolong life are no longer helpful to the person in question is difficult. We wish to avoid saying that a person has "a right to die," as many seem to be doing today, or that human beings exist "to get to heaven," or that one may be allowed to die if "life is useless." All these terms can lead to faulty conclusions. For example, some means of prolonging life may be judged useless, but human life is never useless because of the dignity of the gift and the transcendence of the Giver. Moreover, if one admits there is a right to die, then some would conclude that suicide is licit, which is not to be easily conceded. In discussing the decision to allow oneself or another to die, it is wise to avoid all slogans and spell out completely what one implies by this ethical terminology, recognizing that the distinction is difficult to define.

Although Catholic ethicists in general have little problem approving the decision to allow a person to die in the two above-mentioned situations, that is, if treatment is useless or severely burdensome, many physicians and nurses are not ready to remove life-support systems if it entails allowing a person to die. The reasons for this attitude can be summarized in the following three arguments: (1) it is difficult to know when a patient is terminally ill; (2) even though a patient may be desperately ill, some physicians will not give up hope of doing some good; indeed, they would identify "doing something to help" as their role; and (3) some physicians, wishing to avoid malpractice suits, are hesitant to remove life-sustaining means, even though they may no longer be useful.

Clearly, physicians and ethicists approach the dying patient with different emphases, the ethicist being more concerned with the effect the means have on the person's ability to strive for the spiritual purpose of life and the physician being more concerned with prolonging life. We believe that there need not be any radical disagreement between physicians and moralists, however, if three truths are understood clearly.

1. Physicians and moralists often use the terms *ordinary means* and *extraordinary means* with different connotations. Physicians use the terms ordinary and extraordinary insofar as the means to prolong life is standard and accepted or experimental and unproved. Ethicists, on the other hand, look to

the way in which the therapy will affect the person's ability to function at the spiritual level of human potential. If the therapy is useless or a severe burden insofar as the spiritual function is concerned then it is extraordinary. Thus, one might reject brain surgery to prolong life a few weeks if it might render one comatose for the remainder of one's life.

2. While the physician has the expertise and the right to make decisions concerning the usefulness or medical effects of some particular medical procedure, the patient (or the family of the patient) has the right to determine whether a particular medical procedure is ordinary or extraordinary from an ethical viewpoint.

3. If the means in question from an ethical viewpoint are determined to be ordinary, then they must be employed; if extraordinary, they may or may not be employed, the decision being made by the patient (or the family) in consultation with the physician, but ordinary care should continue.

In maintaining that one is free to decide not to prolong life because a grave burden would result, even though prolonging life is possible, we are affirming that, while human life is a great good, it is not the greatest good. The greatest good is friendship with God, charity. Thus, if prolonging life would seem to interfere with friendship with God, directly or indirectly, life need not be prolonged. This is the practical meaning of the word "burden": making it difficult for one to attain the purpose of life. Pope Pius XII expressed this thought in a statement that is quoted by non-Catholics as well as Catholics:

> Natural reason and Christian morals say that man (and whoever is entrusted with the task of taking care of his fellowman) has the right and duty in case of serious illness to take the necessary treatment for the preservation of life and health. This duty that one has toward himself, toward God, toward the human community, and in most cases toward certain determined persons, derives from a well-ordered charity, from submission to the Creator, from social justice and even from strict justice as well as from devotion toward one's family.
>
> But normally one is held to use only ordinary means—according to the circumstances of persons, places, times and cultures—that is to say, means that do not involve any grave burdens for oneself or another. *A more strict obligation would be too burdensome for most men and would render the attainment of a higher, more important good too difficult. Life, health, all temporal activities are in fact subordinated to spiritual ends.* On the other hand, one is not forbidden to take more than the strictly necessary steps to preserve life and health, as long as he does not fail in some more serious duty.[10] (Emphasis added.)

Is it ever easy to determine when to remove respirators or tube feeding? No. The practical difficulties in applying the ordinary and extraordinary distinction will always remain. Determining whether it is time to allow oneself to die, or to allow another to die, will always be complex. This is especially true if the decision involves discontinuing a means already used or withdrawal of life-support systems from newborns with birth defects, for instance. But following the above-mentioned principles offers the basis for compassionate and ethical decisions in any circumstance. Clearly, the tendency to relegate ethical decisions concerning prolonging life to the courts or the federal government should be resisted.

The Patient Decides

Who decides that life should or should not be prolonged and that a certain means is, ethically speaking, ordinary or extraordinary? Some place the burden primarily on the physician; some believe it should be the courts' duty to protect incompetent patients' rights. Clearly, the physician is deeply involved in the decision and must consider the patient's condition and determine the medical prognosis, that is, whether the means in question will cure, help appreciably, or have no effect on the dying patient. But other circumstances must be considered in addition to the medical effectiveness of the means. What about expense, pain, and inconvenience? Only the patient or the family can decide these circumstances. Hence, the radical right to make a decision on what would be an ordinary means and what would be an extraordinary means from an ethical point of view belongs to the patient. Following the principles of human dignity, informed consent, and professional communication, with the guidance of the physician, and consultation with relatives, the patient decides what actions should be performed and what should be omitted. The physician and patient relationship is expressed aptly in this manner:

> The rights and duties of the doctor are correlative to those of the patient. The doctor, in fact, has no separate or independent right where the patient is concerned. In general, he can take action only if the patient explicitly or implicitly, directly or indirectly, gives him permission.[11]

Proxy Consent

The most difficult problems arise when the patient is incompetent to decide (see Proxy Consent, p. 88). Special care must be taken to defend the right to life of such persons. Some physicians are tempted, for example, to judge too easily that newborns who suffer from a serious handicap are not to be treated despite the fact that parents, once they come to know and love such handicapped children, find their lives very precious. On the other hand, parents who have just been informed that a newborn is handicapped may too quickly decide to allow such children to die. Patients who are severely depressed may also refuse treatment that they would have accepted in a better frame of mind. Treating severe burn victims is difficult because they often ask to be allowed to die, even though many later declare they are happy therapy was instituted. Hence, the norms of proxy consent are not rigid and legalistic and for ethical application must be interpreted in accord with the patient's condition.

What of the patient medically judged to be in an irreversible coma? The guardian of such a patient should insist that this medical prognosis not be quickly made and should be carefully tested, as patients sometimes regain consciousness after a prolonged coma. Moreover, they should make sure that the patient is given ordinary nursing care. Although the comatose person is not conscious of this care, it is required by human dignity and respect for the feelings of others. Does such ordinary care always include the supplying of food and water through gastronasal or intravenous tubes? Some argue that it does because supplying food and water is not a medical treatment but a part of normal life processes. Supplying food and water is a normal life process insofar as persons who have the natural function intact to eat and digest food are concerned, such as infants and senile people. But tube feeding usually is introduced to circumvent or alleviate a pathology which makes natural eating and digestion impossible. Thus the tube feeding is usually a medical procedure. The American Medical Association, through its Council on Ethics and Judicial Affairs, declared that artificial hydration and nutrition may be removed from a patient in irreversible coma, care being taken to verify the diagnosis of this condition. We concur with this statement.[12]

Fear is expressed by some lest permitting the removal of such tubes and thereby allowing comatose people to die becomes a first step toward euthanasia. Certainly it is true that all abuses that lead to the acceptance of euthanasia are to be rejected. Nevertheless, the explanation already given of the meaning of extraordinary means should be followed in such cases. If the person will not be better able to strive for the purpose of life as a result of the therapy then the therapy is extraordinary and may be withheld. Put another way, if the use of gastronasal or intravenous feeding or hydration are proportionately of less benefit to the patient than the burden of prolonged care which is placed on others, then they are extraordinary and nonobligatory. Some might argue that the benefit of continued life outweighs any such burden, but for the irreversibly comatose patient this is not necessarily the case. Feeding of this sort is usually unable to prevent increasing debilitation, and the use of intubation is merely prolonging the dying process for patients unable to use that time for any beneficial activity. Even if the patient can be maintained in a comatose condition indefinitely, it is difficult to claim that a long period of comatose life is of more human value than a short period.

11.6 Pain and Dying

The principle of growth through suffering has been considered in Chapter 6, but a few observations are relevant in regard to pain at time of death.

1. Pain is not an absolute human evil. Although suffering is truly an ontological evil to be alleviated whenever possible, it is not of itself a moral evil nor without supernatural and human benefits when rightly used. Some will scoff at this view of life, but the Christian tradition holds that great good can come out of suffering when this is joined to the suffering of Jesus. Although Christian teaching in this regard is often misrepresented, it does not imply a masochistic desire for pain, nor does it stand in the way of medical progress. As one group of Christians who have investigated the situation maintain, "A terminal illness can be transformed into a time for which everyone concerned is grateful."

2. Alleviating pain by medicine or even by surgery does not constitute active euthanasia, even if the suffering person's life might be shortened by the medical or surgical procedure. In this case, the direct object of the act is to relieve pain; if life is shortened, it is an accidental, even though foreseen, result. This view is expressed succinctly in the *Ethical and Religious Directives for Catholic Health Facilities*: "It is not euthanasia to give a dying person sedatives and analgesics for the alleviation of pain when such measure is judged necessary, even though they may deprive the patient of the use of reason, or shorten his life" (n. 29).

The opportunity to use suffering as a means of spiritual growth is not destroyed if painkilling drugs are used. Rather, the individual and those who care for him have the right to use such drugs to permit the best use of the patient's remaining energies, times of consciousness, and so forth, so that the patient can complete life with maximum composure.

3. In recent years, medical and psychological breakthroughs have occurred in regard to severe pain. Medically speaking, pharmaceutical and surgical procedures make it possible to control and alleviate severe pain in the hospital and at home. Severe and excruciating pain, then, is hardly a realistic excuse for direct euthanasia or suicide. Moreover, an even more startling discovery in the control of pain has been made by people in the hospice movement. Case studies demonstrate that pain is alleviated and controlled when human concern and care are given to the elderly. The ultimate human pain seems to be loneliness and the feeling of dying alone. If these feelings are overcome, it seems that pain is not such a prominent factor, even for those who are dying of debilitating diseases.

4. If the patient is unable to make the pertinent decisions, then the family, in consultation with the physician, should have the right and obligation to determine whether the means in question are ordinary or extraordinary and whether extraordinary means will be used. In making this decision, the family decides as would the patient and for the patient's benefit, not solely for the family's benefit.

5. Such documents as the living will or the *Christian Affirmation of Life* may be used by patients as a means of informing family and physician and as a help in preparing for death. (See page 237.) We do not, however, favor such documents being given legal status by natural death acts. Although such acts are not in themselves wrong, they do not solve any problems and potentially they may lead to disrespect for human life and inhuman care of the dying.

11.7 Care for the Corpse and Cadaver

When a human being dies, the body is no longer unified by the life-giving principle or soul by which it is a human person. The cadaver of a person, then, is not a *human* body in the proper sense of the word. Insofar as is possible, the remains of a person should not be referred to as though the human person existed *in* the human body or was, so to speak, limited by the human body. Language of this nature is misleading because it implies a duality in human existence; in a certain sense, the living human person *is* the living human body. When persons die, they exist in a new form, in a sense incomplete, because they no longer have a body. While existing in this life, the human person is a substantial unity of spirit (form) and body (matter), not an accidental juxtaposition of two distinct entities. Although the remains of a human body may resemble the body of a living person, and although this resemblance may be prolonged through embalming, the remains are not a *human* body but a mass of organic matter, decomposing into constitutive, organic elements.

If the corpse of a human person is not a human body, then why are people so concerned about proper care for the remains of the deceased person? Why treat it with the respect and reverence it usually receives? Respect and reverence are due the remains of a human being because of the sacredness of human life that once informed the now inert mass still bearing the person's bodily image. In order to mourn the fact that the person will no longer be present in the same human manner as before, certain reverential spiritual actions are performed to express the love of the people who remain. Respect for the dead body, then, signifies respect for human life, respect for the author of life, and respect for the person who once subsisted with this now corrupting corpse and who now exists in a different modality. Hence, the actions, the ritual that people follow when caring for the body of a deceased person have a meaning beyond their mere use.

Although the ritual of wake, funeral, and burial has been criticized for its gross and inhuman excesses, fundamentally this process has a meaning and worth in accord with the Judeo-Christian tradition. Having friends share the burden through liturgical services is also a source of strength and support for bereaved people. Hence, the legitimate customs of people at the time of death are not signs of superstition or blind fear; rather they bespeak a noble belief about life, its purpose, and the enduring strength of human love.

In accord with the respect due to the remains of a human person, no organs should be removed from a corpse, nor should the body be dismembered unless a sufficient reason justifies such an action. Usually the next of kin or the person to whom the corpse is committed for care has the legal right to determine if organs may be removed from the body and if an autopsy may be performed. The right of the next of kin in regard to caring for the human body is not absolute. It may be superseded by statements made by the person while still alive, for example, through the Uniform Anatomical Gift Act, or by the needs of society, for example, when an autopsy might help stave off a contagious disease.

The Anatomical Gift Act is "designed to facilitate the donation and use of human tissues and organs for transplantation and other medical purposes and provide a favorable legal environment for such activities."[12] At present, all 50 states have enacted the Gift Act, thus enabling persons who are of sound mind and 18 years of age or more to give all or part of their bodies to persons or institutions authorized to practice or perform research medicine, or to engage in tissue banking, the gift to take effect upon death. This law also recognizes the right of the next of kin to donate the body or any part for the same purpose, but in most states the law declares that if there is a conflict between the donor and the next of kin, the wishes of the donor have precedence. From a Christian point of view, the practice of donating organs and one's body for scientific research is ethical and even to be encouraged if a true need exists. Hence, we are in favor of laws that enable organs to be harvested from dead people who have not signed statements donating the organs. Such laws are common in Europe and have been enacted in some states for people killed in accidents.

Another ethical question, however, does not admit such easy solution: Is it immoral to accept or solicit payment for the gift of certain organs? While some have defended such practices, others maintain that abuses could spring up very quickly if cadaver organs were sold or contracted for money. With this latter opinion we agree. If society is to live in a humane manner, then generosity and charity, rather than monetary gain and greed, must serve as the basis for donation of functioning organs. Recent federal legislation has outlawed sale of human organs for transplant.[13]

Autopsy

Autopsy is the examination of a cadaver performed in order to provide greater medical knowledge concerning the cause of death. Occasionally, the benefit of an autopsy will be to provide knowledge about a rare or contagious disease. In such cases, the good of the community would overrule the rights of the next of kin, and if the next of kin were not willing, the court could order that an autopsy be performed. In cases of violent death or unattended death an autopsy is required by law, no matter what wishes are expressed by the next of kin.

Usually, however, the purpose of an autopsy is not to trace the etiology of a rare disease nor to discover unknown or violent causes of death. More frequently, autopsies are performed in order to help health professionals achieve a higher level of effectiveness in the care of the living. The autopsy rate of a hospital is usually a good sign of concern for excellence and offers a gauge of professional integrity and interest in scientific advancement. Through autopsies, the diagnosis and treatment a person received can be evaluated and staff members persuaded to observe a high level of proficiency. For this reason, autopsies should be encouraged and people should be encouraged to look upon them as an ordinary part of the medical care process. Needless to say, the human remains of a person should always be treated with utmost respect during an autopsy.

In the Judeo-Christian tradition, respect for the dead was usually displayed through burial of the corpse in the ground or in a mausoleum. Cremation of the remains, while not a common part of this tradition, has never been considered as disrespectful treatment. For a long time, however, cremation was forbidden in the Catholic Church because anti-Christian groups in the eighteenth century advocated cremation as a means of denying externally the immortality of the human person and the Resurrection. Thus, not because it was immoral in itself, but rather because of what it might signify, cremation was not an acceptable form of caring for the remains of a person in the Catholic Church.

Because cremation is no longer associated with a denial of religious truth today, while burying the dead is encouraged as the usual procedure, the total remains or an amputated member may be cremated if there is a serious reason: for example, if the custom of the country favors cremation, if there is danger of disease, or if suitable grave sites cannot be obtained at a reasonable cost.

11.8 Conclusion

Because of our weakened nature, death will never be something that we welcome. But through grace, we can accept it as the way to union with God. As we view the health care scene in our country, one is struck by "the denial of death." In order to overcome the fear of death and help oneself as well as other people die well, one must learn to overcome the emotional strain that accompanies suffering and death and deal with the ethical issues often encountered.

It takes more than words to accomplish this transformation of attitude in regard to suffering and death. One must be willing to surrender to God through the person of Jesus Christ every day if one wishes to give new meaning and power to suffering and death. In short, one must enter into a lifelong love affair with God. The small deaths one dies every day prepare a person for the larger and more important deaths and, finally, for the ultimate moment of meaning and power.

The perfection of Christian suffering and death is to accept it with joy. This is not possible unless one works at it faithfully, relying on the unfailing grace of God. To communicate to patients effectively the meaning and power of death, health care professionals must have some experience of its reality themselves. Thus, health care is more than a job, more than knowledge and technique. Basically, in its fullness it is a way of life that sees beyond the hurt, the sickness, the anguish; a way of life that enables one to look beyond the drudgery of daily reality, beyond the suffering in the hospital ward and the emergency room; a way of life that centers in God's love for his children, the suffering of Christ for all human beings, and his victorious resurrection.

Footnotes

1. Pope Pius XII, "Allocution to Italian Medical Society," *The Human Body Papal Teaching* (Boston: St. Paul Editions, 1960), p. 57.

2. Karl Rahner, *On the Theology of Death* (New York: Herder & Herder, 1965).

3. "Refinements in Criteria for the Determination of Death: An Appraisal," *Journal of the American Medical Association* 221 (1973): 48-53.

4. Paul Bryne et al, "Brain Death: An Opposing Viewpoint," *Journal of the American Medical Association* 242 (1979): 1985-1990.

5. Robert Rizzo and Paul Yonder, "Definition and Criteria for Clinical Death," *Linacre Quarterly* 40 (1973): 223-233.

6. Eric Cassell, *The Healer's Art* (Philadelphia: J. B. Lippincott, 1976).

7. Howard Brody, *Ethical Decisions in Medicines* (Boston: Little, Brown, 1976), p. 49.

8. Elizabeth Kübler-Ross, *On Death and Dying* (New York: Macmillan, 1969, p. 183.

9. Congregation for Doctrine, "Declaration on Euthanasia," 6/26/80, (Washington, DC: United States Catholic Conference, 1980).

10. Pope Pius XII, "Prolongation of Life," *The Pope Speaks* 4 pp. 393-398.

11. Pope Pius XII, op. cit. pp. 393-398.

12. American Medical Association, Council on Ethics, V, March 15, 1986.

13. The National Organ Transplant Act PL 98-507, *Congressional Record*, Oct. 19, 1984.

Study Questions

1. How would you respond to a person who maintains that all sickness would be eliminated if people would believe more strongly in Jesus Christ?

2. We know the reality of life and death by observing activities (signs) of the being in question, be it vegetable, animal, or human. What are the activities or signs which indicate that human life is present? What medical criteria enable us to measure these activities?

3. Discuss the statement, "While we may never lie to a patient, in some circumstances medical professionals need not tell patients the whole truth."

4. Distinguish clearly between mercy killling and allowing a patient to die.

5. Distinguish the different connotations of the terms "ordinary and extraordinary means to prolong life" from a medical and ethical perspective.

6. Respond to the statement, "Christians should refrain from alleviating pain at the time of death since God has willed it."

7. In your opinion, why do comparatively few people sign the Anatomical Gift Act on the reverse side of their driver's license?

Cases

1. In the oncology ward at St. Joseph's Hospital, health care professionals experience "burn out" more frequently than in other service areas within the hospital. As a pastoral care person, you are requested to explain this phenomenon and to present a program to alleviate the problem.

2. Carl, a young father with three children, is dying but his life would be prolonged indefinitely through a heart transplant. Tom, injured critically in a motorcycle accident, is admitted to the emergency room. Normal procedure calls for using a respirator on the patient, but the ER physician realizes that Tom will die no matter what care is given. Thus, wishing to provide a heart for Carl, he withholds the respirator from Tom, thinking that this would hasten his death. Is the ER physician acting ethically? What norms would ensure ethical procedures in such cases?

3. Millie is severely depressed and her family feels she may become suicidal if told she is dying. The attending physician does not believe that Millie is clinically depressed and asks you, a fourth-year medical student and a friend of Millie, to inform her of her condition. What ethical norms will you follow in your dialogue with Millie?

4. In the movie, "Whose Life is it Anyway?", Ken, a young artist severely injured in an automobile accident, is quadraplegic and wishes to have a catheter draining his kidneys removed in order to hasten death from uremic poisoning. Evaluate his desire from an ethical viewpoint.

5. Sarah, the teenage daughter of a fundamentalist minister, goes to the hospital with a broken leg and the physicians diagnose a serious lymphoma. Unless surgery and chemotherapy are performed, Sarah will lose her leg and most probably her life within two years. Wishing to express complete dependence upon God, her father refuses all medical care and Sarah agrees with him. Does the physician or the hospital have an ethical obligation to ask the court to appoint a legal guardian for Sarah? What ethical norms should be followed?

6. Federal regulations, known as the Baby Doe regulations, require that the life of each infant be prolonged, no matter how severe the birth defects, unless it can be foreseen that the infant will die in a short time no matter what care is given. Comment on these regulations from an ethical perspective.

7. Your Aunt Ethel is in an irreversible coma, but has been given nourishment and hydration through intravenous (IV) devices. The physician suggests that IV equipment be removed, allowing her to die of natural causes. When you object because Aunt Ethel could suffer pain in this process, the physician replies that analgesics may be given to relieve her pain. What would be your response to removal of IV equipment and administration of analgesics?

8. Patients in some charity hospitals are required to sign a release for autopsy should they die during their hospital stay. When challenged, the medical director defends the practice by saying, "We are a teaching hospital and

society has a right to require that charity patients offer something to society, namely helping educate young physicians, in return for the medical care they receive." Comment on this policy from an ethical perspective.

Chapter 12
Spiritual Ministry and Health Care

Chapter 1 argues that human health involves not only the biological, psychological, and ethical functions of the human person, but also a person's spiritual life, that is, his or her deepest concerns and commitments, his or her world view and value systems. Total health requires the balanced and effective functioning of all these human potentialities. Thus no one is truly healthy if his or her spirutual life is atrophied, stunted, or pathologically conflicted.

In this chapter, we shall consider how health care professionals can contribute to the spiritual well-being and growth of their clients in the process of medical therapy and care. We hope to show that from a spiritual point of view the work of physicians and nurses is truly a healing *ministry* in which they act as ministers of God, who is the author of all life and health. Although in books on medical ethics spiritual care is usually considered as something pertinent only in the care of the dying, we want to stress that it is a dimension of all health care and all sick people need and deserve it. Because they are sick they have special spiritual needs and their spiritual care has special problems.

Although all health care professionals can make a contribution to spiritual care, in this chapter we will give particular attention to the role of the pastoral care personnel who today have a recognized professional role not only in Catholic, Protestant, and Jewish health care facilities but in many secular ones as well, both in counseling and in sacramental ministry. The principles to be applied in this section are mainly those of hope, that is, the principles of stewardship and of growth through suffering, but the principles of human dignity and of well-formed conscience are also operative.

12.1 Purpose of Pastoral Care

Most Catholic and many community health care facilities have a pastoral care department whose staff have a fourfold role: to heal, to sustain, to guide, and to reconcile. Hence, the pastoral care team seeks to afford help at the spiritual and social levels just as other health care professionals offer help at the physiological and psychological levels.

Trained pastoral care staff are a great asset for a health care facility, but their presence also presents a difficulty not often realized by health care personnel and administrators. Because ministers, sisters, priests, and laity trained in pastoral care are present in a hospital, physicians, nurses, and technicians often feel that the patient's spiritual needs are not their concern. Thus, they act as if the patient could be divided effectively into parts and cared for at only one level of personality. As we have indicated, every human act affects each level of human function, even though that act may be primarily concerned with one level of function. Our human faculties and powers are not related as floors in a building but rather as dimensions of a building. Too many health care professionals minister to only one dimension of patient need.

The first task of pastoral care people, then, is to heighten the awareness of other health care professionals so that they are sensitive to patients' social and spiritual needs and that they minister to this level of need whenever possible. True, a nurse or physician may not have the training to respond to spiritual needs, but there is a basic level of spiritual care that any person of faith can offer. A patient being wheeled to surgery may find new courage and a sense of support when they feel very much alone if a technician, nurse, or physician asks, "Would you like to say a prayer with me?" Health care professionals who are not members of the pastoral care team have a wonderful opportunity and a responsibility as well to share in this concern for their patients' spiritual life as part of their total health.

12.2 Spiritual Counseling

Pastoral care professionals contribute to patients' overall health especially in two ways: through spiritual counseling and through sacramental ministry. When offering care, pastoral personnel, in a manner similar to other health care professionals, must realize that there is more to a patient's personality than the dimension to which they minister. Hence pastoral care personnel must be well-trained in their own speciality and able to answer accurately the question, "What do you do to help the patient?" but they must also have some appreciation of medical procedures and practice. On the other hand, pastoral care personnel must be careful not to offer opinions about medical care or give anything resembling medical advice, because they are simply unprepared to do so.

When acting as spiritual counselors, the pastoral care person, like a psychotherapist, is a listener and a reflector through whom the realities of the patient's situation become clearer to the patient and more manageable. Furthermore, like the psychotherapist, the minister listens not just to what the patient seems to be saying superficially but to what the patient, perhaps unconsciously, is trying to say nonverbally and symbolically. The psychotherapist, however, is listening for the message that rises from the patient's subconscious emotional drives, while the minister as a spiritual therapist is listening for a message that comes from a still deeper level, from what the Scripture calls the "heart," that is, from the spiritual interior of the person's being where the person is committed to some sort of ultimate values and to some fundamental insight into reality. In most patients, as in most everyone, this commitment and vision is dim and confused indeed, and yet it is the source of all personal life, where people really live and where they really die. "Out of the depths I call to you O Lord, O Lord hear my voice" (Ps 130). It is this voice *de profundis* to which the minister must listen. Moreover, a spiritual guide is not looking, as is the psychotherapist, for the psychic energies and motivations that flow from human instinctual needs but for the work of the Holy Spirit in the patient, the signs of faith, hope, and charity and the spiritual forces of sin and alienation which oppose these. This is the spiritual level of human functioning that is discussed in Chapter 1.

Questions

The patient may raise these questions directly by saying, "Why has this happened to me? Have I sinned? Am I going to be punished? What will happen to me if I die?" or "I don't seem to be able to pray now that I am sick," and so forth. Today in a secularized society, however, such questions are seldom asked *directly*. Even if they are, the counselor may very well suspect that they do not really come from the spiritual level of personality but are merely the pious language that some people use in speaking of purely physical or psychological problems. Or the patient may think that this is the way you are supposed to converse with a pastoral care person, who is supposed only to talk that kind of religious language. Therefore, the pastoral care person must listen to religious questions inherent in secular language or to secular problems inherent in pseudoreligious language. In both cases counselors must go deeper to find the really spiritual level in the patient.

This requires patience, and certainly it is usually a mistake to begin asking spiritual questions of a patient with whom the needed level of trust has not yet been established. On the other hand, experienced spiritual counselors learn how to cut through other levels of small talk and psychological jargon to the issues with which they must deal. Simple directness is ordinarily not resented by patients. *Directness* is not bluntness or insensitivity. It is, rather, a form of respect for a patient, a refusal to play games.

The counselor as well as the patient must trust in God's providence. God is using the patient's experience of illness as an occasion of possible spiritual growth. The spirit of God is already at work in the sufferer in ways that are not labeled religious. The minister must recognize this growth process and cultivate it, helping patients to understand this in their own terms.

A specific responsibility for ministers is not only to deal with the patient's spiritual problems, but also to help the patient become vividly aware of the real presence of God and of the Church as the People of God in the patient's life in this very event of sickness where the patient may feel abandoned and isolated. Counselors are themselves a visible sign or sacrament of this presence, incarnating God, as it were, in a tangible, human, imperfect, but real form.

Nor is it enough that counselors provide this witness of God's presence only to members of their own church. Too many ministers assume that they have responsibility only to their own parishioners or to those of their own denomination, and that others will resent their presence. Usually, however, this is not the case. Most laity are less ecclesiastically defined than we think. For them any minister, even a rabbi, is still a "man of God" and as such ought to have some interest in them as "children of God." Even the humanist is seldom content with the silence of humanism in the face of the ultimate questions and is resentful if the religious minister writes him or her off as a nonbeliever.

Thus, the spiritual counselor's primary task is really a very simple one. It is to say as much or more by presence, attitude, and nonverbal symbols as by the exhortatory Word, that God is present to sick persons in their fear or suffering, that God as loving, caring Father, as cosuffering Lord Jesus, as Healing Spirit is present and acting, but this presence is in mystery, that is, it exceeds human rational empirical comprehension because it leads to an open future. This implies, of course, a spiritual awe before the *mysterium tremendum*. The sick person, like Job, feels guilty and yet is not clear how he is guilty. There is a sense of *judgment*. The counselor should not deny this. Indeed, a counselor symbolizes this judgment. But the counselor also overcomes judgment by being a sign of mercy and reconciliation.

Sickness may be the time of genuine conversion in which persons truly find God for the first time in their lives or after a long time of forgetfulness and separation. The counselor must affirm the reality of this invitation of divine mercy, but that is not the whole of the minister's responsibility. Conversion is the beginning of a new life, but that life has to be lived authentically or it will be lost again. Consequently, one of the chief aims of spiritual counseling is to assist people to begin to grow daily in the Christian life and to plan practically to continue that growth once they have returned to the routine situations of everyday life.

It is important also that the counselor in helping sick persons realize God's presence also make vivid to them that the counselor's presence is a sign of the concern of God's people, of the Christian community or church, for a suffering brother or sister. Sickness is perceived in Old Testament terms as a kind of "uncleanness," and the patient may be experiencing the "leprosy" of loneliness, alienation, and "excommunication" of the outcast from life and the human community. The minister removes this excommunication and reunites the lonely one with the community that is praying for him or her. Recall how Jesus, healing a leper, sent him to a priest to be readmitted to the Jewish community (Mk 1:44).

12.3 Celebrating the Healing Process

The specific spiritual task of pastoral care, however, is not exhausted simply by the counseling situation. It must not be confined to talking about the presence of God, but it must deepen into *experiencing* that presence in prayer, worship, celebration, and communion.

Today when most chaplains and other ministers as well are training in clinical pastoral education, they sometimes feel a tension between the model of the chaplain as a pastoral counselor whose main task is to engage in a therapeutic psychological process with the patient and the older model of the pastor as the one who reads the Scriptures, prays with and exhorts the patient, and administers the sacraments. These two models seem opposed to each other. In particular, one seems aimed at removing feelings of guilt and giving feelings of interpersonal warmth and confidence and getting clients "in touch with their feelings," while the other tends to generate guilt and to impose a formalized religious response that covers up a patient's real experience.

Actually the two models, when they are well understood, are complementary and can reinforce each other. The Word of God first came to man, not in the text of the Bible that records his coming, but in the incarnation of Jesus Christ, the man who came to the sick and suffering, shared their suffering, and healed them by his touch. Ministers, because they are sent by Jesus, are the living witnesses, "other Christs," as a sign of Christ's care for the patient. Therefore, everything that the minister does to witness this tender concern, this ability to empathize, to listen, and not to judge, is a sacrament of Jesus' presence. Even humor and light banter, if its purpose is precisely to establish real communication, is like the wit that Jesus constantly displayed in his preaching and parables. Above all, the down-to-earthness—the freedom from stuffiness, self-righteousness, and elitism that can be the curse of the clerical status—are in imitation of Jesus, who did not hesitate to eat with sinners in simple fellowship.

Thus, when ministers read the Scripture with patients they should already have placed the Scripture in the kind of human relational context in which the Word of God can be truly understood. Prayer also must grow out of this living context; that is, it should be natural for two people who have come to share a common concern to give it prayerful expression. A minister should not be praying in front of an embarrassed patient who feels as if something is "being laid on him" in which he has no part. An opening for prayer will come, however, only if the patient senses that the minister's concern for him or her goes deep, deeper than mere professional interest.

The Scriptures used should be chosen because they help to make real the presence of Jesus, especially in his power to forgive, heal, and lead on into the fullness of life.

The Catholic priest is more likely than the Protestant minister or the rabbi to be concerned about administering the sacraments in the hospital setting. But these, too, must be understood not as some ritual intruding into a real situation but as a ritualization of a process of healing that is already going on. The primordial sacrament is the touching that Jesus used when he healed the leper. It indicates the intimate presence, the care, the community, the power of life between Jesus and the sick and outcast. When a chaplain gives reassurance that the minister is there, that the patient is not alone, that is the primordial sacramental rite on which all the other sacraments are based—*human bodily contact* as a sign of *spiritual presence*.

Anointing the Sick and Reconciliation

In administering the sacraments, using the new rites that the Catholic Church has recently revised precisely for this purpose, ministers must try to enhance this character of human contact already present in the counseling situation. What ministers have done as good pastoral counselors, they now deepen and intensify by a sign which combines the verbal word of Scripture with the nonverbal sacramental act.

The new rite of anointing of the sick brings this out clearly. It is not merely for the dying, as formerly, but for any person seriously ill. *Serious* should be judged here not merely in physical terms, but also in psychological terms. Thus, when anyone is physically sick enough that the minister suspects that the thought of possible death with its deep anxiety has entered his or her mind and produced fear and the threat of despair, then the spiritual and perhaps physical healing of the sacrament is needed and should be given. Whenever there is question of major surgery or of any disease which patients know sometimes leads to death and thus raises this fear in their own minds, ministers can anoint. They should not anoint when the illness is one in which recovery is assured and which consequently does not appear to contain any serious threat.

What is the meaning of this rite? First, it is not merely something done by a priest to a patient. Even when ministers are alone, they are there to represent not only God, but also the Christian community. In fact, God is the center of the Christian community so the minister is there to represent the Trinitarian community into which all Christians are incorporated in the Second Person Incarnate by their baptism. The anxiety of sick persons is that by their illness they are outcasts, aliens to this community. Patients experience this by their isolation from usual daily life and by the threat of death which might take them away forever. What such patients need is the reassurance that their people and their God are still with them. The priest supplies the sign of this by *touching* a patient. This touch means "presence," "acceptance," and as such is common to all the sacraments. But it is a special kind of touch in this case, a *healing* touch because it is the "anointing with oil," a common kind of healing remedy that has the sense of soothing pain and infusing life and suppleness. Its significance as a spiritual healing is given by the words which are spoken.

But this actual form of the sacrament is also preceded by brief Scriptural passages which can be expanded, in keeping with the general principle of the new rites that each sacrament should begin with a proclamation of the Word of faith, since it is faith that opens the person to God's work and is the beginning of God's gifts.

Misunderstandings

While the sacrament is valid with only the priest and the recipient present, this is not the ideal way to perform it. A recent study made in several public hospitals shows that the doctors and nurses frequently resent the visit of the priest to perform "the Last Rites." There are several reasons for this. One is the notion, now out of date, that these rites seal the fate of the patient and therefore mark the failure of the medical profession, something that health care professionals hate to face. Again, professionals think the rites may frighten and depress the patient. Another reason, however, is that the priest seems like a witch doctor who has been brought in as competition to the medical profession because the family has given up on the doctor's efforts. A fourth reason is the exclusive character of the rite. Even in Catholic hospitals when the priest comes, the physicians, nurses, and family often leave the room. Finally, there is sometimes a simple objection to an outsider coming in to do something for the person, as if the hospital were not all-sufficient.

These misunderstandings can be traced to what is really poor pastoral theology and practice. If one of the aims of the sacrament is to help patients escape their sense of isolation, then obviously it is best if family and friends can be present, and that would include if possible the nurse and the physician. Furthermore, if the sacrament is not to mark the end of life, but to help in the healing process, physical and spiritual, then it is certainly not separated from or in competition with the medical work of the hospital. Rather, it is part of that healing process. In fact, it is a celebration of the healing work of God which God performs not only through the ritual, but also through the *ministry* of the physicians, nurses, and administration. Priests are not the only ministers of health; they are part of a healing team, every member of which is called by God to a healing work and empowered by him through their natural gifts and education. The priest's special role in this team is to make explicit and eucharistic (thankful) the work of all.

It is essential to realize that the sacraments are not performed merely in the ritual moment. Rather, they are the celebration of a culminating moment (not necessarily the last) of the saving work of God that has gone on for some time through what are apparently merely secular events. Therefore, it is fitting not only that physicians and nurses be present at the anointing, but also that they participate in it by reading the Scriptures, or saying some of the prayers and by imposing hands on the patient or signing with the cross. Priests in their instruction and commentary and by additions to some of the prayers, if necessary, should thank God for the healing gifts and work of the medical staff. It would be very appropriate for patients also at this time to express their thanks to the doctors and nurses.

This expansion of the ritual can best be done, of course, when the sacrament takes place at the Eucharist in the hospital chapel, but it can also be done in the hospital room or ward when the physician can be present. The patient's confession when this is necessary would be done privately before the ceremony begins.

The proper rite for the dying patient is not the Anointing of the Sick but the reception of Viaticum, or final communion. This is the expression of the sick person's communion and unity with the Church on earth which prays for his or her swift passage to the eternal banquet. Hence this communion should be shared with others present if possible.

Lay People as Ministers

What should ministers do who are not priests? These days religious sisters and brothers and lay people share in their own way in the sacramental ministry. It is perfectly proper for nonordained persons, sisters, and lay persons to hold a service of healing consisting of Scripture readings, prayers, and the laying on of hands for the sick. It can even make use of blessed oil as a sacramental. It would seem, however, that in such services it should be made clear to all that what is taking place is not a sacrament in the strict sense. By this is not meant that it is inefficacious (all true prayer is efficacious), but that it is *preparatory* to the full public visit of the priest to the sick as a representative of the Christian community. Just as the arrival of the physician completes the care given to patients by nurses, even when in fact the physician has little to do except to approve and confirm what has already been done, so the priest approves and confirms the healing prayer of a local group and of auxiliary ministry. This is not a mere formality but an expression of the unity and public witness of the Church.

The Sacrament of Reconciliation for the sick can also take place in the form of a penance service in the hospital chapel or even in the ward, with the invitation to all who wish to make individual confessions and receive absolution. Such a service is an opportunity for the priest to deal with the question of sin and true guilt and the meaning of suffering and to alleviate *neurotic* guilt. When confession is made on a ward, it should be remembered that if it is difficult to achieve sufficient privacy the penitent can be instructed simply to make a general acknowledgement of sins and to speak of them in detail in a future confession.

It should be remembered too that deacons, sisters, brothers, and other visitors, although they cannot give absolution, can truly help a sick person to conversion and reconciliation with God and neighbor in an efficacious way. We are not proposing revival of the "confession to a layman," which was common enough in the Middle Ages when a priest was not available, but are emphasizing that today in pastoral counseling such confession often takes place spontaneously. When it does, the ministers who are not priests should help such patients make an act of contrition and then encourage them to go to the sacrament when it becomes possible, but should also assure them here and now that the mercy of God is truly present in prayer, and that with this trust in God's mercy they should be at peace. The reason for confession later is to ratify and complete by the public acknowledgement of the priest as a representative of the Church a conversion which has already taken place. There is no reason for nonordained ministers to feel that because they are not ordained they cannot help patients achieve this reconciliation here and now.

12.4 Baptism and Eucharist

Today, some Catholics are raising doubts about infant baptism. Such doubts, however, seem to have Pelagian overtones because they imply that the grace of God can only be received on one's initiative. Baptism, however, is a sign of the pure gift of God, the gift of faith and justification that comes to people without any merit on their part if they do not reject it. Before an infant is born it is already subject to the grace of God through the prayers of the Church. Infant baptism is the public ratification of this drawing of the infant, alienated from God through no fault of its own by the sins of society (original sin), who is now being drawn by the Holy Spirit through Jesus Christ and his redeemed community of the Church into union with the Father. This act of incorporating the infant into the life of the human community begins biologically and sociologically from the moment of conception and birth. Why then should not the infant also be incorporated into the redeemed community of the Church? Consequently, it is certain that baptism can be validly conferred on the child from the moment of conception and probable that it can be conferred on any unconscious adult (although not with the same certitude, because the person may have refused the grace of God that he offers to all).

From this some theologians in the past concluded that it is essential that all children in danger of death, even *in utero*, should be baptized or they could not enter heaven, and encouraged the baptism of all doubtfully baptized adults who had not actually refused baptism.

Today theologians still maintain the principle that persons can only be saved by Christ through the Church, but they see the *prayer* of the Church as efficacious even when it cannot be ritually expressed in the sacraments (cf. I Co 7:14). Thus, it is very probable that the infant dying before baptism has already been sanctified through the prayer of the Church (especially of the child's family) and will enter into the intimate mystery of God. The *Instruction of the Congregation for the Doctrine of the Faith on Infant Baptism*, Oct. 20, 1980, says, "As for infants who have died without baptism, the Church can do nothing but commend them to the mercy of God," as in fact she does in the funeral rite designed for them. Nevertheless, it still is important and seriously obligatory to administer baptism in order to obey the command of Christ and manifest the concern of the Church and thus to keep alive the consciousness of the dignity of the human person from the first moment of existence. Consequently, nurses and physicians should baptize infants who are in danger of death and even miscarried fetuses who exhibit human form and some sign of life (Canons 867-868; 871). They should pour water on the child (on the head, if possible) so as to wash the skin and should say, "I baptize you in the name of the Father, Son, and Holy Spirit." In this way they have expressed Christian reverence and fellowship with this little person who will forever be part of the Trinitarian community.

For the dying unconscious person, it is permissible also to perform such a baptism with the condition, "If you are not baptized, I baptize you." Clearly this is not a grave obligation unless the person has asked to be baptized before lapsing into unconsciousness and should not be done in a merely mechanical manner (trying to baptize everyone in the hospital, and so forth), but as part of the nurses' care for particular persons in their charge whom they believe have given some indication that they might wish such an administration. Again, the reason is to show the Church's concern for a person who has providentially come under the care of the Catholic community.

The Eucharist

The Eucharist is the supreme sacrament and sign of the Christian community, indicating that such patients remain a part of that community, even when absent from the public worship assembly, and that they are destined for eternal life with the community. It is a life-giving, health-giving sacrament, since the eating of bread and drinking of wine are the basic symbols of the power to live. After Jesus raised the daughter of Jairus, "He told them to give her something to eat" (Lk 8:55). Again St. Paul believed (I Co. 11:27-31) the unworthy reception of the Eucharist leads to sickness and death because this hypocrisy cuts a person off from the God of the living.

Today the Eucharist is often distributd by auxiliary ministers, not by the priest. This is not inappropriate, since in the earliest days communion was taken from the public assembly to the homes of the sick. In a hospital it would be proper when possible (and the current leniency with regard to the fast before communion makes this easy) to have the patients who wish to listen to the Mass in the chapel on closed-circuit radio or television then to be brought communion immediately after the Mass. Ambulatory patients who attended the Mass could be the auxiliary ministers. In this way the union between Mass and communion would be emphasized. It is essential in any case that communion in the hospital should not be reduced to a routine in which someone pops in and out of a room to place a wafer in a sleepy patient's mouth. We would suggest at least a card containing Scripture reading and prayers that a patient can use while preparing for communion should be available.

What we have been saying may sound liturgical rather than ethical, but it sums up the ethical message of this book, namely, that medical ethics has to do not merely with certain rules about forbidden procedures, but with a healing process by which the dignity of every human person in all its dimensions is respected by the community and the sick person is restored to full life in community. Unethical behavior tends to exclude persons from the deepest sharing of communal life centered in the Trinity. Ethical behavior fosters this communion. This ethical vision with its perception of the true scale of values is summed up and expressed in the sacraments, especially in the Eucharist. The sacraments represent for us how Jesus went about treating suffering people.

12.5 Conclusion

In order to be fully healthy, we must fulfill human needs in an integrated and balanced manner. Caring for the spiritual needs of sick and dying people is the work of the pastoral care team. Other health care professionals should contribute to this effort, but the primary responsibility for spiritual care lies with the pastoral care team. Ministering adequately in the service of pastoral care requires more than a degree in theology or training in clinical pastoral education. Like all forms of health care, pastoral care requires a knowledge and love of the person to whom care is being given. Only if the patient is recognized and valued as a unique and worthwhile individual is health care truly human and humanizing. Thus the person who is a pastoral care worker is an integral member of the health care team, and counseling and sacramental celebration are integral elements of health care.

Study Questions

1. Why would a priest or minister need special preparation, in addition to the preparation required for ordination, to offer pastoral care in a health care facility?

2. Why are most people reluctant to speak about spiritual realities, even though those realities are important in our lives?

3. What can the pastoral minister do to help the patient "experience the presence" of God when receiving the sacraments?

4. Explain the healing potential of the Eucharist.

Cases

1. Research indicates that many physicians look upon pastoral care as an intrusion in the healing process. Other physicians look upon pastoral care as another form of psychotherapy or social work. In your capacity as CEO of a Catholic hospital, how would you respond to those opinions?

2. Jane, a lay minister of the pastoral care department, does not wish to administer to AIDS patients. Though she realizes there is no danger of contagion, she feels that her inability to accept homosexual activity makes her a poor counselor for such patients. Analyze her attitudes from an ethical perspective.

3. Albert, a young Protestant minister serving in a home for retired people, find that the people make him uneasy because of the respect they offer him. Albert wishes they would look upon him as a friend rather than a clergyman. What thoughts can you offer to help Albert feel more at home in his ministry?

4. Though Fred is on a respirator, he is declared brain dead. His parents want you, as a priest, to give him the last rites of the Church. In addition to the Sacraments of Anointing, they wish you to administer Viaticum to him, arguing that he can still digest the host. What is your response?

Epilogue

"Wherever Jesus put in an appearance, in villages, in towns, or at crossroads, they laid the sick in the marketplace and begged him to let them touch just the tassel of his cloak. All who touched him got well" (Mk 6:36). Jesus is the Great Physician of body and soul, and he came to show us that his father wants health for all his children. That means God wants us, with all the science and technology we can develop through research, to share in Jesus' ministry of healing of body and of mind, and with the same attitudes of compassion and of respect for the dignity of every child of God that he had. Thus, we share in Jesus' ministry mainly by internalizing the values Jesus presented in the Gospels, which makes following the teaching of the Church more of a benefit than a burden.

This vocation to health is given to every one of us, and we all have personal responsibility for the health of our own minds and bodies. But we are also called to help one another to achieve health and to care for one another in times when health fails. As Christians, we realize the communal aspect of every human endeavor; as citizens, we have a great responsibility to do what we can to bring about peace and justice not only in our own country but throughout the world. We must seek to preserve the ecology of our planet and to cleanse it of the pollution it has suffered from unwise technology so that our environment may be healthy. And we must strive to establish economic and political conditions where famine, poverty, contagious disease, and destructive violence will be overcome so that healthy life for all may be possible. We must strengthen families through responsible parenthood achieved in ways that respect the gift of sexuality and the gift of children as God has given these gifts, since only out of healthy families will a healthy future develop.

As Christians we know that this better, healthier world cannot be achieved simply by human power. Our sins as a human community and as individuals go very deep, and we cannot heal ourselves, because we are like surgeons operating with diseased hands. Even in trying to do good we do much harm. Yet, there is good news and certain hope. If we faithfully follow our vocation to share in the healing work of Jesus, the great physician, we can accomplish all these works of healing with ultimate success.

Nevertheless, if we are to achieve success through him, we must also share his Cross, and that means that in the work of health care we must be ready to meet scorn and opposition from the sin-sick society in which we live. In our society, far beyond the limits of the Christian community, the Spirit of God is at work, and there are many waiting for our witness to give them courage to speak up for the values that the Spirit has led them to appreciate in their own hearts but that they feel very much alone in defending. We must have the courage to rally all these men and women of good will who stand for a deep respect for human dignity and human rights, so that we may stand together against the self-destructive spirit of a world that today seems bent on polluting the environment, wasting its resources, breaking up the family, denying the value of children, destroying life in the womb, exalting lust and violence, wasting the powers of science on instruments of destruction, producing luxuries rather than necessities, prolonging dying, and neglecting the poor and powerless—a sick world that must reach out to touch Jesus if it is ever to be healed.

APPENDIX 1

THE UNIVERSAL DECLARATION OF HUMAN RIGHTS OF THE UNITED NATIONS

Article 1. All human beings are born free and equal in dignity and rights. They are endowed with reason and conscience and should act toward one another in a spirit of brotherhood.

Article 2. Everyone is entitled to all the rights and freedoms set forth in this Declaration, without distinction of any kind, such as race, colour, sex, language, religion, political or other opinion, national or social origin, property, birth or other status. Furthermore, no distinction shall be made on the basis of the political, jurisdictional or international status of the country or territory to which a person belongs, whether it be independent, trust, non-self-governing or under any other limitation of sovereignty.

Article 3. Everyone has the right to life, liberty and security of a person.

Article 4. No one shall be held in slavery or servitude; slavery and the slave trade shall be prohibited in all their forms.

Article 5. No one shall be subjected to torture or to cruel, inhuman or degrading treatment or punishment.

Article 6. Everyone has the right to a recognition everywhere as a person before the law.

Article 7. All are equal before the law and are entitled without any discrimination to equal protection of the law. All are entitled to equal protection against any discrimination in violation of this Declaration and against any incitement to such discrimination.

Article 8. Everyone has the right to an effective remedy by the competent national tribunal for acts violating the fundamental right granted him by the constitution or by law.

Article 9. No one shall be subjected to arbitrary arrest, detention or exile.

Article 10. Everyone is entitled in full equality to a fair and public hearing by an independent and impartial tribunal, in the determination of his rights and obligations and of any criminal charge against him.

Article 11. (1) Everyone charged with a penal offence has the right to be presumed innocent until proved guilty according to law in a public trial at which he has had all the guarantees necessary for his defense. (2) No one shall be held guilty of any penal offence on account of any act or omission which did not constitute a penal offence, under national or international law, at the time when it was committed. Nor shall a heavier penalty be imposed than the one that was applicable at the time the penal offence was committed.

Article 12. No one shall be subjected to arbitrary interference with his privacy, family, home or correspondence, nor to attacks upon his honour and reputation. Everyone has the right to the protection of the law against such interference or attacks.

Article 13. (1) Everyone has the right to freedom of movement and residence within the borders of each state. (2) Everyone has the right to leave any country, including his own, and to return to his country.

Article 14. (1) Everyone has the right to seek and to enjoy in other countries asylum from persecution. (2) This right may not be invoked in the case of prosecutions genuinely arising from non-political crimes or from acts contrary to the purposes and principles of the United Nations.

Article 15. (1) Everyone has the right to a nationality. (2) No one shall be arbitrarily deprived of his nationality nor denied the right to change his nationality.

Article 16. (1) Men and women of full age, without any limitation due to race, nationality or religion, have the right to marry and to found a family. They are entitled to equal rights as to marriage, during marriage and at its dissolution. (2) Marriage shall be entered into only with the free and full consent of the intending spouses. (3) The family is the natural fundamental group unit of society and is entitled to protection by society and the state.

Article 17. (1) Everyone has the right to own property alone as well as in association with others. (2) No one shall be arbitrarily deprived of his property.

Article 18. Everyone has the right to freedom of thought, conscience and religion; this right includes freedom to change his religion or belief, and freedom, either alone or in community with others and in public or private, to manifest his religion or belief in teaching, practice, worship and observance.

Article 19. Everyone has the right to freedom of opinion and expression; this right includes freedom to hold opinions without interference and to seek, receive and impart information and ideas through any media, regardless of frontiers.

Article 20. (1) Everyone has the right to freedom of peaceful assembly and association. (2) No one may be compelled to belong to an association.

Article 21. (1) Everyone has the right to take part in the government of his country, directly or through freely chosen representatives. (2) Everyone has the right of equal access to public service in his country. (3) The will of the people shall be the basis of the authority of government; this will shall be expressed in periodic and genuine elections which shall be by universal and equal suffrage and shall be held by secret vote or by equivalent free voting procedures.

Article 22. Everyone, as member of a society, has the right to social security and is entitled to realization, through national effort and international cooperation and in accordance with the organization and resources of each State, of the economic, social and cultural rights indispensable for his dignity and the free development of his personality.

Article 23. (1) Everyone has the right to work, to free choice of employment, to just and favourable conditions of work and to protection against unemployment. (2) Everyone, without any discrimination, has the right to equal pay for equal work. (3) Everyone who works has the right to just and favourable remuneration ensuring for himself and his family an existence worthy of human dignity, and supplemented, if necessary, by other means of social protection. (4) Everyone has the right to form and to join trade unions for the protection of his interests.

Article 24. Everyone has the right to rest and leisure, including reasonable limitation of working hours and periodic holidays with pay.

Article 25. (1) Everyone has the right to a standard of living adequate for the health and well-being of himself and of his family, including food, clothing, housing and medical care and necessary social services, and the right to security in the event of unemployment, sickness, disability, widowhood, old age or other lack of livelihood in circumstances beyond his control. (2) Motherhood and childhood are entitled to special care and assistance. All children, whether born in or out of wedlock, shall enjoy the same protection.

Article 26. (1) Everyone has the right to education. Education shall be free, at least in the elementary and fundamental stages. Elementary education shall be compulsory. Technical and professional education shall be made generally available and higher education shall be equally accessible to all on the basis of merit. (2) Education shall be directed to the full development of the human personality and to the strengthening of respect for human rights and fundamental freedoms. It shall promote understanding, tolerance and friendship among all nations, racial or religious groups, and shall further the activities of the United Nations for the maintenance of peace. (3) Parents have a prior right to choose the kind of education that shall be given to their children.

Article 27. (1) Everyone has the right freely to participate in the cultural life of the community, to enjoy the arts and to share in scientific advancement and its benefits. (3) Everyone has the right to the protection of the moral and material interests resulting from any scientific, literary, or artistic production of which he is the author.

Article 28. Everyone is entitled to a social and international order in which the rights and freedoms set forth in this Declaration can be fully realized.

Article 29. (1) Everyone has duties to the community in which alone the free and full development of his personality is possible. (2) In the exercise of his rights and freedoms, everyone shall be subject only to such limitations as are determined by law solely for purpose of securing due recognition and respect for the rights and freedoms of others and of meeting the just requirements of morality, public order and the general welfare in a democratic society. (3) These rights and freedoms may in no case be exercised contrary to the purposes and principles of the United Nations.

Article 30. Nothing in this Declaration may be interpreted as implying for any State, group or person any right to engage in any activity or to perform any act aimed at the destruction of any of the rights and freedoms set forth herein.

General Assembly resolution 217 A (III) of 10 December 1948.

ETHICAL AND RELIGIOUS DIRECTIVES FOR CATHOLIC HEALTH FACILITIES

The *Ethical and Religious Directives for Catholic Health Facilities*, dated September, 1971, were approved by the Committee on Doctrine of the National Conference of Catholic Bishops (letter from chairman, dated October 30, 1971). In the judgment of the Committee on Doctrine these *Directives* contain nothing contrary to Catholic teaching or morality.

At the annual meeting of the National Conference of Catholic Bishops and the United States Catholic Conference, November, 1971, the *Directives* were approved as the national code, subject to the approval of the bishop for use in the diocese.

Preamble

Catholic health facilities witness to the saving presence of Christ and His Church in a variety of ways: by testifying to transcendent spiritual beliefs concerning life, suffering, and death; by humble service to humanity and especially to the poor; by medical competence and leadership; and by fidelity to the Church's teachings while ministering to the good of the whole person.

The total good of the patient, which includes his higher spiritual as well as his bodily welfare, is the primary concern of those entrusted with the management of a Catholic health facility. So important is this, in fact, that if an institution could not fulfill its basic mission in this regard, it would have no justification for continuing its existence as a Catholic health facility. Trustees and administrators of Catholic health facilities should understand that this responsibility affects their relationship with every patient, regardless of religion, and is seriously binding in conscience.

A Catholic-sponsored health facility, its board of trustees, and administration face today a serious difficulty as, with community support, the Catholic health facility exists side by side with other medical facilities not committed to the same moral code, or stands alone as the one facility serving the community. However, the health facility identified as Catholic exists today and serves the community in a large part because of the past dedication and sacrifice of countless individuals whose lives have been inspired by the Gospel and the teachings of the Catholic Church.

And just as it bears responsibility to the past, so does the Catholic health facility carry special responsibility for the present and future. Any facility identified as Catholic assumes with this identification the responsibility to reflect in its policies and practices the moral teachings of the Church, under the guidance of the local bishop. With the community the Catholic health facility is needed as a courageous witness to the highest ethical and moral principles in its pursuit of excellence.

The Catholic-sponsored health facility and its board of trustees, acting through its chief executive officer, further, carry an overriding responsibility in conscience to prohibit those procedures which are morally and spiritually harmful. The basic norms delineating this moral responsibility are listed in these *Ethical and Religious Directives for Catholic Health Facilities.* It should be understood that patients and those who accept board membership, staff appointment or privileges, or employment in a Catholic health facility will respect and agree to abide by its policies and these *Directives.* Any attempt to use a Catholic health facility for procedures contrary to these norms would indeed compromise the board and administration in its responsibility to seek and protect the total good of its patients, under the guidance of the Church.

These *Directives* prohibit those procedures which, according to present knowledge, are recognized as clearly wrong. The basic moral absolutes which underlie these *Directives* are not subject to change, although particular applications might be modified as scientific investigation and theological development open up new problems or cast new light on old ones.

In addition to consultations among theologians, physicians, and other medical scientific personnel in local areas, the Committee on Health Affairs of the United States Catholic Conference, with the widest consultation possible, should regularly receive suggestions and recommendations from the field, and should periodically discuss any possible need for an updated revision of these *Directives*

The moral evaluation of new scientific developments and legitimately debated questions must be finally submitted to the teaching authority of the Church in the person of the local bishop, who has the ultimate responsibility for teaching Catholic doctrine.

Section I

ETHICAL AND RELIGIOUS DIRECTIVES

1. General

Directive

1. The procedures listed in these *Directives* as permissible require the consent, at least implied or reasonably presumed, of the patient or his guardians. This condition is to be understood in all cases.

2. No person may be obliged to take part in a medical or surgical procedure which he judges in conscience to be immoral; nor may a health facility or any of its staff be obliged to provide a medical or surgical procedure which violates their conscience or these *Directives*.

3. Every patient, regardless of the extent of his physical or psychic disability, has a right to be treated with a respect consonant with his dignity as a person.

4. Man has the right and the duty to protect the integrity of his body together with all of its bodily functions.

5. Any procedure potentially harmful to the patient is morally justified only insofar as it is designed to produce a proportionate good.

6. Ordinarily the proportionate good that justifies a medical or surgical procedure should be the total good of the patient himself.

7. Adequate consultation is recommended, not only when there is doubt concerning the morality of some procedure, but also with regard to all procedures involving serious consequences, even though such procedures are listed here as permissible. The health facility has the right to insist on such consultations.

8. Everyone has the right and the duty to prepare for the solemn moment of death. Unless it is clear, therefore, that a dying patient is already well-prepared for death as regards both spiritual and temporal affairs, it is the physician's duty to inform him of his critical condition or to have some other responsible person impart this information.

9. The obligation of professional secrecy must be carefully fulfilled not only as regards the information on the patients' charts and records but also as regards confidential matters learned in the exercise of professional duties. Moreover, the charts and records must be duly safeguarded against inspection by those who have no right to see them.

10. The directly intended termination of any patient's life, even at his own request, is always morally wrong.

11. From the moment of conception, life must be guarded with the greatest care. Any deliberate medical procedure, the *purpose* of which is to deprive a fetus or an embryo of its life, is immoral.

12. Abortion, that is, the directly intended termination of pregnancy before viability, is never permitted nor is the directly intended destruction of a viable fetus. Every procedure whose sole immediate effect is the termination of pregnancy before viability is an abortion, which, in its moral context, includes the interval between conception and implantation of the embryo. Catholic hospitals are not to provide abortion services based upon the principle of material cooperation.

13. Operations, treatments, and medications, which do not directly intend termination of pregnancy but which have as their purpose the cure of a proportionately serious pathological condition of the mother, are permitted when they cannot be safely postponed until the fetus is viable, even though they may or will result in the death of the fetus. If the fetus is not certainly dead, it should be baptized.

14. Regarding the treatment of hemorrhage during pregnancy and before the fetus is viable: Procedures that are designed to empty the uterus of a living fetus still effectively attached to the mother are not permitted; procedures designed to stop hemorrhage (as distinguished from those designed precisely to expel the living and attached fetus) are permitted insofar as necessary, even if fetal death is inevitably a side effect.

15. Caesarean section for the removal of a viable fetus is permitted, even with risk to the life of the mother, when necessary for successful delivery. It is likewise permitted, even with risk for the child, when necessary for the safety of the mother.

16. In extrauterine pregnancy the dangerously affected part of the mother (e.g., cervix, ovary, or fallopian tube) may be removed, even though fetal death is foreseen, provided that: (a) the affected part is presumed already to be so damaged and dangerously affected as to warrant its removal, and that (b) the operation is not just a separation of the embryo or fetus from its site within the part (which would be a direct abortion from a uterine appendage); and that (c) the operation cannot be postponed without notably increasing the danger to the mother.

17. Hysterectomy, in the presence of pregnancy and even before viability, is permitted when directed to the removal of a dangerous pathological condition of the uterus of such serious nature that the operation cannot be safely postponed until the fetus is viable.

2. Procedures Involving Reproductive Organs and Functions

Directive

18. Sterilization, whether permanent or temporary, for men or for women, may not be used as a means of contraception.

19. Similarly excluded is every action which, either in anticipation of the conjugal act, or in its accomplishment, or in the development of its natural consequences, proposes, whether as an end or as a means, to render procreation impossible.

20. Procedures that induce sterility, whether permanent or temporary, are permitted when: (a) They are immediately directed to the cure, diminution, or prevention of a serious pathological condition and are not directly contraceptive (that is, contraception is not the purpose); and (b) a simpler treatment is not reasonably available. Hence, for example, oophorectomy or irradiation of the ovaries may be allowed in treating carcinoma of the breast and metastasis therefrom; and orchidectomy is permitted in the treatment of carcinoma of the prostate.

21. Because the ultimate personal expression of conjugal love in the marital act is viewed as the only fitting context for the human sharing of the divine act of creation, donor insemination and insemination that is totally artificial are morally objectionable. However, help may be given to a normally performed conjugal act to attain its purpose. The use of the sex faculty outside the legitimate use by married partners is never permitted even for medical or other laudable purpose, e.g., masturbation as a means of obtaining seminal specimens.

22. Hysterectomy is permitted only when it is sincerely judged to be a necessary means of removing some serious uterine pathological condition. In these cases, the pathological condition of each patient must be considered individually and care must be taken that a hysterectomy is not performed merely as a contraceptive measure, or as a routine procedure after any definite number of Caesarean sections.

23. For a proportionate reason, labor may be induced after the fetus is viable.

24. In all cases in which the presence of pregnancy would render some procedure illicit (e.g., curettage), the physician must make use of such pregnancy tests and consultation as may be needed in order to be reasonably certain that the patient is not pregnant. It is to be noted that curettage of the endometrium after rape to prevent implantation of a possible embryo is morally equivalent to abortion.

25. Radiation therapy of the mother's reproductive organs is permitted during pregnancy only when necessary to suppress a dangerous pathological condition.

3. Other Procedures

Directive

26. Therapeutic procedures which are likely to be dangerous are morally justifiable for proportionate reasons.

27. Experimentation on patients without due consent is morally objectionable, and even the moral right of the patient to consent is limited by his duties of stewardship.

28. Euthanasia ("mercy killing") in all its forms is forbidden. The failure to supply the ordinary means of preserving life is equivalent to euthanasia. However, neither the physician nor the patient is obliged to use extraordinary means.

29. It is not euthanasia to give a dying person sedatives and analgesics for the alleviation of pain, when such a measure is judged necessary, even though they may deprive the patient of the use of reason, or shorten his life.

30. The transplantation of organs from living donors is morally permissible when the anticipated benefit to the recipient is proportionate to the harm done to the donor, provided that the loss of such organ(s) does not deprive the donor of life itself nor of the functional integrity of his body.

31. Post-mortem examinations must not be begun until death is morally certain. Vital organs, that is, organs necessary to sustain life, may not be removed until death has taken place. The determination of the time of death must be made in accordance with responsible and commonly accepted scientific criteria. In

accordance with current medical practice, to prevent any conflict of interest, the dying patient's doctor or doctors should ordinarily be distinct from the transplant team.

32. Ghost surgery, which implies the calculated deception of the patient as to the identity of the operating surgeon, is morally objectionable.

33. Unnecessary procedures, whether diagnostic or therapeutic, are morally objectionable. A procedure is unnecessary when no proportionate reason justifies it. A *fortiori*, any procedure that is contra-indicated by sound medical standards is unnecessary.

Section II

THE RELIGIOUS CARE OF PATIENTS

Directive

34. The administration should be certain that patients in a health facility receive appropriate spiritual care.

35. Except in cases of emergency (i.e., danger of death), all requests for baptism made by adults or for infants should be referred to the chaplain of the health facility.

36. If a priest is not available, anyone having the use of reason and proper intention can baptize. The ordinary method of conferring emergency baptism is as follows: The person baptizing pours water on the head in such a way that it will flow on the skin, and, while the water is being poured, must pronounce these words audibly: *I baptize you in the name of the Father, and of the Son, and of the Holy Spirit.* The same person who pours the water must pronounce the words.

37. When emergency baptism is conferred, the chaplain should be notified.

38. It is the mind of the Church that the sick should have the widest possible liberty to receive the sacraments frequently. The generous cooperation of the entire staff and personnel is requested for this purpose.

39. While providing the sick abundant opportunity to receive Holy Communion, there should be no interference with the freedom of the faithful to communicate or not to communicate.

40. In wards and semi-private rooms, every effort should be made to provide sufficient privacy for confession.

*41. Special care and concern should be shown that those who are seriously ill or are dangerously ill due to sickness or old age receive the Sacrament of Anointing. A prudent or probable judgment about the seriousness of the sickness is sufficient. If necessary a doctor may be consulted, although there should be no reason for scruples.

A sick person should be anointed before surgery whenever a dangerous illness is the reason for the surgery. Old people may be anointed if they are in weak condition although no dangerous illness is present. Sick children may be anointed if they have sufficient use of reason to be comforted by this sacrament.

The sacrament may be repeated if the sick person recovers after anointing or, during the same illness, the danger becomes more serious.

Normally the sacrament is celebrated when the sick person is fully conscious. It may be conferred upon the sick who have lost consciousness or the use of reason, if, as Christian believers, they would have asked for it if they were in control of their faculties.

*41a. All baptized Christians who can receive communion are bound to receive viaticum. Those in danger of death from any cause are obliged to receive communion. The administration of this sacrament is not to be delayed for the faithful are to be nourished by it while still in full possession of their faculties.

*41b. For special cases, when sudden illness or some other cause has unexpectedly placed one of the faithful in danger of death, the continuous rite should

*Revisions — 1975

be used by which the sick person may be given the sacraments of penance, anointing, and eucharist as viaticum in one service.

42. Personnel of a Catholic health facility should make every effort to satisfy the spiritual needs and desires of non-Catholics. Therefore, in hospitals and similar institutions conducted by Catholics, the authorities in charge should, with the consent of the patient, promptly advice ministers of other communions of the presence of their communicants and afford them every facility for visiting the sick and giving them spiritual and sacramental ministrations.

43. If there is a reasonable cause present for not burying a fetus or member of the human body, these may be cremated in a manner consonant with the dignity of the deceased human body.

Sources
Final paragraph of Preamble: Vatican II, *Constitution on the Church,#27.*

Directive
 3 *Pacem in Terris, #11.*
11 Vatican II, *The Church Today, #51.*
18 *Humanae Vitae, #14.*
19 *Humanae Vitae, #14.*
20 *Humanae Vitae, #15.*
28 Vatican II, *The Church Today, #27.*
42 *Directory for the Application of the Decisions of the Second Ecumenical Council of the Vatican Concerning Ecumenical Matters, #63.*
43 *Canon Law Digest,* Vol. 6, p. 669.

CHRISTIAN AFFIRMATION OF LIFE

Many people have expressed a desire not to have their lives prolonged by extraordinary medical procedures when they are terminally ill. The Christian Affirmation of Life (CAL) is designed for such people. In addition, it helps people understand death in relation to other Christian mysteries and to prepare for death well before the appointed time. Expressing truths of the Christian faith concerning human and eternal life, *The Christian Affirmation of Life is not a legal document.* Rather, it is a document for reflection and meditation which can help people inform physicians and loved ones concerning preferred medical treatment at the time of terminal illness.

To my family, friends, physician, lawyer, and clergyman: I believe that each individual person is created by God our Father in love and that God retains a loving relationship to each person throughout human life and eternity.

I believe that Jesus Christ lived, suffered, and died for me and that his suffering, death, and resurrection prefigure and make possible the death-resurrection process which I now anticipate.

I believe that each person's worth and dignity derives from the relationship of love in Christ that God has for each individual person, and not from one's usefulness or effectiveness in society.

I believe that God our Father has entrusted to me a shared dominion with him over my earthly existence so that I am bound to use ordinary means to preserve my life but I am free to refuse extraordinary means to prolong my life.

I believe that through death life is not taken away but merely changed, and though I may experience fear, suffering, and sorrow, by the grace of the Holy Spirit, I hope to accept death as a free human act which enables me to surrender this life and to be united with God for eternity.

Because of my belief:

I, _____

request that I be informed as death approaches so that I may continue to prepare for the full encounter with Christ through the help of the sacraments and the consolation and prayers of my family and friends.

I request that, if possible, I be consulted concerning the medical procedures which might be used to prolong my life as death approaches. If I can no longer take part in decisions concerning my own future and there is no reasonable expectation of my recovery from physical and mental disability, I request that no life-support systems be used to prolong my life.

I request, though I wish to join my suffering to the suffering of Jesus so I may be united fully with him in the act of death — resurrection, that my pain, if unbearable, be alleviated. However, no means should be used with the intention of shortening my life.

I request, because I am a sinner and in need of reconciliation and because my faith, hope, and love may not overcome all fear and doubt, that my family, friends, and the whole Christian community join me in prayer and mortification as I prepare for the great personal act of dying.

Finally, I request that after my death, my family, my friends, and the whole Christian community pray for me, and rejoice with me because of the mercy and love of the Trinity, with whom I hope to be united for all eternity.

Signed _____

Date _____

Witness_____

Date _____

Selected and Annotated Bibliography

General Resources

Institutes

The Hastings Center (Institute of Society, Ethics and the Life Sciences), 360 Broadway, Hastings-on-Hudson, NY. Publishes the *Hastings Center Report*, an excellent journal on current developments in bioethics, and other materials.

The Joseph and Rose Kennedy Institute of Ethics, Georgetown University, Washington, DC 20057. Publishes the bibliography edited by Leroy Walters and the encyclopedia edited by Warren T. Reich, listed below.

The Pope John Center (Pope John XXIII Medical-Moral Research and Education Center), 186 Forbes Rd., Braintree, MA 02184. This center is dedicated to applying Catholic Church teaching to bioethics and especially to serving as a resource for the U.S. Catholic bishops. It publishes a newsletter, *Ethics and Medics*, and numerous monographs on particular issues, many of which are included in this bibliography.

The Society for Health and Human Values, Sixth Floor, 925 Chestnut St., Philadelphia 19107. Publishes *Journal of Medicine and Philosophy*.

Bibliographies

Andrews, Theodora, *A Bibliography of the Socioeconomic Aspects of Medicine* (Littleton, CO: Libraries Unlimited, 1975).

Annotated Bibliography of Bioethics (Rockville, MD: Information Planning Associates, 1977).

Culyer, A.J., Wiseman, J., and Walker, A., *An Annotated Bibliography of Health Economics: English Language Sources* (New York: St. Martin's Press, 1977).

The Hastings Center's Bibliography of Ethics, Biomedicine, and Professional Responsibility (Frederick, MD: University Publications of America, 1984).

Litman, Theodor J., *The Sociology of Medicine and Health Care: A Bibliography* (San Francisco: Boyd and Fraser, 1976).

McCormick, Richard A., SJ, *Note on Moral Theology: 1965 through 1980* (Washington, DC: University Press of America, 1981). These notes review books and articles, both in English and foreign languages, on current moral theology and often on medical-moral topics. McCormick's own point of view is proportionalist.

Walters, Leroy, *Bibliography of Bioethics*. (Detroit: Gale Research Co., 1975). The most complete bibliography, published annually, systematically classified. A selection from its items can be found in:

Goldstein, Doris Mueller, ed., and Leroy Walters, consulting ed., *Bioethics: a Guide to Information Sources* (Detroit: Gale Research Co., 1982).

Periodicals

Bioethics Quarterly (Northwest Institute of Ethics and the Life Sciences, 6241 31st Ave., NE, Seattle 98115).

Ethics and Medics (see under Institutes).

Hastings Center Report (see under Institutes).

Journal of the American Medical Association (535 N. Dearborn St., Chicago 60610).

Journal of Medicine and Philosophy (see under Institutes).

Linacre Quarterly (National Federation of Catholic Physicians' Guilds, 8430 W. Capitol Drive, Milwaukee 53222).

New England Journal of Medicine (10 Shattuck St., Boston, 02115).

Church Documents

Catholic Social Teaching and the U.S. Economy (second draft), *Origins* 15 (Oct. 1, 1985): 257-296. Catholic attitude to capitalism and socialism. Notes contain references to the many papal documents on the subject.

Paul VI, *On the Regulation of Birth (Humanae Vitae)*, and John Paul II, *The Role of the Christian Family in the Modern World (Familiaris Consortio)* (Washington, DC: U.S. Catholic Conference, 1969 and 1981), are essential to understanding the theology of sexuality.

Pius XII, *The Human Body* (Boston: St. Paul Editions, 1960). Systematic selection of texts from this pope's extensive writings on bioethics, which anticipated many current problems.

United States Catholic Conference, *Ethical and Religious Directives for Catholic Health Facilities*. Approved by the National Conference of Catholic Bishops and the U.S. Catholic Conference in 1971 as "the national code, subject to approval of the bishop for use in the diocese," (Washington, DC: United States Catholic Conference, United States National Conference of Catholic Bishops).

Vatican II: The Conciliar and Post Conciliar Documents and *More Post Conciliar Documents* (vol. 1, 1975, and vol. 2, 1982), trans. and ed. by Austin Flannery, OP (New York: Costello). *The Church in the Modern World (Gaudium et Spes)* (vol. 1:903-1002) shows the Church's positive attitude to medical technology. The declarations on *Regulation of Birth*, *Procured Abortion* (vol. 2:441-453), and *Euthanasia* (vol. 2:510-517) are especially important. See also the *Declaration on Certain Questions Concerning Sexual Ethics*, under the bibliography for Chapter 8 that follows.

Encyclopedia

Reich, Warren T., *The Encyclopedia of Bioethics*, 4 vols. (New York: The Free Press, 1978). This is the most comprehensive reference work on bioethics. When researching a topic, students are advised to begin with its articles for statement of issues, historical background, and basic bibliography. The articles are well informed on Catholic teaching but do not always conform to it.

Historical Studies

Burns, Chester R., ed., *Legacies in Ethics and Medicine* (New York: Science History Publications, 1977). Values in ancient, medieval, and modern medicine.

Burns, Chester R., *Medical Ethics in the United States Before the Civil War* (Ann Arbor, MI: University Microfilms, 1969).

Kelly, David F., *The Emergence of Roman Catholic Medical Ethics in North America* (New York: Edwin Mellen Press, 1979). Useful account but colored by author's advocacy of recent "dissenting" Catholic theologians.

Konold, Donald E., *A History of American Medical Ethics: 1847-1912* (Madison: Department of History, University of Wisconsin, 1962). History of ethical codes of American Medical Association up to 1912.

Newman, Lucile F., et al., "Medical Ethics, History of," in Reich, pp. 876-1007. No book exists in English on the general history of medical ethics, but the other studies listed here give some American background.

General Treatises and Readings in Medical Ethics

Collections of readings and essays are often arranged systematically and cover the main topics of bioethics. Consequently they often are used as textbooks and thus are included here.

Recommended

The following are recommended as consistent with the *Ethical and Religious Directives for Catholic Health Facilities.*

Ashley, Benedict, OP, and O'Rourke, Kevin, OP, *Health Care Ethics; a Theological Analysis*, 2d rev. ed. (St. Louis: Catholic Health Association, 1982). A more extensive, reference version with detailed documentation of the present work.

McCarthy, Donald G., and Bayer, Edward J., *Handbook on Critical Life Issues.* (St. Louis: The Pope John Center, 1982). A recommended brief handbook on the major issues in line with Catholic teaching.

McFadden, Charles J., *Medical Ethics*, 6th ed. (Philadelphia: F.A. Davis Co., 1967). A standard Catholic work, now dated but still of value for discussion of many topics.

————, *Challenge to Morality: Life Issues, Moral Answers*, (Huntington, IN: Our Sunday Visitor Press, 1978).

May, William F., *Human Existence: Medicine and Ethics* (Chicago: Franciscan Herald Press, 1977). A clear and readable discussion of principles and bioethical cases from a Catholic perspective. Highly recommended.

O'Donnell, Thomas, SJ, *Medicine and Christian Morality* (Staten Island, NY: Alba House, 1976). A sound and reliable Catholic medical ethics text, especially well informed on medical facts.

O'Rourke, Kevin, OP, and Brodeur, Dennis, *Medical Ethics: Common Ground for Understanding*. (St. Louis: Catholic Health Association, 1986). A series of essays considering many ethical issues in health care, based on the goals of medicine. Prepared for a pluralistic audience.

Other

Abernethy, Virgina, ed., *Frontiers in Medical Ethics: Applications in a Medical Setting* (Cambridge, MA: Ballinger Publishing Co., 1980).

Abrams, Natalie, and Buckner, Michael D., eds., *Medical Ethics: A Clinical Textbook and Reference for the Health Care Professions* (Cambridge: MIT Press, 1983). Over 100 short articles with cases.

Arras, John, and Hunt, Robert, *Ethical Issues in Modern Medicine*, 2d ed. (Palo Alto, CA: Mayfield Publishing Co., 1983). This edition emphasizes social aspects of medical ethics.

Bandman, Elsie L., and Bandman, Bertram, eds., *Bioethics and Human Rights: A Reader for Health Professionals* (Boston: Little, Brown & Co., 1978). Over 50 articles. A secular approach based on the principle of human rights.

Barry, Vincent, *Moral Aspects of Health Care* (Belmont, CA: Wadsworth Publishing Co., 1982). Text includes exercises and case studies and deals with several topics sometimes neglected.

Beauchamp, Tom L., and Childress, James F., *Principles of Biomedical Ethics*, 2d ed. (New York and Oxford: Oxford University Press, 1983). An important effort to develop a systematic deontological bioethics, based on the principles of autonomy, nonmaleficence, beneficence, and justice. Contains 29 cases and 9 major ethical codes.

_____, and Walters, Leroy, eds., *Contemporary Issues in Bioethics*, 2d ed. (Belmont, CA: Wadsworth Publishing Co., 1982). Introductory chapter on theory. Method is dialectical; point of view humanist.

Brody, Howard, *Ethical Decisions in Medicine*, 2d ed. (Boston: Little, Brown & Co., 1981). Contains 66 cases.

Childress, James F., *Who Should Decide?* (New York: Oxford University Press, 1982). Examines paternalism as a source of decision and limits it through beneficence and respect of persons in case studies.

Cohen, Marshall, Nagel, Thomas, and Scanlon, Thomas, eds., *Medicine and Moral Philosophy* (Princeton, NJ: Princeton University Press, 1981). Collection of papers from *Philosophy and Public Affairs*.

Culver, Charles M., and Gert, Bernard, *Philosophy in Medicine: Conceptual and Ethical Issues in Medicine and Psychiatry* (New York: Oxford University Press, 1982).

Curran, Charles E., *Politics, Medicine and Christian Ethics* (Philadelphia: Fortress Press, 1973).

————, *Issues in Sexual and Medical Ethics* (Notre Dame, IN: University of Notre Dame Press, 1978).

————, *Transition and Tradition in Moral Theology* (Notre Dame, IN: University of Notre Dame Press, 1979).

————, *Moral Theology: A Continuing Journey* (Notre Dame, IN: University of Notre Dame Press, 1982).

————, *Critical Concerns in Moral Theology* (Notre Dame, IN: University of Notre Dame Press, 1984). Curran's many essays on the methodology of moral theology and its application to medical-ethical problems is always thought provoking in showing the many interdisciplinary facets of an issue. However, his own "theology of compromise" leads to dissent from Church teachings on many issues.

David, Anne J., and Aroskar, Mila, *Ethical Dilemmas and Nursing Practice* (New York: Appleton-Century-Crofts, 1978). Nurses' point of view; contains cases.

Fletcher, Joseph, *Morals and Medicine* (Boston: Beacon Press, 1954). Influential exposition of situationalism.

Glover, Jonathan, *Causing Death and Saving Lives* (New York: Penguin Books, 1977).

Gorovitz, Samuel, *Doctors' Dilemma: Moral Conflict and Medical Care* (New York: Macmillan Publishing Co., Inc. 1982).

————, et al., eds., *Moral Problems in Medicine.* 2d ed. (Englewood Cliffs, NJ: Prentice-Hall, Inc., 1983). Readings emphasizing philosophical approach.

Haring, Bernard, *Medical Ethics*, ed. by Gabrielle L. Joan (Notre Dame, IN: Fides, 1973).

————, *Ethics of Manipulation: Issues in Medicine, Behavior Control and Genetics* (New York: Seabury Press, 1975). Haring is a noted Catholic moral theologian who stresses the primacy of charity, but in his antilegalism he sometimes dissents from accepted Church teaching.

Heyer, Robert, *Medical/Moral Problems* (Ramsey, NJ: Paulist Press, 1977).

Hollis, Harry, ed., *A Matter of Life & Death: Christian Perspective* (Nashville: Broadman Press, 1977). Readings with a Protestant approach.

Humber, James M., and Almeder, Robert F., eds., *Biomedical Ethics and the Law*, 2d ed. (New York: Plenum Press, 1979). Readings on abortion, mental illness, human experimentation, genetics, and death and dying.

Jakobvitz, Immanuel, *Jewish Medical Ethics* (New York: Bloch Publishing Co., 1959). Standard work on Orthodox Jewish tradition.

Jonsen, Albert R.; Siegler, Mark; and Winslade, William J., *Clinical Ethics* (New York: Macmillan Publishing Co., Inc. 1982). A work by a physician, a lawyer, and an ethicist. Valuable bibliography.

Kieffer, George H., *Bioethics: A Textbook of Issues*, (Reading, MA: Addison-Wesley Publishing Co., 1979).

Leach, Gerald, *The Biocrats: Implications of Medical Progress*, rev. ed. (Baltimore: Penguin Books, 1972). Readable, somewhat out-of-date, but provocative raising of issues.

Lovett, Ethelbert, *An Approach to Ethics* (Baltimore: University of Maryland, 1963). Useful because written specifically for dentists.

Mappes, Thomas, and Zembaty, Jane S., eds., *Biomedical Ethics* (New York: McGraw-Hill Book Co., 1981).

McConnell, Terrance C., *Moral Issues in Health Care: an Introduction to Medical Ethics*, (Monterey, CA: Wadsworth Health Sciences Division, 1982).

McCormick, Richard A., SJ, *How Brave a New World: Dilemmas in Bioethics* (Garden City, NY: Doubleday Publishing Co., 1981).

_____, *Health and Medicine in the Catholic Tradition* (New York: Crossroads, 1984). These works apply proportionalist methodology to a number of problems, with some dissent from Church teaching.

Meyers, David W., *The Human Body and the Law: a Medico-Legal Study*, (Chicago: Aldine Publishing Co., 1970).

Munson, Ronald, *Intervention and Reflection: Basic Issues in Medical Ethics.* (Belmont, CA: Wadsworth Series in Social Philosophy, Wadsworth Publishing Co., 1979). Essays on major topics, each with a case study.

Nelson, James B., *Human Medicine: Ethical Perspectives on New Medical Issues* (Minneapolis: Augsburg Publishing House, 1973). Protestant perspective.

_____, *Rediscovering the Person in Medical Care* (Minneapolis: Augsburg Publishing House, 1976).

Ponce, Gregory E., *Ethical Options in Medicine* (Oradel, NJ: Medical Economics Co., 1980).

President's Commission for the Study of Ethical Problems in Medicine and Biomedical Behavioral Research, *Summing Up* (Washington, DC, U.S. Government Printing Office, 1983). Summary of commission's publications.

Purtilo, Ruth, and Cassel, Christine, *Ethical Dimensions in the Health Professions* (Philadelphia: W.B. Saunders Co., 1981). Useful as representing the nurses' point of view.

Ramsey, Paul, *The Patient as Person* (New Haven, CT: Yale University Press, 1970).

_____, *Ethics at the Edge of Life: Medical and Legal Intersections* (New Haven, CT: Yale University Press, 1978). The first of these is a classical and very influential work by an outstanding Protestant moralist. The methodology is deontological.

Reiser, Stanley J., Dyck, Arthur J., and Curran, William J., eds., *Ethics in Medicine: Historical Perspectives and Contemporary Concerns* (Cambridge: MIT Press, 1977). An important reference source, with many documents and cases.

Restak, Richard M., *Pre-Meditated Man: Bioethics and the Control of Future Human Life* (New York: Viking Press, 1975). Emphasis on futuristic developments.

Rosner, Fred, *Modern Medicine and Jewish Law* (New York: Yeshiva University Press, 1971). Orthodox Jewish perspective by a physician who is also a rabbinic scholar.

Rosner, Fred, and Bleich, J. David, eds. *Jewish Bioethics* (New York: Sanhedrin Press; Hebrew Publishing Co., 1979). Collection of essays from conservative and orthodox points of view.

Shannon, Thomas A., ed., *Bioethics*, rev. ed. (Ramsey, NJ: Paulist Press, 1981). Collection of essays by various authors. Catholic viewpoint but does not always support Church teaching.

Varga, Andrew C., SJ, *The Main Issues in Bioethics* (Ramsey, NJ: Paulist Press, 1980). A concise, clear textbook that states controversial issues well but sometimes leaves the answers ambiguous.

Visscher, Maurice B., ed., *Humanistic Perspectives in Medical Ethics* (Buffalo, NY: Prometheus Books, 1972). The editor of these readings works from an explicitly humanist viewpoint.

Cases

Many of the previous texts contain numerous cases, but the following collections are especially useful.

Levine, Carol, and Veatch, Robert M., eds., *Cases in Bioethics from the Hastings Center* (Hastings-on-Hudson, NY: The Hastings Center, 1982).

Veatch, Robert M., *Case Studies in Medical Ethics* (Cambridge, MA: Harvard University Press, 1977).

Wojcik, Jan, *Muted Consent: A Casebook of Modern Medical Ethics* (West Lafayette, IN: Purdue University Press, 1978).

Chapter 1: The Person and Health Care

Donceel, J.F., SJ, *Philosophical Anthropology* (New York: Sheed and Ward, 1967). Philosophical analysis of human personality.

Fletcher, Joseph, *Humanhood: Essays in Biomedical Ethics* (Buffalo, NY: Prometheus Books, 1979). A humanist effort to define the human person. Fletcher goes so far as to accept infanticide in some cases.

Gelin, Albert, SS, *The Concept of Man in the Bible* (London: Geoffrey Chapman, 1968). The biblical basis for an understanding of the human person.

Goetz, Joseph, SJ, *A Christian Anthropology* (St. Meinrad, IN: Abbey Press, 1974). An article translated from the *Dictionnaire de Spiritualite* on the history of the development of the Christian concept of person.

"The Humanist Manifesto I and II," *The Humanist* 33 (January-February 1973):13-14.

Krapiec, Mieczystaw Albert, *Man: An Outline of Philosophical Anthropology* (New Britain, CT: Mariel Publications, 1983). Difficult reading but an important update of Catholic thinking.

Lawler, Ronald D., *The Christian Personalism of John Paul II* (Chicago: Franciscan Herald Press, 1982).

Maslow, Abraham H., *Religion: Values and Peak Experiences* (Columbus, OH: Ohio State University Press, 1964).

————, *Motivation and Personality*, 2d ed. (New York: Harper & Row, Publishers, Inc. 1970). An influential psychologist studies the manifold dimensions of human personality and, unlike some psychologists, gives recognition to the spiritual dimension.

Roth, Robert J., SJ, ed., *Person and Community* (New York: Fordham University, 1975). Essays on relation of community to its members as persons.

Technological Powers and the Person, part III, "The Human Person" (St. Louis: The Pope John Center, 1983) pp. 187-350. Essays by several authors given at a workshop for U.S. Catholic bishops.

Woznicki, Andrew N., *A Christian Humanism* (New Britain, CT: Mariel Publications, 1980). A study of the "existential personalism" of Pope John Paul II (Karol Wojtyla).

Chapter 2: Defining Human Health

Ahmed, Paul I., and Coelho, George V., eds., *Toward a New Definition of Health: Psychosocial Dimensions* (New York: Plenum Press, 1979). Essays on newer thinking about nature of human health in holistic terms.

Blum, Henrik L., *Planning for Health* (New York: Behavioral Publishers, 1974). Discusses the various ways of defining health.

Freidson, Eliot, *Profession of Medicine: a Study of the Sociology of Applied Knowledge* (New York: Dodd, Mead & Co., 1971). Freidson criticizes the medical professions' understanding of health and disease because (he thinks) physicians ignore the social factor and social attitudes.

Guttmacher, Sally, "Whole in Body, Mind and Spirit: Holistic Health and the Limits of Medicine," *Hastings Center Report* 9 (1979):15-21. The controversy about holistic medicine.

Kelman, Sander, "Social Organization and the Meaning of Health," *Journal of Medicine and Philosophy* 5 (1980):133-144. Philosophical analysis of different definitions of health and disease.

Temkin, Owsei, "Health and Disease," in *Dictionary of the History of Ideas*, Philip P. Weiner, ed. (New York: Scribner's, 1973) vol. 2:395-407. Temkin is an authority on the history of the different notions of health in different cultures.

Tillich, Paul, "The Meaning of Health", in *Religion and Medicine*, David Belgum, ed. (Ames, IA: Iowa State University Press) pp. 3-12. A classic essay by a distinguished Protestant theologian.

Chapter 3: Personal Responsibility for Health

Belski, Marvin S., and Gross, Leonard, *How to Choose and Use Your Doctor* (New York: Arbor Publishing Co., 1975).

Cassel, Eric J., *The Healer's Art*. (Philadelphia: J.B. Lippincott Co., 1975). A very sensitive and profound study of the patient-physician relationship.

Cousins, Norman, *Anatomy of an Illness as Perceived by the Patient* (Toronto: Bantam Books, 1981). A vivid and moving account by a famous journalist.

Freedman, Benjamin, "The Case for Preventive Medicine, Inefficient or Not," in *Hastings Center Report* 7 (1977):31-39. The future of medicine probably lies in prevention rather than cure.

Hendry, George S., *The Theology of Nature* (Philadelphia: Westminister Press, 1980). Corrects mistaken notions that the Bible and Christianity are responsible for anti-ecological attitudes.

Illich, Ivan, *Medical Nemesis* (New York: Pantheon Books, 1976). The author's thesis is that modern medicine, except for its work against contagious diseases, probably does more harm than good, and the profession needlessly monopolizes knowledge about health. One sided but thought provoking.

Lewis, Charles E., et al., *A Right to Health—the Problem of Access to Medical Care* (New York: John Wiley & Sons, Inc., 1976).

Menninger, Karl, *Man Against Himself* (New York: Harcourt Brace, 1938). A noted psychoanalyst shows how unconscious self-destructive attitudes often underlie illness and neglect of health.

Chapter 4: Responsibilities of Health Care Professionals

Annas, George J., *The Rights of Hospital Patients: the Basic American Civil Liberties Guide to a Hospital Patient's Rights* (New York: Avon Books, 1975). A lawyer codifies patients' rights in legal terms. Opposes idea that these rights can be left to peer discipline by physicians.

Annas, George J., Glanz, Leonard H., and Katz, Barbara F., *The Rights of Doctors, Nurses, and Allied Health Professionals* (Cambridge, MA: Ballinger Publishing Co., 1981). A primer of legal rights and responsibilities from abandonment to zoning.

Bosk, Charles, *Forgive and Remember, Managing Medical Failure* (Chicago: University of Chicago Press, 1979). Outstanding account of social systems used to improve care, dissipate guilt, and punish error among surgeons in large teaching hospitals.

Carlton, Wendy, *In Our Professional Opinion: the Primacy of Clinical Judgement Over Moral Choice* (Notre Dame, IN: University of Notre Dame Press, 1978). Brilliant sociological study of process used in decision making for value issues in large urban teaching hospitals.

Crane, Diana, *The Sanctity of Social Life: Physicians' Treatment of Critically Ill Patients* (New York: Sage Foundation, 1979).

Freidson, Eliot, *Profession of Medicine: a Study of the Sociology of Applied Knowledge* (New York: Dodd, Mead & Co., 1971). Sociologist stresses tendency of physicians to overemphasize professional autonomy.

Glaser, William A., *Paying the Doctor: Systems of Renumeration and Their Effects* (Baltimore: John Hopkins University Press, 1970).

May, William F., *The Physician's Covenant: Images of The Healer in Medical Ethics* (Philadelphia: Fortress Press, 1983). Examines the physician's various roles as healer, technocrat, and teacher and considers the goals and activities pertinent to each.

Pellegrino, Edmund D., *Humanism and the Physician* (Knoxville, TN: University of Tennessee Press, 1979). The need of health care professionals for a wide educational background.

Pendleton, David, and Hasler, John, eds., *Doctor-Patient Communication* (New York: Academic Press, 1983).

Siegler, Miriam, and Osmond, Humphrey, *Models of Madness, Models of Medicine* (New York: Macmillan Publishing Co., 1974). The different models of therapy and the therapeutic relationship.

Chapter 5: Social Responsibility for Health Care

Alford, Robert R., *Health Care Politics: Ideological and Interest Group Barriers to Reform* (Chicago: University of Chicago Press, 1975). Why it is so difficult to develop an adequate national policy.

Crawford, R., MD, and Douders, E., JD, *Institutional Ethics Committees and Health Care Decision Making* (Ann Arbor: Health Administration Press). A collection of essays from legal, ethical, and medical perspectives assessing the genesis and values of ethics committees.

Enthoven, Alan C., *Health Plan* (Menlo Park, CA: Addison-Wesley Publishing Co., 1980). One of the more influential works on health care planning and financing, focusing on the rewards for physicians for providing costly services.

Freymann, John Gordon, *The American Health Care System: Its Genesis and Trajectory* (New York: Medcom, 1974). Now somewhat dated, this study remains important for understanding our pluralistic system.

Fuchs, Victor, *Who Shall Live: Health, Economics, and Social Choice* (New York: Basic Books, 1974). One of the first studies to point out the effects of a faulty financing system for health care and its social ramifications.

Kelly, S. Margaret John, and McCarthy, Donald G., eds., *Ethics Committees: a Challenge for Catholic Health Care* (St. Louis: Pope John Center and Catholic Health Association, 1984)

O'Rourke, Kevin D., OP, JCD, *Reasons for Hope* (St. Louis: Catholic Health Association, 1984). Analyzes the future of the Catholic hospital system. Demonstrates need for lay involvement and management.

President's Commission for the Study of Ethical Problems in Medicine and Biomedical and Behavioral Research, *Securing Access to Health Care*, vols. I, II, and III (Washington, DC: U.S. Government Printing Office, 1983). A comprehensive study concerning the availability of health care in the United States and the legal, ethical, and social implications.

Starr, Paul, *The Social Transformation of American Medicine* (New York: Basic Books, 1982). Analysis of development of medical professionals and hospitals in the nineteenth and twentieth centuries. The best sociological analysis of the U.S. health care system today.

Chapter 6: Norms of Christian Decisions in Bioethics

We recommend the following for the beginner's reference in the vast field of ethical theory.

Codes

The major bioethical codes can be found in Beauchamp & Childress, previously cited under General Treatises. . . .

Ethics

Bourke, Vernon J., *History of Ethics*, 2 vols. (Garden City, NY: Doubleday Image Books, 1968).

Frankena, William, *Ethics*, 2d ed. (Englewood Cliffs, NJ: Prentice-Hall, Inc., 1973). A clearly written example of the Kantian, deontological methodology in its contemporary form.

Grisez, Germain, and Shaw, Russell, *Beyond the New Morality* (Notre Dame, IN: University of Notre Dame Press, 1974). An excellent textbook in the Catholic tradition. Highly recommended.

McCabe, Herbert, OP, *What Is Ethics All About?* (Washington: Corpus Books, 1969). A series of essays examining human behavior as a means of communication. Demonstrates against situationism that love is suitable norm for ethical behavior only if properly understood.

Christian Ethics

Ashley, Benedict M., OP, *Theologies of the Body: Humanist and Christian* (Braintree, MA: Pope John Center, 1985). This work provides a scientific, historical, philosophical, and theological background to the understanding of the relation of the human body to the human person.

Curran, Charles E., and McCormick, Richard A., SJ, *Readings in Moral Theology, no.1: Moral Norms and Catholic Tradition* (New York: Paulist Press, 1979). Essays on issue of proportionalist methodology, mainly in its favor.

Grisez, Germain, et al., *The Way of the Lord Jesus, vol. 1, Christian Moral Principles* (Chicago: Franciscan Herald Press, 1983). This important theological ethics contains extensive discussion of various controversial issues concerning ethical methodology and principles. Highly recommended.

Gustafson, James M., *Ethics from a Theocentric Perspective*, 2 vols. (Chicago: University of Chicago Press, 1981). Leading Protestant ethician.

Haring, Bernard, CSSR, *Free and Faithful in Christ*, 3 vols. (New York: Seabury, 1982). A comprehensive study of Catholic moral teachings by a European moral theologian. Contains sections on medical ethics and technology. Sometimes vague and ambiguous.

Hauerwas, Stanley, *A Community of Character* (Notre Dame, IN: University of Notre Dame Press, 1981). Stresses the often neglected topic of virtue and character in ethics as against overemphasis on decision making.

McCormick, Richard A., SJ, ed., *Doing Evil to Achieve Good* (Chicago: Loyola University Press, 1978). An influential set of essays on the proportionalist methodology.

Ramsey, Paul, *Deeds and Rules in Christian Ethics* (New York: Charles Scribner's Sons, 1967). Protestant criticism of situationism.

Schnackenburg, Rudolf, *The Moral Teachings of the New Testament* (New York: Herder and Herder, 1965). An extensive and well-balanced presentation of the biblical basis for a Christian ethics.

Critiques of Bioethics

The following raise some critical questions about the nature of bioethics.

Branson, Roy, "Bioethics as Individual and Social: the Scope of a Consulting Profession and Academic Discipline," *Journal of Religious Ethics* 3 (Spring, 1975):111-139.

Callahan, Daniel, "Bioethics as a Discipline," *Hastings Center Studies* 1(1) (1973):66-73.

————, "The Ethics Backlash," *Hastings Center Report* 5 (August 1975):18.

Camenisch, Paul F., "Progress in Medical Ethics: How the Ethicist Can Help," *Linacre Quarterly* 43 (November 1976):169-179.

Churchill, Larry R., "Tacit Components of Medical Ethics: Making Decisions in the Clinic," *Journal of Medical Ethics* 3 (September 1977):129-132.

Clouser, K. Danner, "Medical Ethics, Some Uses, Abuses, and Limitations," *New England Journal of Medicine* 293 (Aug. 21, 1975).

————, "Bioethics," in Reich, Encyclopedia..., vol. 1:115-127. An important attempt to define bioethics' relation to other disciplines.

Freedman, Benjamin, "A Meta-Ethics for Professional Morality," *Ethics* 89 (October 1978):1-19.

Hardison, O.B., Jr., "Problems of Value in Medicine and the Humanities, or Will the Real Doctor Please Stand Up?" *Perspectives in Biology and Medicine* 20 (Spring 1977).

Kass, Leon R., "The New Biology: What Price Relieving Man's Estate?" *Science* 174 (Nov. 19, 1971):779-788.

_____, "Regarding the End of Medicine and the Pursuit of Health," *Public Interest* 40 (Summer 1975):779-788.

Masters, Roger D., "Is Contract an Adequate Basis for Medical Ethics?" *Hastings Center Report* 5(6) (December 1975):24-28.

Mitchell, Basil, "Is Moral Consensus in Medical Ethics Possible?" *Journal of Religious Ethics* 2 (March 1976):18-23, 27.

Ogletree, Thomas W., "Values, Obligations, and Virtues: Approaches to Bio-Medical Ethics," *Journal of Religious Ethics* 4 (Spring 1976):105-130.

Pellegrino, Edmund, and Thomasma, David. *A Philosophical Basis of Medical Practice* (New York: Oxford University Press, 1981). An extensive and perceptive examination of the philosophical foundations of ethical medical practice. A basic and important work.

Rachels, James, "Can Ethics Provide Answers?" *Hastings Center Report* 10(3) (June 1980):32-40.

Ruddick, William, Fleischman, A.R., Siegler, M., and Freedman, B., "Physicians and Philosophers," *Hastings Center Report* 11(2) (April 1981):12-22.

Spicker, Stuart F., and Engelhardt, H. Tristram, Jr., eds., *Philosophical Medical Ethics: Its Nature and Significance* (Boston: D. Reidel Publishing Co., 1977). A symposium.

Szasz, Thomas, *The Theology of Medicine: the Political-Philosophical Foundation of Medical Ethics* (Baton Rouge: Louisiana State University Press, 1977). Misleading title. A work by the leading antipsychiatrist and critic of the modern medical model of therapy.

Veatch, Robert M., *A Theory of Medical Ethics* (New York: Basic Books, 1981). Interesting effort to build a deontological, three-way contract theory (patient, physician, society) of medical ethics. Aptly considers cases in light of this theory.

Chapter 7: Human Research and Triage

Annas, George J., Glanz, Leonard H., and Katz, Barbara F., *Informed Consent to Human Experimentation: the Subject's Dilemma* (Cambridge, MA: Ballinger Publishing Co., 1977). Legal, human rights point of view.

Berg, Kare, and Tranoy, Knut Erik, eds., *Research Ethics* (New York: Alan R. Liss, Inc., 1983). Readings.

Bok, Sissela, "The Ethics of Giving Placebos," *Scientific American* 231 (November 1974):17-23. Interesting analysis of deception in experimentation and therapy.

Hatfield, Frank, "Prison Research: the View from Inside," *Hastings Center Report* 7 (February 1977):11-12. What prisoners think of their freedom to volunteer.

Katz, Jay, and Capron, Alex, *Experimentation with Human Beings* (New York: Sage, 1972). An extensive examination of ethical principles and legal decisions concerning human experimentation.

Levy, Charlotte L., *The Human Body and the Law* (Dobbs Ferry, NY: Oceana Publications, 1975). Legal aspects of experimentation with human subjects.

Lucas, George R., Jr., "Triage," *Inquiries into Medical Ethics*, Donald G. McCarthy, ed., vol. 3, *Medicine and Society* (Houston, TX: Institute of Religion and Human Development, 1975).

McCarthy, Donald, and Moraczewski, Albert, OP, *An Ethical Evaluation of Fetal Experimentation: an Interdisciplinary Study* (St. Louis: Pope John Center, 1976). Catholic perspective.

President's Commission for the Study of Ethical Problems in Medicine and Biomedical and Behavioral Research, *Implementing Human Research Regulations* (Washington, DC: U.S. Government Printing Office, 1983).

Ramsey, Paul, *Fabricated Man: the Ethics of Genetic Control* (New Haven, CT: Yale University Press, 1972). An early exposition of the principles that govern experimentation in human subjects.

————, *The Ethics of Fetal Research* (New Haven, CT: Yale University Press, 1975).

Rosenthal, Robert, and Rosnow, Ralph L., *The Volunteer Subject* (New York: Wiley-Interscience, 1975).

U.S. National Commission for the Protection of Human Subjects of Biomedical and Behavioral Research, *The Belmont Report: Ethical Principles and Guidelines for the Protection of Human Subjects of Research* (Washington, DC: U.S. Government Printing Office, 1978).

Chapter 8: Sexuality and Reproduction

Ashley, Benedict, OP, "A Critique of the Theory of Delayed Hominization," Appendix I in *An Ethical Evaluation of Fetal Experimentation*, Donald G. McCarthy and Albert Moraczewski, OP (St. Louis: Pope John Center, 1976), pp. 113-133. Shows that attempts to revive the medieval theory of the infusion of the human soul after conception, although based on sound principles, leads to the opposite conclusion when these principles are applied to modern embryology.

Billings, E., MD, and Billings, W., *The Billings Method* (Victoria, Australia: O'Donovan Publishing Co., 1981). An analysis of the simplest effective method of family planning by the method's developers.

Boyle, John P., *The Sterilization Controversy: a New Crisis for the Catholic Hospital?* Presents the problem well but does not seem to support the Church's position on contraceptive sterilization.

Catholic Bishops Joint Committee on Bioethics (for Bishops of Great Britain), "Use of 'Morning After Pill' in Cases of Rape," *Origins* 13 (March 1986):634-638. Holmes, Helen B., ed., *The Custom-Made Child?* (Clifton, NJ: Humana Press, 1981).

Grisez, Germain, *Contraception and the Natural Law* (Milwaukee: Bruce, 1964). A married lay theologian, previous to *Humanae Vitae*, wrote this classical, brief, and powerful refutation of efforts by some theologians to justify contraception.

Hess, Loyd, "Treatment for Rape Victims in Catholic Health Facilities" *Ethics and Medics* 10(11), 10(12), 11(1). Up-to-date information on this difficult problem.

John Paul II (Karol Wojtyla), *Love and Responsibility* (New York: Farrar, Strauss & Giroux, 1981).

————, "The Role of the Christian Family in the Modern World" (Apostolic Exhortation *Familaris Consortio*) (Boston: St. Paul Editions, 1981). The first of these works is a profound meditation on the Christian atttitude toward married love. The second sums up the conclusions of the 1980 World Synod of Catholic Bishops and is the most complete statement of Catholic Church teaching on sexuality.

Kippley, John, MD, and Kippley, Sheila, *The Art of Natural Family Planning*, 3d ed. (Cincinnati: The Couple-to-Couple League, 1985). Most complete and up-to-date book on all aspects of family planning by noncontraceptive methods.

Lawler, Ronald, OFMCap., Boyle, Joseph, and May, William F., *Catholic Sexual Ethics* (Huntington, IN: O.S.V. Press, 1985). Two married laymen and a priest present Catholic Church teaching on sexuality, discussing its biblical roots, authentic interpretation by pope and bishops, and pastoral applications. Useful and complete account both of theoretical and practical issues.

Lucas, George R., Jr., and Ogletree, Thomas W., eds., *Lifeboat Ethics: The Moral Dilemmas of World Hunger* (New York: Harper & Row, Publishers, Inc., 1976). Readings on population explosion.

Noonan, John T., Jr., *Contraception: a History of Its Treatment by the Catholic Theologians and Canonists* (New York: Harvard University Press, Belknap Press, 1965). Although somewhat biased by its unsuccessful effort to prove (before *Humanae Vitae*) that the Church could change its teaching to accept some forms of contraception, this is the most complete history of Church teaching on sexual ethics now available.

————, *Human Sexuality and Personhood* (St. Louis: Pope John Center, 1981). A workshop for North American Catholic bishops.

Pope John Center, *Sex and Gender: a Theological and Scientific Inquiry* (St. Louis: Pope John Center, 1982). A consultation between leading scientists in the field of sexual research and theologians on the moral, psychological, and medical aspects of the development of sexual identity, gender, and orientation.

————, *The Family Today and Tomorrow: the Church Addresses Her Future.* (Braintree, MA: Pope John Center, 1985). A workshop for North American Catholic Bishops.

S. Congregation for the Doctrine of the Faith, *Declaration on Certain Questions Concerning Sexual Ethics (Persona Humana)*, (Washington, DC: United States Catholic Conference). Catholic moral teachings with commentaries by leading theologians. This declaration has been roundly criticized by dissenting American theologians, but it is clearly in line with Catholic tradition.

Sterilization, Implications for Mentally Retarded and Mentally Ill Persons (Ottawa, Canada: Law Reform Commission of Canada, 1979). A legal and ethical evaluation of sterilization; well-thought-out analysis of political issues.

Abortion

Burtchaell, James, *Rachel Weeping and other Essays on Abortion* (Kansas City, MO: Andrews and McMeel, 1982). A powerful critique of abortion, the abortion movement and mentality.

Connery, John R., SJ, *Abortion: the Development of the Roman Catholic Perspective* (Chicago: Loyola University Press, 1977). The most complete, accurate history of Church teaching on the subject.

Denes, Magda, *Necessity and Sorrow: Life and Death in an Abortion Hospital* (New York: Basic Books, 1976). A sensitive account of the pressures that lead women to accept and justify abortion.

Germain, Grisez, *Abortion: the Myths, the Realities and the Arguments* (New York: Corpus Books, 1970). The most complete treatment of this issue from a Catholic point of view, considering all its aspects.

Mall, David, and Watts, Walter F., MD, eds., *The Psychological Aspects of Abortion* (Washington, DC: University Publications of America, 1979).

Nathanson, Bernard, *Aborting America* (Garden City, NY: Doubleday Publishing Co., 1979). The account of how the physician who led the campaign to repeal restrictive abortion laws came to see the immorality of abortion.

Noonan, John T., Jr., *A Private Choice: Abortion in America in the Seventies* (New York: The Free Press, 1979). The legal fallacies and social effects of the Supreme Court decision.

Ramsey, Paul, *Ethics at the Edge of Life: Medical and Legal Intersections* (New Haven, CT: Yale University Press, 1978). A Protestant theologian and medical ethicist who rejects pro-choice arguments.

Thomasma, David, *An Apology for the Value of Human Life* (St. Louis: Catholic Health Association, 1983). A defense of life and a critique of our life-destroying culture. The first work to feature the "seamless robe" of moral principles in the affirmation of life.

Artificial Reproduction

Flynn, Eileen P., *Human Fertilization in Vitro: a Catholic Moral Perspective* (Lanham, MD: University Press of America, 1984). A dissertation that provides analysis of issues but a proportionalist methodology.

Hess, Loyd, "Assisting the Infertile Couple," *Ethics and Medics* 10(8), 10(10), 11(2).

Singer, Peter, and Wells, Deane, *Making Babies: the New Science of Conception* (New York: Charles Scribner's Sons, 1985). Discusses the medical possibilities, but its ethical analysis is not recommended.

Wakefield, John, *Artificial Childmaking: Artificial Insemination in Catholic Teaching* (St. Louis: Pope John Center, 1978). Well-constructed study asking the right questions about Catholic teaching in regard to artificial insemination.

Chapter 9: Reconstructing Human Beings

Surgical Reconstruction

Benjamin, Harry, *Standards of Care: The Hormonal and Surgical Sex Reassignment of Gender Dysphoric Persons* (Galveston, TX: The Harry Benjamin International Gender Dysphoria Association, Inc., 1980). On this problem, see also Pope John Center, *Sex and Gender.*

Kelly, Gerald, SJ, "Pope Pius XII and the Principle of Totality," *Theological Studies* 16 (1955):373-396; and "The Morality of Mutilation: Toward a Revision of the Treatise," 322-344. The classical articles on transplantation from a Catholic perspective.

Levine, Stephen B., MD, and Lothstein, Leslie, PhD, "Transsexualism or the Gender Dysphoria Syndromes," *Journal of Sex and Marital Therapy* 12 (1981):69-82.

Lyons, Catherine, *Organ Transplants: the Moral Issues* (Philadelphia: Westminister Press, 1970).

Mack, Eric, "Bad Samaritanism and the Causation of Harm," *Philosophy and Public Affairs* 9 (1980):230-259. The dangers of excessive pressure on potential organ donors.

Miller, George W., *Moral and Ethical Implications of Human Organ Transplants* (Springfield, IL: Charles C Thomas, Publisher, 1971).

Titmus, Richard, *The Gift Relationship: From Human Blood to Social Policy* (New York: Penguin Books, 1973). Discusses sale of blood, etc.

Genetic Reconstruction

Catholic Bishops Joint Committee on Bioethics (for Bishops of Great Britain), "Report: In Vitro Fertilization: Morality and Public Policy," (Abbots Langley: Catholic Information Service, May 1983).

Hilton, Bruce, and Callahan, Daniel, eds., *Ethics Issues in Human Genetics* (New York: Plenum Press, 1973). Collections of essays, visionary when published, discussing genetic manipulation in interdisciplinary fashion.

Lappe, Marc, ed., *Ethical and Scientific Issues Posed by Human Uses of Molecular Genetics* (New York: The New York Academy of Sciences, 1976).

Ludmerer, Kenneth M., *Genetics and American Society: a Historical Appraisal* (Baltimore: John Hopkins University Press, 1972). Ideological factors in promoting the illusion that eugenics can solve our social problems.

Pope John Center, *Genetic Counseling: The Church and the Law*, ed. by Gary M. Atkinson and Albert Moraczewski, OP (St. Louis: Pope John Center, 1980). A short study of the ethical issues in genetic counseling and of the moral responsibilities of genetic counselors.

_____, *Handbook on Critical Sexual Issues* (St. Louis: Pope John Center, 1983), Chapters 11 and 12. A clear presentation of the moral responsibilities in genetic research and experimentation.

President's Commission for the Study of Ethical Problems in Medicine and Biomedical and Behavioral Research, *Screening and Counseling for Genetic Conditions* (Washington, DC: U.S. Government Printing Office, 1983).

_____, *Splicing Life* (Washington, DC: U.S. Government Printing Office, 1982). Concise statement of the principal scientific facts.

Smith, George, *Genetics, Ethics and the Law.* (Gaithersburg, MD: Associated Faculty Press, 1981). The law on genetic questions is developing rapidly and must be followed in the journals.

Chapter 10: Psychotherapy and Behavior Modification

Bloch, Sidney, and Chodoff, Paul, eds., *Psychiatric Ethics* (New York: Oxford University Press, 1981).

Clinebell, Howard, *Understanding and Counseling the Alcoholic* (Nashville: Abingdon Press, 1956). A standard textbook dealing with the diagnosis, treatment, and care of the alcohol-dependent person.

De Ropp, Robert S., *Drugs and the Mind*, rev. ed. (New York: Delacorte Press, 1976).

Johnson, Vernon, *I'll Quit Tomorrow* (New York: Harper & Row, Publishers, Inc., 1973). A classic study of the psychodynamics of alcoholism and leading therapies.

London, Perry, *Behavior Control*, 2d ed. (New York: New American Library, 1977). A standard introduction.

Rieff, Philip, *The Triumph of the Therapeutic: Uses of Faith after Freud* (New York: Harper & Row Torchbooks, 1968). A reliable and readable study of the responsible uses of psychotherapeutic procedures.

Valenstein, Elliot S., ed., *The Psychosurgery Debate: Scientific, Legal, and Ethical Perspectives* (San Francisco: W.H. Freeman Co., 1980). Gives a good view of the controversy.

Vitz, Paul, *Psychology as Religion: the Cult of Self Worship* (Grand Rapids, MI: Eerdmans, 1977). An analysis of the proper roles of psychology and spirituality in Christian life.

Chapter 11: Suffering and Death

Becker, Ernest, *The Denial of Death* (New York: Macmillan Publishing Co., 1973). A very moving analysis of our avoidance of the inevitable.

Corr, Charles A., and Donna M., eds., *Hospice Care: Principles and Practice* (New York: Springer Publishing Co., 1983).

Grisez, Germain, and Boyle, J., *Life, Death with Liberty and Justice* (Notre Dame, IN: University of Notre Dame Press, 1979). A complete examination of euthanasia and allied ethical issues form a perspective of Catholic teaching.

Horan, Dennis, and Mall, David, *Death, Dying and Euthanasia* (Washington, DC: University of America Press, 1977). A comprehensive study of the moral issues of defining death, euthanasia, suicide, and allowing to die.

Horan, Dennis, and Delahoyde, Melinda, eds., *Infanticide and the Handicapped Newborn* (Provo, UT: Brigham Young University Press, 1982). Horan is a lawyer who has carried on an extensive struggle against euthanasia.

Kohl, Marvin, ed., *Beneficient Euthanasia* (Buffalo, NY: Prometheus Books, 1975). The humanist arguments for euthanasia.

Kübler-Ross, Elisabeth, *On Death and Dying.* (New York: Macmillan Publishing Co., 1969). A classical study of the psychological experiences of dying patients and their care.

McCarthy, Donald, and Moraczewski, Albert, OP, eds., *Moral Responsibility in Prolonging Life Decisions* (St. Louis: Pope John Center, 1981).

President's Commission for the Study of Ethical Problems in Medicine and Biomedical and Behavioral Research, *Defining Death* (Washington, DC: U.S. Government Printing Office, 1981).

Walton, Douglas N., *Ethics of Withdrawal of Life-Support Systems: Case Studies on Decision Making in Intensive Care* (Westport, CT: Greenwood Press, 1983).

Chapter 12: Spiritual Ministry and Health Care

Browning, Don, *The Moral Context of Pastoral Care* (Philadelphia: Westminster Press, 1976). Pastoral care is not merely psychological.

Cobb, John B., *Theology and Pastoral Care* (Philadelphia: Fortress Press, 1977). A Protestant perspective.

LaPlace, Jean, *Preparing for Spiritual Direction* (Chicago: Franciscan Herald Press, 1975).

Ling, Richard, *The Rite of Anointing the Sick and Their Pastoral Care: a Pastoral, Theological, and Liturgical Commentary* (Yonkers, NY: New York Clergy Conference, 1973).

Nouwen, Henry, *The Wounded Healer: Ministry in Contemporary Society* (New York: Doubleday, 1979). A popular work that considers the need for healing the professional as well as the patient.

O'Rourke, Kevin D., OP, *The Mission of Healing: Readings in the Christian Values of Health Care* (St. Louis, Catholic Health Association, 1974).

Pruyser, Paul, *The Minister as Diagnostician: Personal Problems in Pastoral Perspective* (Philadelphia: Westminster Press, 1976). Proposes a methodology for accountability in pastoral care.

Schanz, John P., *Introduction to the Sacraments* (New York: Pueblo Publishing Co., 1983). A contemporary theology of the sacraments as saving acts of Christ.

Smith, Eaymond K., "Training and Certification for Pastoral Care: Is It a Success?" *Hospital Progress* 58 (February 1977):74-75.

Studies in the Reformed Rites of the Catholic Church, 7 vols., (New York: Pueblo Publishing Co., 1985), by Aidan Kavanagh, Gerard Austin, James Dallen, Nathan Mitchell, Charles W. Gusmer, and Richard Rutherford. Each volume is a careful analysis of one of the sacraments. Especially useful is Gusmer's vol. 6, *And You Visited Me: Sacramental Ministry to the Sick and Dying.*

Index